I0056031

Handbook of
SORGHUM

The Authors

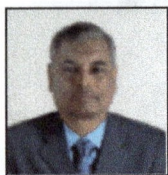

Dr. J.V. Patil obtained his M.Sc. (Agri.) from, MPKV, Rahuri. He completed his course work for Ph.D. at CCSHAU, Hisar and research at MPKV, Rahuri in 1992. He rendered his research and teaching services at MPKV Rahuri as Geneticist, Associate Professor, Plant Breeder and Professor of Genetics & Plant Breeding and Head, Genetics and Plant Breeding Department, MPKV, Rahuri (Maharashttra). He also delivered many administrative responsibilities in the university. Dr. Patil joined as the Director, Directorate of Sorghum Research, Hyderabad in August 2010.

He has vast expertise in conventional plant breeding in pulses and rabi sorghum. He has, to his credit, several varieties in Safflower - Girna (Safflower), Pulses - Vaibhav (Mungbean), Varun (French bean), Vipula, Rajashree (Pigeonpea), Vihar, Kripa, Virat, Digvijay, Rajas (Chickpea) and Sorghum - Phule Anuradha, Phule Chitra, Phule Suchitra, Phule Vasudha, Phule Revati, CSV 19SS, CSV 22R, Phule Amrutha, Phule Uttara, Phule Panchami and CMS 1409 A/B. He developed and popularized several crop production technologies such as sowing methods, seed treatment, foliar nutrient application and IPM in chickpea and *in situ* moisture conservation, soil type-based cultivars, protective irrigation, nutrient supply and intercultural time schedule in sorghum. He taught post-graduate courses in Genetics and Plant Breeding since 1994 and he had been instrumental in course curriculum designing and created laboratory facilities with modern teaching aids in MPKV, Rahuri. He has guided 15 M.Sc. and 15 Ph.D students as a major guide in Plant Breeding. He has to his credit 115 peer reviewed foreign and national journal papers, 25 books and 53 other technical publications. He delivered 27 Radio Talks and 11 TV shows for the benefit of farmers cultivating sorghum and pulses.

Dr. Patil is the recipient of *NAAS Fellowship award, Baliraja' Late Annasaheb Shinde Smruti Krishi Sanshodhan Gaurao Purskar* and *Vasantrao Naik krishi Puraskar* for outstanding research in crop improvement, Maharashtra state's *Vasantrao Naik award for Best Marathi literature - 2010 and 2012* and *Bharat Krishak Samaj Award -2012*. He received team awards - *CGIAR's Baudouin Award 2002* and *ICRISAT's Doreen Mashler Award 2002*.

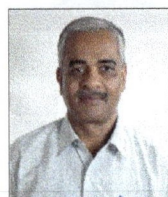

Dr. J.S. Mishra, born on 31st March 1967 in district Sultanpur, Uttar Pradesh, Dr J S Mishra has obtained his M. Sc. (Ag.) from NDUAT, Faizabad and Ph D (Agronomy) from JNKVV, Jabalpur. He started his career as Scientist in Agricultural Research Service (ARS) in 1991, and served for 18 years in the Directorate of Weed Science Research (DWSR), Jabalpur in various positions. He moved to the Directorate of Sorghum Research, Hyderabad in 2008 as Principal Scientist (Agronomy). He has made outstanding contributions in the field of Weed Management Research and Popularization of Sorghum Cultivation in Rice-fallows of Coastal Andhra Pradesh. His pioneering contributions are in the area of Biology of parasitic weed *Cuscuta campestis* and its management, conservation tillage and weed management in rice/soybean-based cropping systems, influence of tillage systems on weed seedbank dynamics, and identification and popularization of sorghum hybrids for rice-fallows. He has published 90 research papers, 7 reviews, 8 books, 22 book chapters, 25 technical/extension bulletins, 68 popular articles and 31 technical articles and reports. He has also presented over 70 papers in national and international forum. Dr. Mishra is a recipient of PS Deshmukh Young Agronomist Award (1999) for Outstanding Contributions in Agronomy Research and Best Scientist Award (2007) of DWSR, Jabalpur. He is also the Fellow of Indian Society of Weed Science (2007) and Indian Society of Agronomy (2010).

Handbook of SORGHUM

Dr. J.V. Patil
Director,
Directorate of Sorghum Research,
Rajendranagar,
Hyderabad – 500 030.

Dr. J.S. Mishra
Principal Scientist (Agronomy)
Directorate of Sorghum Research,
Hyderabad - 500 030

2014
Daya Publishing House®
A Division of
Astral International Pvt. Ltd.
New Delhi – 110 002

© 2014 AUTHORS
ISBN 9789351302933

Publisher's note:
Every possible effort has been made to ensure that the information contained in this book is accurate at the time of going to press, and the publisher and author cannot accept responsibility for any errors or omissions, however caused. No responsibility for loss or damage occasioned to any person acting, or refraining from action, as a result of the material in this publication can be accepted by the editor, the publisher or the author. The Publisher is not associated with any product or vendor mentioned in the book. The contents of this work are intended to further general scientific research, understanding and discussion only. Readers should consult with a specialist where appropriate.
Every effort has been made to trace the owners of copyright material used in this book, if any. The author and the publisher will be grateful for any omission brought to their notice for acknowledgement in the future editions of the book.
All Rights reserved under International Copyright Conventions. No part of this publication may be reproduced, stored in a retrieval system, or transmitted in any form or by any means, electronic, mechanical, photocopying, recording or otherwise without the prior written consent of the publisher and the copyright owner.

Published by   : **Daya Publishing House®**
A Division of
Astral International Pvt. Ltd.
– ISO 9001:2008 Certified Company –
4760-61/23, Ansari Road, Darya Ganj
New Delhi-110 002
Ph. 011-43549197, 23278134
E-mail: info@astralint.com
Website: www.astralint.com

Laser Typesetting   : **Classic Computer Services**, Delhi - 110 035

Printed at   : **Replika Press Pvt. Ltd.**

PRINTED IN INDIA

Acknowledgements

Our special thanks are due to Dr. S. Ayyappan, Secretary, DARE and Director General, ICAR, and Dr. S.K. Datta, Deputy Director General (Crop Science), ICAR for their kind encouragement and for writing Forewords to this handbook. The authors express sincere thanks to Dr. C.V. Ratnavathi (Principal Scientist), Dr. R. Madhusudana (Principal Scientist), Dr. Sanjana Reddy (Senior Scientist) and Dr. Hariprasanna (Senior Scientist) of Directorate of Sorghum Research, Hyderabad for providing valuable scientific inputs for this handbook. We are also grateful to Mr. H.S. Gawali, Technical Officer, DSR for cover designing of the book.

Dr. J.V. Patil
Dr. J.S. Mishra

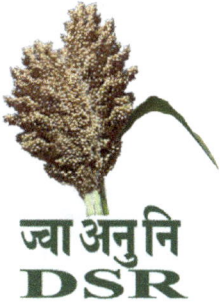

Directorate of Sorghum Research (DSR)

Directorate of Sorghum Research (DSR) is a premier agricultural research institute engaged in basic and strategic research on sorghum under Indian Council of Agricultural Research (ICAR). Besides the basic and strategic research on various areas, it coordinates and facilitates sorghum research at national level through All India Coordinated Sorghum Improvement Project (AICSIP), and provides linkages with various national and international agencies. DSR was established by the ICAR on 16 November, 1987 with main center at Hyderabad, and the two regional stations at Solapur (for *Rabi* sorghum) and Warangal (Off Season Nursery). DSR's primary vision and goals encompass the objective to promote economic growth by generating and disseminating ready-to-use technologies which create markets, respond to current and future economic demands, and maintain the long-term sustainability, value-addition and marketing to meet significant food, feed, fodder, fuel (bio-energy) requirements of the country. Sorghum being a rainfed crop, grown with limited inputs, varietal improvement leading to high yielding hybrids and varieties forms the core of major research achievements along with the development of crop production technologies. Through its network centres located across the country in various geographical zones, 32 hybrids (CSH 1 to CSH 32) and 30 varieties (CSV 1 to CSV 30F) have been released at the national level. These exemplary achievements are a standing testimony highlighting the success story of Indian sorghum improvement programme in terms of yield enhancement, diversification of parental lines, incorporation of resistance against major pests and diseases, developing production technologies for dry land agriculture, and enhancing diversification, utilization and alternate uses of sorghum.

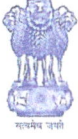

भारत सरकार
कृषि अनुसंधान और शिक्षा विभाग एवं
भारतीय कृषि अनुसंधान परिषद्
कृषि मंत्रालय, कृषि भवन, नई दिल्ली 110 001

GOVERNMENT OF INDIA
DEPARTMENT OF AGRICULTURAL RESEARCH & EDUCATION
AND
INDIAN COUNCIL OF AGRICULTURAL RESEARCH
MINISTRY OF AGRICULTURE, KRISHI BHAVAN, NEW DELHI 110 001
Tel.: 23382629; 23386711 Fax: 91-11-23384773
E-mail: dg.icar@nic.in

डा. एस. अय्यप्पन
सचिव एवं महानिदेशक
Dr. S. AYYAPPAN
SECRETARY & DIRECTOR GENERAL

Foreword

In order to match the rapidly increasing food demand in ways that are environmentally and socially sustainable, there is need to double the global food production by 2050. Good agronomic practices must judiciously inter-mix the applications of soil and plant sciences to produce food, feed, fodder and of late fuel while ensuring sustainability of the system in as much possible environment and eco-friendly manner.

In arid and semi-arid regions of the World, dry land cereals play a major role in the economy. Sorghum is a traditional dry land crop grown on marginal lands with low inputs. It plays a significant role in food, fodder and nutritional security especially resource poor populations in dry land areas. Due to its unique trait for sustaining in adverse climatic conditions, sorghum is a preferred crop under changing climate scenario. In spite of the multiple uses of sorghum, its area and consumption declined considerably in past 2 decades. However, in view the increased diabetic patients, malnourished women and children, especially in rural areas, declining fodder availability and threat to climate change, there is a need to increase the demand of sorghum through popularization as health food, nutritive fodder, value addition and commercialization.

The *Handbook of Sorghum* provides exhaustive information on all aspects of sorghum production and utilization. I believe this book will prove useful to all stakeholders, who strive for ensuing the food and nutritional security of the resource-poor farmers of India. I congratulate the authors for bringing out this publication.

S. Ayyappan

Foreword

प्रो॰ स्वपन कुमार दत्ता
उपमहानिदेशक (फसल विज्ञान)
Prof. Swapan Kumar Datta
Deputy Director General
(Crop Science)

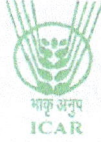

भारतीय कृषि अनुसंधान परिषद्
कृषि भवन, डा. राजेन्द्र प्रसाद मार्ग, नई दिल्ली - 110001
INDIAN COUNCIL OF AGRICULTURAL RESEARCH
KRISHI BHAWAN, DR. RAJENDRA PRASAD ROAD, NEW DELHI-110001

भाकृ अनुप
ICAR

Foreword

Sorghum is one of the most important cereal crops grown in the semi-arid tropics of the world. It is traditionally grown for food and fodder at subsistence levels by resource-poor farmers with limited inputs. Of late, sweet sorghum is emerging as a potential feedstock for biofuels. With the threat of climate change looming large on the crop productivity, sorghum being a temperature and drought resilient crop will play an important role in sustaining food, fodder and nutritional security in dry land regions.

In India sorghum is cultivated during both *Kharif* (rainy) and *Rabi* (post-rainy) seasons, mainly as a rainfed crop. It was known as "great millet" till early eighties with an area of more than 18 million ha. However, the area has declined drastically from 18.6 m ha in 1969-70 to 6.25 m ha in 2011-12. The total production also declined from 9.72 m t to 6.01 m t. But, the productivity has increased from 522 kg/ha to 962 kg/ha during the same period mainly due to adoption of improved production technologies by the farmers. In recent years, sorghum cultivation is gaining popularity in non-traditional areas like rice-fallows in coastal Andhra Pradesh with a very high productivity.

Sorghum is grown in the regions challenged by number of biotic and abiotic stresses. Developing cultivars and appropriate production technologies resilient to these challenges, value addition and commercialization is the key to improving sorghum productivity in farmers' fields. The efforts made by the authors to put valuable information on recent advances in soil and crop management, varietal improvement, pest management, biotechnology, food and industrial uses, fodder quality and bio-energy potential is a step forward in dissemination of knowledge.

This book provides exhaustive information on all aspects of sorghum production and utilization. I would like to congratulate the authors of this book Drs. J.V. Patil and J.S. Mishra for bringing out this publication timely. I am sure that this book will be of immense value to sorghum researchers, extension workers, students and farmers involved in sorghum research and development.

Swapan K. Datta

Preface

Under the changing climatic scenario, there is an urgent need of sustainable food production to feed the vast growing population. Sorghum, the fifth most important cereal crop on the globe and native to Sub-Sarahan Africa, is traditionally grown for grain both as food (Africa and India) and as animal feed (developed countries like USA, China, Australia, etc) and stalks as animal fodder. Of late, sweet sorghum is emerging as a potential feedstock for bio-fuels. The crop has potential to sustain under extreme weather conditions. Thus, it is the key for the sustenance of human and livestock population in the semi-arid tropics.

Sorghum in India is cultivated as a rainfed crop during both rainy (*kharif*) and post-rainy (*rabi*) seasons. Maharashtra is the largest sorghum grower and producer followed by Karnataka, Madhya Pradesh and Andhra Pradesh. Known as "great millet" till early eighties, the sorghum area has declined from 18 million ha in 1969-70 to 6.25 m ha in 2011-12 primarily due to introduction of more remunerative crops like soybean, cotton and maize in rainy season. However, due to adoption of improved production technologies by the farmers, the productivity has increased from 522 kg/ha to 962 kg/ha. Although the productivity of *rabi* sorghum is low i.e. 741 kg/ha as compared to 1267 kg/ha in *kharif*, it has better economic value for farmers because of its better grain quality for food as well as very good source for fodder for animals during lean summer period. Enhanced productivity leading to better income is the way to improve the livelihoods of small and marginal farmers.

Sorghum production is however, constrained by several biotic and abiotic stresses depending on the production environment. Developing production technologies resilient to these challenges, diverse end uses, value addition and commercialization as a health food are the key issues for improving sorghum productivity and making sorghum cultivation a profitable and attractive venture. This handbook provides exhaustive information on all aspects of sorghum production, value addition and commercialization. We believe that this handbook will be highly useful to the end-users and policy makers to promote sorghum farming.

Dr. J.V. Patil

Dr. J.S. Mishra

Contents

Chapter 1

Introduction, Origin and History

SORGHUM is the fifth most important cereal crop in the world. It is a native to Sub-Saharan Africa and is traditionally grown both as food (in Africa and India) and as animal feed (in developed countries like USA, China, Australia, etc). Its stalks are used as animal fodder, building material and fuel. The oldest cultivation record dates back to 3000 B.C. Egypt. Sorghum is known by various names in different parts of the world. In Western Africa, it is called great millet, *kafir* corn or guinea corn, which represents a connection with corn or millet. It is called *jowar* in India, *kaolian* in China and *milo* in Spain. It is the dietary staple for more than 500 million people in 30 countries (Kumar *et al.*, 2011). Sorghum grain is mostly used for food purpose (55 per cent) followed by feed grain (33 per cent). Lately, sweet sorghum is emerging as a potential feedstock for biofuels. Its drought adaptation capability, makes it a preferred crop in tropical, warmer and semi-arid regions of the world that witness high temperature and water stress (Paterson, *et al.*, 2009). With the threat of climate change looming large on the crop productivity, sorghum,for being a drought hardy crop, will play an important role in producing food, feed and fodder security in dryland economy.

Sorghum grain has high nutritive value. It has, 70-80 per cent carbohydrate, 11-13 per cent protein, 2-5 per cent fat, 1-3 per cent fiber, and 1-2 per cent ash. Protein in sorghum is gluten free and, thus, it is a specialty food for people who suffer from celiac disease, as well as for diabetic patients (Prasad and Staggenborg, 2009). Sorghum fibers are used in wallboard, fences, biodegradable packaging materials, and solvents. Its dried stalks are used as cooking fuel, and dye can be extracted from the plant to colour leather (Maunder, 2000).

Numerous factors have contributed to the wide acceptance of sorghum as a grain and forage crop. These factors are;

1. Versatile planting dates
2. Tolerance to drought
3. Relatively shorter growing season

4. Suitability for double cropping and rotation systems
5. Ability to grow in areas with marginal soil, scanty rainfall and high temperature, when other cereals often fail there.

Area and Spread

In 2012, sorghum was grown on 37.85 million ha area in the entire world, producing about 58.10 million tonnes of grain with an average yield of 1535 kg/ hectare (Table 1.1). USA, India, Mexico, Nigeria, Sudan, Ethiopia and Australia are the major producers of sorghum in the world (FAO, 2012) while India and Africa account for the largest share (>70 per cent) of global sorghum area. Over 55 per cent of the global sorghum production is in the semi-arid tropics (SAT); of the total SAT production, Asia and Africa contribute about 65 per cent, of which 34 per cent is harvested in India (Sahrawat *et al.*, 1996). However, though the sorghum area declined globally from 51 m ha in 1980s to 38 m ha in 2012, the productivity increased from 1300 kg/ha to 1535 kg/ha during the same period due to adoption of improved sorghum cultivars and management practices.

Table 1.1: Area, Production and Productivity of Sorghum in World (2012)

Continent/Country	Area (million ha)	Production (million tonnes)	Yield (kg/ha)
Asia	7.93	9.50	1198
India	6.32	6.01	951
China	0.47	2.00	4245
Africa	22.63	23.44	1036
Burkina faso	1.62	1.92	1188
Cameroon	0.74	1.11	1499
Chad	0.90	1.2	1333
Ethiopia	1.92	3.95	2054
Mali	0.86	1.21	1412
Niger	2.50	1.00	400
Nigeria	5.50	6.90	1254
Sudan	6.61	2.63	469
America	6.42	22.14	3447
Argentina	1.15	5.20	4522
Brazil	0.69	2.04	2948
USA	2.00	6.27	3128
Europe	0.22	0.78	3516
Australia and New Zealand	0.65	2.24	3445
World	**37.85**	**58.10**	**1535**

Source: FAO 2014. http://faostat.fao.org verified on January 8, 2014.

Unlike in other parts of the world, sorghum in India is cultivated both during rainy (*kharif*) and post-rainy (*rabi*) seasons, mainly as a rainfed crop (92 per cent of the area). The area, production and productivity of sorghum in different states of India are given in Tables 1.2–1.5. In India, Maharashtra is the largest cultivator and producer of sorghum followed by Karnataka, Madhya Pradesh and Andhra Pradesh. It was known as "great millet" till early eighties with an area of more than 18 million ha. The area has declined drastically from 18.6 m ha in 1969-70 to 6.25 m ha in 2011-12. The total production also declined from 9.72 m t to 6.01 m t. However the productivity has increased from 522 kg/ha to 962 kg/ha during the same period mainly due to adoption of improved production technologies by the farmers. The reduction of the area has been mainly in the *kharif* (rainy) season (Figure 1.1) primarily due to introduction of more remunerative crops like soybean, cotton and maize. *Kharif* sorghum is grown in most of the states while *rabi* (post-rainy) sorghum is largely confined to contiguous Deccan plateau regions of Maharashtra, Karnataka and Andhra Pradesh. Although the productivity of *rabi* sorghum is low (741 kg/ha as compared to 1267 kg/ha in *kharif*), yet it has better economic value for farmers as compared to *kharif* sorghum because its grain quality for food is better as well as it is a very good source of fodder for animals during lean summer period. In recent years, sorghum cultivation is gaining popularity among the farmers in rice-fallows of coastal Andhra Pradesh, especially in Guntur and adjoining Krishna, East Godavari and Prakasam districts. The area of sorghum in rice-fallows has increased from 1000 ha during 2008-09 to >24,000 ha area in 2012-13. The average productivity has also increased from 5.7 t/ha to 6.5 t/ha during the same period.

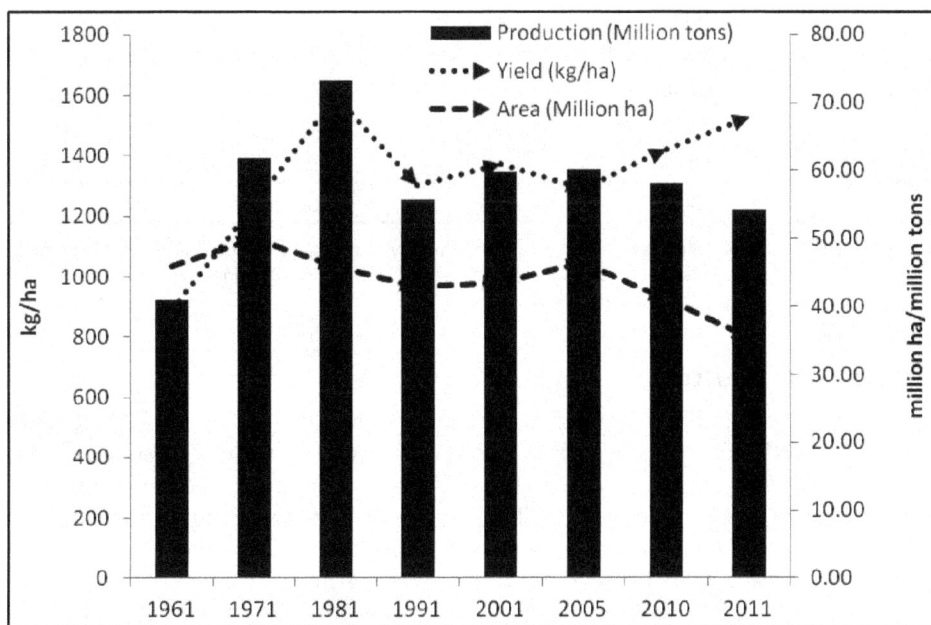

Figure 1.1: Trends in Area, Production and Productivity of World Grain Sorghum.

Table 1.2: State-wise Area, Production and Productivity of Sorghum in India (2010-11)

State	Season	Area (million ha)	Production (million tonnes)	Productivity (kg/ha)
Andhra Pradesh	Kharif	0.11	0.11	1000
	Rabi	0.14	0.19	1386
	Total	0.25	0.30	1213
Gujarat	Kharif	0.12	0.17	1331
	Rabi	0.05	0.04	860
	Total	0.17	0.21	1049
Haryana	Kharif	0.07	0.04	500
Karnataka	Kharif	0.21	0.35	1597
	Rabi	1.03	1.11	1093
	Total	1.24	1.46	1180
Madhya Pradesh	Kharif	0.43	0.61	1426
Maharashtra	Kharif	1.03	1.36	1325
	Rabi	3.03	2.09	689
	Total	4.06	3.45	850
Orissa	Kharif	0.01	0.01	644
Rajasthan	Kharif	0.72	0.10	145
Tamil Nadu	Kharif	0.20	0.15	715
	Rabi	0.06	0.07	1185
	Total	0.26	0.22	929
Uttar Pradesh	Kharif	0.19	0.17	885
Others	Kharif	0.02	0.02	870
All India	Kharif	3.07	3.44	1119
	Rabi	4.31	3.56	827
	Total	7.38	7.00	949

Source: Directorate of Millet Development (DMD), Ministry of Agriculture, GoI, Jaipur, 2012, State of Indian Agriculture 2012-13. Government of India, Ministry of Agriculture, Department of Agriculture and Cooperation, New Delhi.

Origin and History

Sorghum originated in Africa, more precisely in Ethiopia, nearly 5000 to 7000 years ago (ICRISAT, 2005). Sorghum's center of origin is believed to be near Lake Chad in Africa. From there it was further distributed along the trade and shipping routes around the African continent. Through the Middle East Sorgghum first came to India at least 3000 years ago. It then further journeyed along the Silk Route into China (Dicko *et al.*, 2006). It was first taken to North America in the 1700-1800's AD through the slave trade, from West Africa and was re-introduced in Africa in the late 19th century for commercial cultivation. From there it spread to South America and Australia. There is evidence of sorghum being found in Assyria by 700 BC and in

Table 1.3: Area, Production and Productivity of *Kharif* Grain Sorghum (India)

Year	Area (Million ha)	Production (Million tons)	Yield (Kg/ha)
1969-70	11.52	6.46	560
1974-75	10.25	6.11	598
1979-80	10.17	8.18	803
1984-85	9.82	7.96	810
1989-90	9.1	8.28	911
1994-95	6.76	7.45	1092
1999-00	5	5.02	1005
2004-05	4.07	3.95	967
2005-06	3.94	4.16	1055
2006-07	3.77	3.95	1048
2007-08	3.50	4.11	1176
2008-09	3.21	2.82	879
2009-10	3.31	3.25	978
2010-11	3.07	3.44	1119
2011-12	2.62	3.32	1267

Table 1.4: Area, Production and Productivity of *Rabi* Grain Sorghum (India)

Year	Area (Million ha)	Production (Million tons)	Yield (Kg/ha)
1969-70	7.06	3.4	482
1974-75	5.89	2.72	454
1979-80	6.21	3.54	729
1984-85	6.43	3.4	528
1989-90	6.04	3.47	574
1994-95	5.68	3.67	644
1999-00	5.33	3.25	611
2004-05	5.23	3.12	597
2005-06	4.84	3.82	788
2006-07	4.79	3.78	840
2007-08	4.26	3.81	894
2008-09	4.45	4.16	935
2009-10	4.39	4.04	921
2010-11	4.31	3.56	827
2011-12	3.62	2.69	741

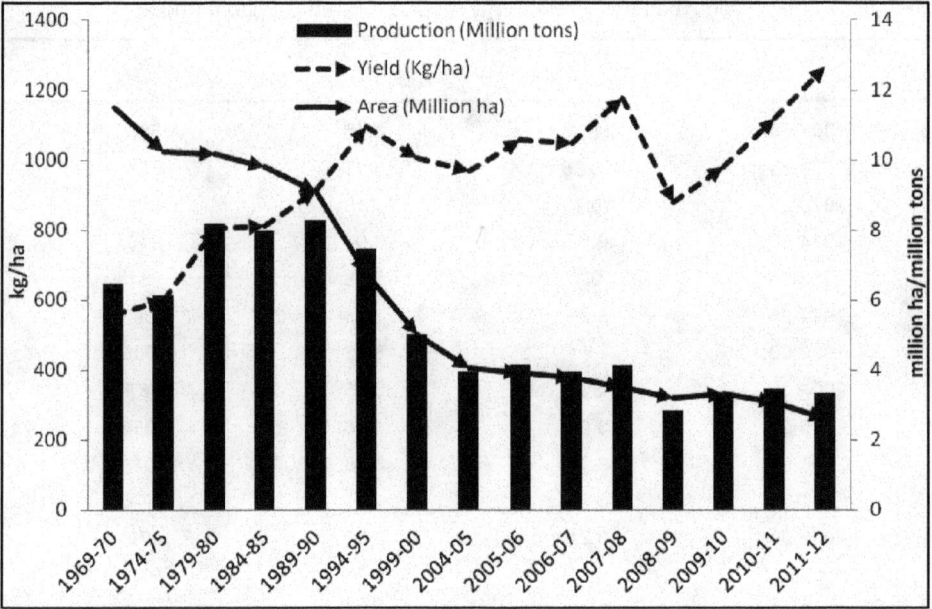

Figure 1.2: Trends in Area, Production and Productivity of *Kharif* Grain Sorghum in India.

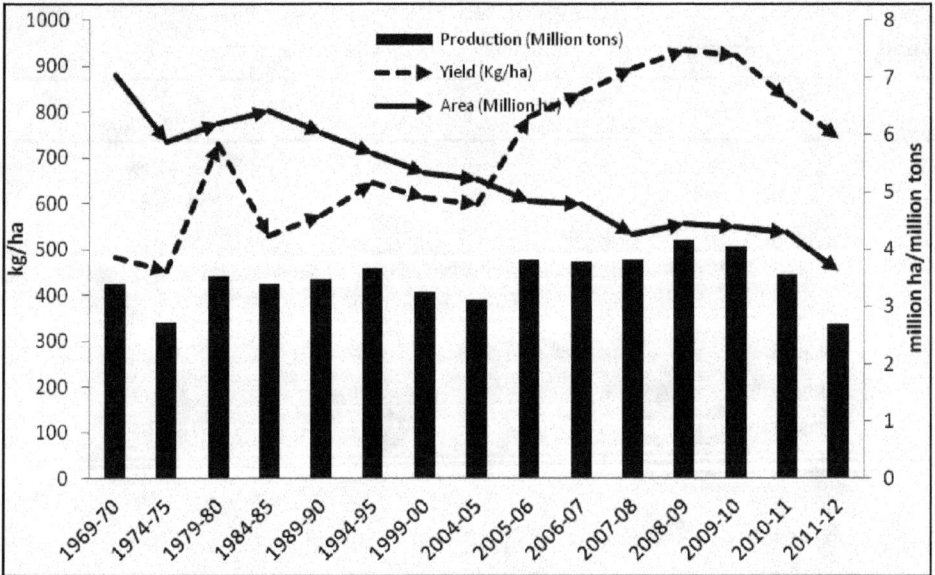

Figure 1.3: Trends in Area, Production and Productivity of *Rabi* Grain Sorghum in India.

India and Europe by I AD (Eastin, 1983). This crop is now widely found in the dry areas of Africa, Asia (India and China), the Americas and Australia (Dicko *et al.*, 2006). Grain sorghum belongs to the family of Poaceae (grass), tribe Andopogoneae, sub-tribe Sorghinae, genus Sorghum. In 1794, Moench established the genus Sorghum

Table 1.5: Area, Production and Productivity of Total Grain Sorghum (*Kharif* + *Rabi*) in India

Year	Area (Million ha)	Production (Million tons)	Yield (Kg/ha)
1969-70	18.61	9.72	522
1974-75	16.19	10.41	643
1979-80	16.67	11.65	699
1984-85	15.94	11.40	715
1989-90	14.84	12.90	869
1994-95	11.51	8.97	779
1999-00	10.25	8.68	847
2004-05	9.09	7.24	797
2005-06	8.67	7.24	880
2006-07	8.47	7.15	844
2007-08	7.76	7.93	1021
2008-09	7.53	7.25	962
2009-10	7.79	6.70	860
2010-11	7.38	7.00	949
2011-12	6.25	6.01	962

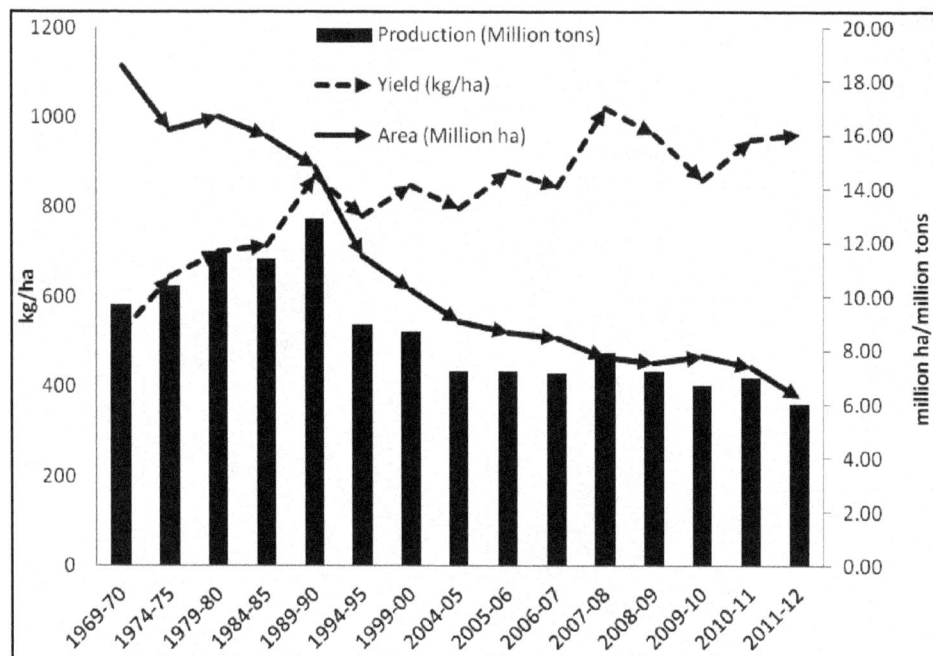

Figure 1.4: Trends in Area, Production and Productivity of Total Grain Sorghum in India.

and brought the sorghums under the name *S. bicolor*. All cultivated sorghum belongs to *Sorghum bicolor* subsp. Bicolor (Dicko *et al.*, 2006). There are five basic races: bicolor, guinea, caudatum, kafir, durra; and ten intermediate races under *S. bicolor*. It is a cereal of a remarkable genetic variability, with more than 30,000 selections present in the world genetic collections (Assefa and Staggenborg, 2010). The morphological characteristics change with genotype and growing conditions. Most of the tropical sorghums are short day plants and their response to day length is an important adaptation. However, the selection of early-maturing varieties and hybridation helped its spread in the USA (Prasad and Staggenborg, 2009).

Historical Background of Sorghum Research in India

In India, while sorghum research was being carried out since pre-independence years, organized research was initiated only in 1962, with the establishment of Accelerated Sorghum and Millet Improvement Project (ASMIP). Later, in 1969 All India Coordinated Sorghum Improvement Project (AICSIP) was established which had 18 main centres spread over 13 State Agricultural Universities in 11 major sorghum growing states. First commercial sorghum hybrid 'CSH 1' was released in 1964 for all India cultivation, using the parental line bred in USA and supplied by the Rockefeller Foundation. Since then, Indian sorghum breeding steadily gained competence and moved to the vanguard. In 1970, AICSIP was shifted from New Delhi to IARI Regional Station Hyderabad. In 1972 the International Crops Research Institute for Semi-Arid Tropics (ICRISAT) was established in Hyderabad, which further spurred sorghum improvement research. National Research Centre for Sorghum was established in 1987 in Hyderabad by upgrading IARI Regional Station. During 1960's and 1970's, sorghum was cultivated through highly traditional mode of agriculture, and there was very little impact of modern technologies in terms of high yielding varieties, adequate fertilization and plant protection. The agronomic research in sorghum during the last 50 years was mostly concentrated on nutrient and water management and sorghum-based intercropping systems.

Chapter 2

The Grain Sorghum Plant

Sorghum is often a cross pollinated C_4 plant of *Poaceae* family. It is a cereal, grown widely as food, animal feed, fibre and fuel. Tolerant to hot and dry conditions, it is a staple for large populations in the West African Sahel region and semi-arid tropical areas in India. The morphological characteristics change with genotype and

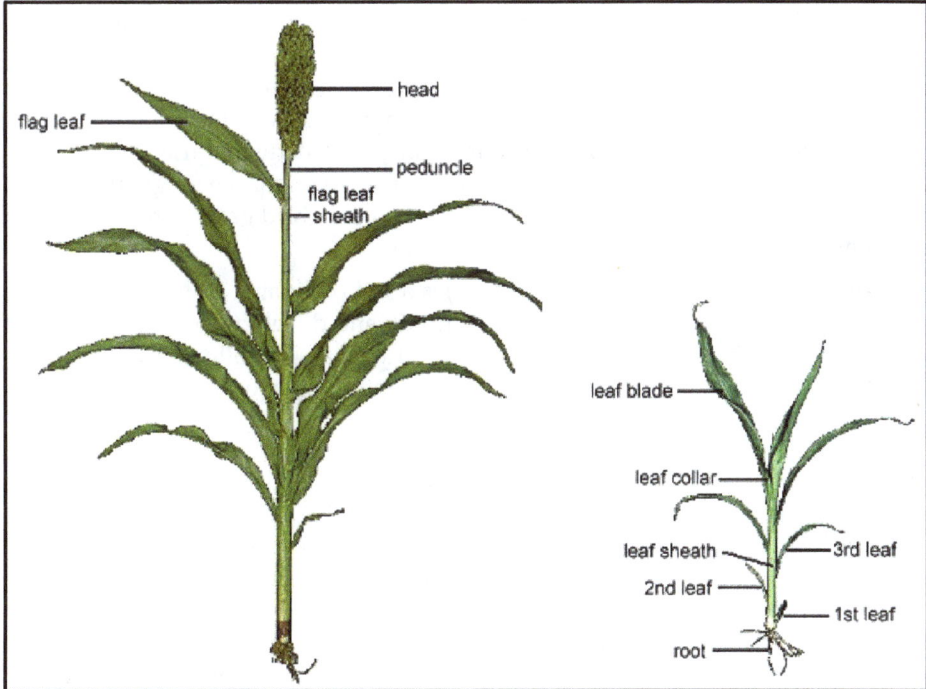

Figure 2.1: The Grain Sorghum Plant.
Source: http://www.soilcropandmore.info

growing conditions. Most of the tropical sorghums are short day plants and their response to day length is an important adaptation.

2.1 Morphology

Taxonomy and Characteristics

All sorghums belong in the *Poaceae* grass plant family and in the *Sorghinae* sub-tribe within the *Andropogoneae* plant tribe (Dahlberg, 2000). The genus *Sorghum* includes three species: *bicolor*, *propinquum*, and *halepense*. *Sorghum bicolor* contains all of the cultivated sorghums. Both *Sorghum propinquum* and *Sorghum halepense* are rhizomatous wild, weedy perennials that are able to cross with *Sorghum bicolor* (de Wet, 1978). *Sorghum bicolor* (L.) Moench. is further divided into three subspecies, *Sorghum bicolor* subsp. *bicolor*, *drummondii*, and *verticilliforum* (formerly known as *Arundinaceum*). The latter two subspecies are annual weeds (Dahlberg, 2000; de Wet, 1978). The cultivated subspecies *bicolor* consists of five different races, which can combine with each other to produce ten hybrid intermediate races, totaling 15 races all together (Dahlberg, 2000; de Wet, 1978). The race *bicolor* is large and complex, consisting of many different sub-races that produce small amounts of grain and that are mainly used as forage. One of the most important sub-races of the race *bicolor* is sorgo, which contains many of the sweet sorghum cultivars that are used for syrup production. Another race – guinea - is well adapted to high-rainfall environments and is very important in West Africa where it is widely grown for human consumption. The race durra contains the most drought tolerant cultivars that are grown in the Near East, Ethiopia, and India, and were once popular in the United States where they were commonly called milo (Harlan and de Wet, 1972). A fourth race, caudatum, is known for its high grain yield potential and high seed quality (Dahlberg, 2000; Harlan and de Wet, 1972). The last race, kafir, is agronomically important due to its high yield potential and closed to semi-open panicle structure (Harlan and de Wet, 1972). The 'kafir-caudatum' intermediate race is the most important for grain sorghum production in the United States today, because most hybrid grain sorghums are of this intermediate race (Harlan and de Wet, 1972).

Sorghum (*Sorghum bicolor* L. Moench.) is a self pollinated C_4 plant of poaceae family. It is important to understand the growth and developmental behaviour of sorghum plant to manage the crop for better productivity. The following section gives a brief description of germination, growth and reproduction of sorghum plant.

Germination and Seedling Development

Germination is defined as the emergence of radical from the seed coat. The process involves uptake of water (imbibation), mobilization of food reserves stored within the seed; and the resumption of growth and development of the embryo to form the root and shoot structures of the seedling (Fisher, 1984). Temperature and soil moisture are the two most important environmental requirements for germination. At optimum temperature (25-30°C) and moisture, sorghum seed germinates in 3-5 days. The seed absorbs water and swells, this breaks the seed coat and a small coleoptile and radicle (primary root) emerges (House, 1985). The young seedling takes its nutrients from the endosperm. Secondary roots develop in 3-7 days. The germination and seedling development phase is more sensitive to cold temperature (Tiryaki and Andrews, 2001a, b). Poor emergence and seedling death due to cold temperatures results in reduced plant populations and grain yields.

Root System

Sorghum roots are adventitious and fibrous. The early temporary/embrionic root is the single radicle of the germinating seedling. The remaining of the fibrous root system develop from lowest node of the stem. Mature roots are adventitious. Sorghum root system could

Figure 2.2: Germination of Sorghum Seed. **Source**: R. L. Vanderlip, *How a Sorghum Plant Develops*, Kansas State University, January 1993.

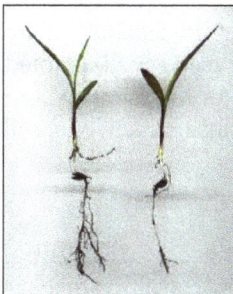

be described under seminal, adventitious and nodal roots (Maiti, 1996a). Seminal or primary roots develop directly from the elongation of the radicle and can easily be distinguished by its continuity with the base of the culm. These roots are mainly responsible for the establishment of seedlings and are reported to survive up to 4-5 days by which time the other roots systems. Primary roots have a limited growth and their functions are soon taken over by the secondary roots. The adventitious or secondary roots developed from the base of the coleoptiles to form the extensive root system. These roots become active in about 30 days of plant age and are found to be active up to anthesis. The nodal/crown roots develop from the lowest node of the stem after 30-40 days of emergence and are heavily branched. These roots are strong and slightly green in colour. Depending on the cultivar, crown root development may extend to several nodes. Nodal roots are active from anthesis up to maturity and support the stem, but they are not effective in water and nutrient uptake. The cultivated sorghums are either non-rhizomatous or very weakly rhizomatous. The root system survives to support the tillers and ratoon crop from adventitious buds at the base of the parent stem. Well developed rhizomes are found in the subspecies *halepense* (House, 1985).

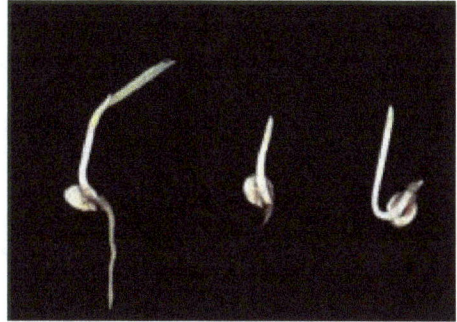

| Seminal Roots | Adventitious Roots | Crown Roots |

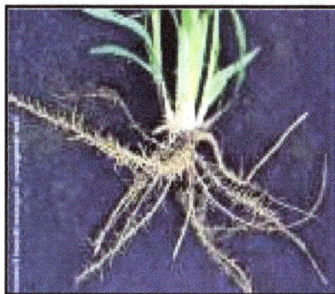

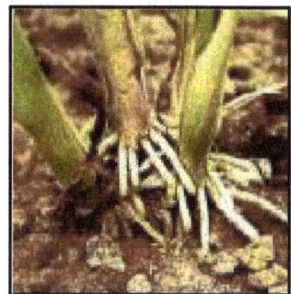

Figure 2.3: Root Systems in Sorghum.

Stem

The stem or culm is erect and made up of a series of alternating nodes and inter-nodes encircled by leaf sheaths. Sorghum stems are solid, though the centre may become spongy, with spaces in the pith. It measures 0.5 to 5.0 cm in diameter near the plant base, becoming narrower towards peduncle. It grows to a height of 0.5-4.0 m at maturity depending up on the cultivar. The nodes appear as a ring at the base of the leaf sheath. A bud is present at each node except at the flag leaf, and sprouts on alternate sides of the stem. Sometimes these buds develop into auxiliary tillers, while basal tillers are formed at the first node (House, 1980). Vascular bundles are scattered throughout the stem, but they are more near the peripheral area. The vascular bundles in the central portion of the stem are larger than those at the periphery, and these central bundles branch into leaf midribs, while the peripheral bundles branch to form the smaller veins in the leaf blade. The pith may be sweet or insipid, juicy or dry. Sweet sorghum and certain fodder varieties are juicier and sweeter than the grain sorghum.

Leaf

Sorghum has four embryonic leaves. The leaves on the main stem vary from 14 to 17 depending on cultivar. Generally, young leaves are erect and the older leaves are curved. Mature leaves may attain a maximum length of >100 cm and width 10-15 cm. The terminal leaf is called flag leaf. The leaf sheath is attached to the node and surrounds the internodes. The leaf sheath is often covered with a waxy bloom. The angle of attachment of leaves to the stem varies. The arrangement of leaves on the stem is usually alternate in two ranks on opposite side of the stem. Leaves are glabrous with smooth or scabrid leaf margin. The leaf blade is long, narrow and pointed. It may be straight or bent like an arc. The tip of the leaf may even drop down. The length and width of leaf blade varies widely. Most leaf growth occurs between the growing point differentiation stage and the boot stage. Generally, young leaves are erect and the older leaves are curved. Mature leaves may attain a maximum length of >100 cm and width 10-15 cm. The terminal leaf is called flag leaf. The arrangement of leaves on the stem is usually alternate in two ranks on opposite side of the stem. Leaves are glabrous with smooth or scabrid leaf margin. The midrib is prominent, greenish or white in colour, flattened or slightly concave on the upper surface and convex on the lower one. There is a short membranous ligule at the junction of the leaf blade with the sheath. The number of leaves vary depending on the genotype. In a well-adapted plant there will be usually 14-17 leaves (House, 1985). The stomata is present on both surfaces of the leaf and there are also lines of motor cells which cause the leaves to roll inwards under drought conditions.

Panicle

The inflorescence of sorghum is a panicle (also known as 'head') with a central rachis from which primary branches arise. The panicle consists of several spikelets in pairs, one of them being sessile and fertile, the other being pedicelled and male or sterile. The size of panicle ranges from 7.5-50 cm in length and 4-20 cm in width. They may be compact or loose. The rachis, central axis of the panicle may be completely hidden by dense panicle branches or exposed, and differs greatly in shape and length. The rachis may be striated, hairy or glabrous. Several primary branches are borne at each node and these branches vary in length and strength. Each primary branch bears secondary branches, which in turn bear spikelets. The panicle usually grows erect at the apex of the culm, but may be recurved depending on the genotype. The wild and forage type sorghums have a rather loose pyramidal panicle with spreading branches (House, 1985).The raceme always consists of one or several spikelets. One of the spikelets is always sessile (fertile) and the other pedicellate (sterile), except the terminal sessile spikelet, which is accompanied by two pediceled spikelets. The racemes vary in length in accordance with the number of nodes and length of internodes. On the pediceled spikelet, the pedicels vary in length from 0.5 to 3.0 mm, and usually are very similar to the internodes.

Sessile spikelet has two glumes of roughly equal length, which might be coriaceous (leathery) or charlaceous (papery) at maturity. The lower glume partially envelops the upper one and they may be roughly grouped in to ovate, elliptic or obovate shapes. The glumes enclose two florets, the upper being perfect the lower being sterile. The fertile floret has a membranous lemma with a two toothed, cleft at the apex. There are three stamens and a single-celled ovary with two long styles ending in plumose stigmas. Due to the second floret being fertile, certain sorghum varieties regularly produce twin seeds in each spikelet.

Grain

Sorghum grain is 'Caryopsis'. Grain is a ripened ovary with attached glumes. It is usually partially enclosed by glumes, which are removed during threshing. The shape of the seed is oval to round, from 4 to 8 mm in diameter (Purseglove, 1972) and varying in size, shape and colour depending on the cultivar. The grains are pointed at the base and have a slight

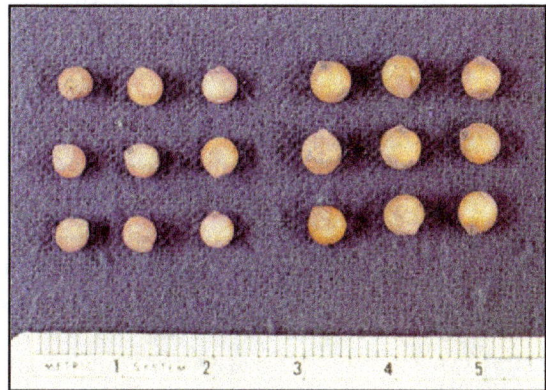

depression near the end. The grain colour may be white, yellow or brownish-yellow. The pigment is confined to seed coat layer with the exception of yellow shade, which can be present in the endosperm. Sorghum grain consists of endosperm, pericarp, testa and germ. Twin seeds are is also found in some genotypes. The 1000-grain weight varies from 25-30 g.

2.2 Physiology

Yield Limitations

A survey made by Peacock (1980) to investigate yield-reducing factors in different sorghum-growing regions of the world indicated that drought, stand establishment, soil fertility, weeds and grain quality are the most serious problems limiting sorghum production in semi-arid tropical countries. Drought was the major constraint reported in 14 countries. However, sorghum is relatively more tolerant to drought as compared to other cereals crops. Mechanisms of drought resistance in sorghum include escape, avoidance and tolerance (Seetharama *et al.*, 1982). Three escape mechanisms that enable crop plants to resist drought are early maturity, developmental plasticity and remobilization of stem reserves stored before anthesis to the developing grains (Turner, 1979). The replacement of traditional 130- to 180- day sorghum cultivars with earlier hybrids (100-110-day cultivars) in India allowed the crop to avoid moisture stress by maturing before the end of the rains or before soil moisture was depleted. This simple performance approach modification resulted in remarkable increase in sorghum production in India (Rao *et al.*, 1979).

Factors Affecting Maturity

Larson and Thompson (2011) studied the effects of planting populations on seed maturation, on dryland trials in southeast Colorado and found that, increasing the seeding rate of grain sorghum decreased the amount of time that it took for the grain to reach maturation. As plant populations are increased, fewer tillers are produced due to the increased plant competition and limiting resources during the vegetative growth stages (Lafarge *et al.*, 2002; Larson and Thompson, 2011). In a plant population study done by Gerik and Neely (1987), a decreased number of tillers with increased plant populations shortened the overall maturity since the tillers flowered about seven to ten days later than the main culms. A similar effect on maturity was found by Bandaru *et al.* (2006) when they conducted a dryland study on growing sorghum in clumps. Plants grown in the clumps had fewer tillers and matured faster than those grown in traditional rows.

Studies have been carried out on row spacing and orientation to see if they play any role in sorghum maturity. The study revealed that, light interception by plants is affected by row direction and it was found that the interception was lower in rows planted east and west than in rows planted north and south (Steiner, 1986; Witt *et al.*, 1972). In a study done by Witt *et al.* (1972) in Manhattan, Kansas, light meters above and below the crop were used to determine the amount of light intercepted by the plants in the 300-450 nm range in the different treatments. Light interception by the plants was lower in the wide rows (1 m spacing) than in the narrow rows (0.5 m spacing) in both row orientations. This was attributed to a decrease within row population from the row spacing, which allowed more light to be intercepted by the plants in the narrow rows. The light interception data was collected every five or seven days, beginning around mid-July. Up to 40 per cent of light, reached the soil surface between the rows going north and south, which helped to heat the surface. Less light reached the soil surface in the mid-point between the rows in the east/west orientation and more light on the south side of rows in the wide row spacing (1 m). At the same row spacing but north/south orientation, more light was accumulated at the mid-point than next to the rows. In a study using the SORKAM model, increasing row widths decreased the number of tillers due to within row plant densities increasing which would shorten the time to maturity since fewer tillers were produced (Baumhardt *et al.*, 2005).

Plant genetics and cultivar selection might have the biggest effect on the amount of thermal time that the plants take to reach full maturity (Croissant, 1969). Long season hybrids generally produce more tillers than short season hybrids, and the grain fill period is also extended in long season cultivars, both of which increase the total time to maturity (Baumhardt *et al.*, 2005; Schaffer, 1980). Photoperiod during the growing season affects time to maturity as different sorghum hybrids have varying levels of photoperiod sensitivity. Photoperiod sensitive hybrids are more sensitive to temperature fluctuations than photoperiod insensitive hybrids. They will only flower when a certain photoperiod is reached during the growing season (Quinby and Schertz, 1970; Rooney and Aydin, 1999).

Other important factors that affect the time to maturity are soil fertility, temperature, water availability, and solar radiation (Vinall and Reed, 1918; Croissant, 1969; Roozeboom and Fjell, 1998). When important macronutrients such as nitrogen and phosphorus are at adequate level in the soil, maturity in sorghum can be hastened due to faster leaf development and more efficient photosynthetic capabilities of the plant (Srivastava and Singh, 1969). Cool temperatures can prolong the growth of the plant at all growth stages, as grain sorghum is very sensitive to cold temperatures during different development stages (Doggett, 1970). This is the reason a base temperature is used when calculating GDD for reaching development stages. Plants that are drought stressed will mature faster or slower depending on the growth stage of the plants, as drought will shorten the duration of grain filling, and will extend maturity if flowering has not occurred (Schaffer, 1980). A study by Vinall and Reed (1918), found that solar radiation intercepted by the plant was an important factor for the development rate of sorghum in addition to temperature. They discovered this when they observed significant growth differences at two locations where the thermal time based on the air temperature was similar.

Factors Affecting Yield

Unlike maturity, much research has been done on the effects of agronomic factors on the overall yield of grain sorghum. Steiner (1986) found that high plant populations (18 compared to 6 and 12 plants m^{-2}) decreased yield during dry years, and Wade and Douglas (1990) had similar results in their study when late maturing hybrids in high plant densities yielded much lower under water stress than when adequate water was available. In 1995, a study by Jones showed that yield in a dry year was higher in treatments with low plant populations and wide rows, than treatments with high populations and narrow rows. Bandaru *et al.* (2006) investigated the effects of growing sorghum plants in clumps as compared to the traditional (75 cm) row spacing to reduce vegetative growth (including tillers). They found that the yield was higher in the clump treatments since water was preserved early in the season and this made more water available during flowering and grain filling. Tillers that were produced when water was limited did not increase or contribute to the overall final yield.

Bond *et al.* (1964) noted that during a drought year sorghum grown in wide rows (1 m) yielded higher than when those grown in narrow rows (0.51 m). Steiner (1986) also found that plants in wide rows used less water during the vegetative growth stage, and subsequently–more water was available later in the season during critical growth stages. Vigil *et al.* (2008) noted that the skip-row yield was higher than traditional 0.76 m row spacings during years when moisture was limited. Skip-row also showed an advantage when the yield was lower than 3.5 Mg/ha. Abunyewa *et al.* (2008) noted in a grain sorghum study in Nebraska that, skip-row yield was increased as compared to yield in traditional row spacings which were less than 4.5 Mg/ha. Baumhardt *et al.* (2005) used the SORKAM crop model to simulate the dryland sorghum yield in Bushland, Texas from 1958 to 1998, and observed that sorghum planted in narrow rows tillered more than in wide rows due to a lower within row population. Therefore, yield was higher in the narrow row spacings as more tillers were produced. Another dryland study conducted in the Texas High Plains concluded that, row spacings of 1.5 m produced less grain than rows that were half as wide. They suggested the use of a lower seeding rate in the narrow rows, to increase tillering and overall yield during wet years (Jones and Johnson, 1991). Stickler and Laude (1960) conducted a dryland study in Manhattan, Kansas and found no significant difference among row widths at a low seeding population, but as the population was increased, the yield increased in the narrow rows.

Steiner's study in 1986 investigated the effects of row orientation on yield and found that row direction had no significant effects on either yield or water consumption by the plants. In a light interception and yield study done by Witt *et al.* (1972), there saw no significant yield difference between two different row orientations of north/south and east/west planted rows. Lugg (1974) found that north and south oriented rows yielded higher than rows planted in the other three orientations of east/west, northwest/southeast, and northeast/southwest. He attributed the difference in yield mainly to differences in water availability and distribution within the trial area rather than to row orientation.

Late maturity hybrids tend to yield higher than shorter season sorghum hybrids due to the longer grain-filling period and increased vegetative growth (Baumhardt *et al.*, 2005). Earlier maturing hybrids are generally more stable for yield than later maturing ones since the grain-filling period is shorter and less variable (Saeed and Francis, 1983). If the growing season is long enough, late maturity hybrids will almost always yield higher than early maturing hybrids, as long as both are well adapted for the growing conditions (Roozeboom and Fjell, 1998). If the growing season is short, late maturity hybrids will have a much higher chance of a reduced yield and test weight due to frost damage before physiological maturity (Staggenborg and Vanderlip, 1996).

Major environmental factors that can affect yield are, water availability, soil fertility, and temperature. Yield can be negatively affected by water stress caused by prolonged drought conditions, especially during critical development stages such as flowering (Doggett, 1970; Kramer and Ross, 1970; Vanderlip, 1993). Adequate levels of important nutrients, such as nitrogen, phosphorus, and potassium ensure that, the yield potential of hybrids is attainable, as more nutrients are needed as the yield potential increases (Cothren *et al.*, 2000). Extreme high or low temperatures can negatively affect yield and excessively high temperatures, before or during flowering, can decrease the grain yield dramatically (Staggenborg and Vanderlip, 1996; Vanderlip, 1993; Vinall and Reed, 1918). Low temperatures can also decrease the yield during flowering, and it can also be detrimental during the grain fill period when the plants are still accumulating dry matter (Staggenborg and Vanderlip, 1996).

Physiological Maturity

Sorghum grains mature in 30-35 days after fertilization. At physiological maturity, a dark brown callus tissue is formed at the base where the seed is attached to the spikelet. This callus tissue stops the translocation of nutrients from the plant to the seed. Grain sorghum is almost ready to harvest at this stage, and the length of time between physiological maturity and harvest depends on the climate conditions. At this stage, the seed contains 25-30 per cent moisture and fully viable. If grain-drying facilities are not available, then the sorghum should be harvested when the kernel moisture has dropped to 14-15 per cent or lower (McClure *et al.*, 2010).

Growth Stages

Grain sorghum is perennial, but it is treated as an annual plant in many parts of the world where it is grown. It has ten distinct growth stages, that were defined by Vanderlip and Reeves in 1972, by using predominate characteristics for each stage. The emergence of the seedling is denoted as growth stage zero and is defined as when the coleoptiles becomes visible above the soil surface. Stages one and two occur when the third and fifth leaf collars, respectively, become visible on the culm. The third stage occurs when the growing point shifts from vegetative growth to reproductive growth and this is when the main stem begins to elongate in order form the peduncle (Vanderlip and Reeves, 1972). This stage marks the beginning of the critical growth period as any environmental stresses such as drought or extreme temperatures will negatively affect the final yield (Downes, 1972; Gerik *et al.*, 2003; McClure *et al.*, 2010). Stages four and five occur when the last leaf (flag leaf) is visible and when all leaves have fully emerged and expanded. Stage six, or half bloom, occurs when half of the panicle has started to flower as panicles start to flower from the top and progress downward (Poehlman, 1987; Vanderlip and Reeves, 1972). Stages seven and eight are the soft and hard dough stages, and the last stage is physiological maturity, which occurs when the plant has finished accumulating dry matter and maximum dry weight is achieved (Vanderlip and Reeves, 1972). The time that the grain sorghum plant will take to complete its entire life cycle largely depends on the maturity class of the hybrid and the growing conditions (Gerik *et al.*, 2003).

The growth period of sorghum has three distinct phases: seedling development, panicle initiation and reproduction (Table 2.1).

Growth Stage (GS) 1: (Seedling Development)

It consists of seedling stage and starts from the date of seedling emergence to the onset of the reproductive phase (panicle initiation stage). Most of the leaves initiate during this stage.

Growth Stage 2: (Panicle Initiation)

It is the panicle development stage and starts from panicle initiation (PI) to anthesis (or 50 per cent flowering). The duration ranges from 35 to 40 days. This stage is also paralleled by stem elongation.

Growth Stage 3: (Reproduction)

It is the grain-filling stage and starts from anthesis to physiological maturity. Formation of the black layer at the base of grain, signals the end of this stage. The duration usually ranges between 40 and 45 days depending upon genotype and environment.

Table 2.1: Developmental and Physiological Growth Stages of Sorghum and Approximate Time Required for each Stage (Vanderlip and Reeves, 1972; Maiti, 1996; Rao *et al.*, 2004).

Developmental Stage	Growth Stage	Identifying Characters	Days after Emergence*
0	–	Seedling emergence: Coleoptile leaf visible	0
1	1	Three leaf: collar of third leaf visible	5-6
2	1	Five leaf: collar of fifth leaf visible	10-16
3	1	Panicle initiation: growing point differentiation (approximately 8th leaf visible), potential number of kernels per head determined. Might have lost 1-3 leaves from bottom of the plant.	25-32
4	2	Flag leaf: Tip of final leaf visible in the leaf whorl	35-50
5	2	Booting: head extended into the flag leaf sheath; potential head size has been determined.	50-55
6	2	Half bloom (50 per cent flowering): half of the plant at bloom stage.	55-65
7	3	Soft dough: milky stage, grain can be easily squeezed between fingers; 8-10 functional leaves; one half of the grain weight accumulated.	65-80
8	3	Hard dough: milky stage converted to hard dough stage; grains cannot be squeezed between fingers; three-fourths of the grain dry weight has accumulated	80-90
9	3	Physiological maturity: dark spot at the tip of the kernel; black hilar layer formed at the hilar region of the seed, maximum of total dry weight accumulated; grain has 25 to 35 per cent moisture.	90-110

* Planting to emergence takes about 4 days.

2.3. Plant Nutrition

Nitrogen, phosphorus and potassium are the essential elements required in relatively large amounts for proper growth and development of sorghum plant. Besides, sorghum requires iron, zinc, calcium, magnesium and manganese in smaller quantities based on soil test values. Roy and Wright (1974) reported that Nitrogen and P accumulation by whole plants increased almost linearly until maturity, but K accumulation was more rapid, early in the season. Nitrogen, P, and K accumulation rates were higher during the 35th to 42nd day and 70th to 91st day which coincide with the peak vegetative growth period and the grain-filling stage, respectively. In unfertilized plants relatively higher translocation of N and P from the vegetative parts to the developing grain occurred. Little K was translocated. A much smaller percentage of total K was found in the head and more K accumulated in the stem than N and P. A grain crop of 8.5 t/ha contains (in the total aboveground plant) 207 kg of N, 39 kg of P and 241 kg of K (Vanderlip, 1972). Pal *et al.* (1982) reported that in the early stages of crop growth, N and P were accumulated slowly as compared to the rapid accumulation of K. In later stages, uptake of K decreased, relatively to that of N and P.

2.4. Plant Composition

The plant composition values in sorghum were found to be quite similar in seedling whole plant samples, but major differences were demonstrated in vegetative, bloom, and fruiting stage leaf samples. There is a need for specific grain sorghum nutrient sufficiency values.

At harvest, the grain sorghum stubble contains 50-70 per cent moisture; it can be made into silage. The crude protein content will be about 6-7 per cent (3-5 per cent if irrigated) in the stubble.

Grain sorghum is mostly used as a cereal grain energy source and is a good feedstuff for poultry, pigs and ruminants. Its composition is roughly similar to that of maize and it is particularly rich in starch (more than 70 per cent of the dry matter). Crude protein content in sorghum grain ranges from 9 to 13 per cent DM and is slightly higher than that of maize, though much more variable, depending on growing conditions. Like maize, it has a low lysine content and its utilization may require amino acid supplementation. Fat content is also slightly lower in sorghum grain than in maize. Sorghum grain is devoid of xanthophyllin and 70 per cent of its phosphorus is bound in phytate (Sauvant *et al.*, 2004).

Sorghum is the chief cereal grain consumed in Asia and Africa. It is used to prepare foods for adults and children. In the tropical regions, baby foods are made from sorghum and maize gruels with addition of sugar (Obizoba, 1988). The protein quality of sorghum grain is poor because of the low content of essential amino acids such as lysine, tryptophan and threonine (Badi *et al.*, 1990). Malting improves protein quality of cereals because of an increase in lysine (Dalby and Tsai, 1976). Sorghum is poorly digested by infants, but if it is supplemented with foods high in lysine, it can be a satisfactory weaning food (MacLean *et al.*, 1981). Sorghum proteins become less digestible after cooking. Sorghum, like the other cereals, is a good source of B vitamins such as thiamin, riboflavin, vitamin B6, biotin and niacin, but refining produces, losses it of all such B vitamins (Hegedus *et al.*, 1985). Mineral composition of sorghum is similar to that of pearl millet. The chief minerals present in sorghum grain are potassium and phosphorus, while calcium is low. Sorghum contains polyphenolic compounds called condensed tannins, which are antinutritional factors. Condensed tannins decrease the nutritional value of the sorghum grain because they are able to bind to dietary proteins, digestive enzymes, minerals such as iron and B vitamins like thiamin and vitamin B6. They are present in sorghums that have a pigmented testa and are absent in white and coloured sorghums which are without a pigmented testa (see Anglani, 1998). A comparison of nutrients in various cereals is presented in Table 2.2 (Leder, 2004).

Table 2.2: Comparison of Nutrients in 100-g Edible Portions of Various Cereals at 12 per cent Moisture.

Cereal	Protein (g)	Fat (g)	CHO (g)	Crude Fiber (g)	Ash (g)	Energy (kcal)	Calcium (mg)	Iron (mg)	Thiamin (mg)	Niacin (mg)	Riboflavin (mg)
Wheat	11.6	2.0	71	2.0	1.6	348	30	3.5	0.405	5.05	0.101
Brown rice	7.9	2.7	76	1.0	1.3	362	33	1.8	0.413	4.31	0.043
Maize	9.2	4.6	73	2.8	1.2	358	26	2.7	0.378	3.57	0.197
Sorghum	10.9	3.2	73	2.3	1.6	329	27	4.3	0.300	2.83	0.138
Pearl millet	11.0	5.0	69	2.2	1.9	363	25	3.0	0.3	2.0	0.15
Foxtail millet	9.9	2.5	72	10.0	3.5	351	20	4.9	0.593	0.99	0.099
Finger millet	6.0	1.5	75	3.6	2.6	336	350	5.0	0.3	1.4	0.10
Kodo millet	11.5	1.3	74	10.4	2.6	353	35	1.7	0.15	–	–
Japanese barnyard millet	10.8	4.5	49	14.7	4.0	–	22	18.6	–	–	–
Proso millet	10.6	4.0	70	12.0	3.2	364	8	2.9	0.405	4.54	0.279

2.5 Water Requirement

Sorghum is drought tolerant crop. Its water requirement varies from 350 to 700 mm depending on, the season, crop duration, soil, nutrition and other environmental conditions. For optimum yields on good soil, short-growth, average-growth, and long-growth varieties requires 500 to 600 mm, 650 to 800 mm, and 950 to 1100 mm of well distributed rainfall, respectively. Raheja (1961) reported that sorghum crop requires about 610 mm water for optimum yield, whereas Chandramohan (1970) stated that 488 mm water was adequate for sorghum under Tamil Nadu conditions. Water requirement of main and ratoon sorghum was assessed at 520 and 293 mm, respectively when irrigation was scheduled at 50 per cent available soil moisture (Subbarayalu, 1982). Higher grain yield of 4.92 t/ha was obtained by applying 45 kg N/ha with a water requirement of 425 mm (Sharma and Neto, 1986). The water requirement for pure sorghum was less than sorghum + groundnut intercropping systems respectively (Shinde and Umrani, 1988).

2.6 Drought Resistance

The great advantage of sorghum is that it can become dormant under adverse conditions and can resume growth even after a relatively severe drought. However, shoot removal, lowers its capacity to withstand drought. Early drought stops growth before floral initiation and the plant remains vegetative; it will resume leaf production and flower when conditions again become favourable for growth. Late drought stops leaf development but not floral initiation (Whiteman and Wilson, 1965).

The dormancy strategy is one of many strategies that the drought-hardy plant employs. Sorghum also generates more roots in dry conditions, to enhance the plant's ability to search for water. It has wax on its leaves and stems to reduce moisture loss. It has narrow leaves that have the ability to fold the in on themselves. All these are strategies to conserve moisture in both heat and drought stress. It is reported that sorghum uses one-third of less moisture than corn and it takes one-half the water required by sugarcane.

The crop faces frequent drought spells during its growth and reproductive periods. Early withdrawal of monsoon by mid-September many a times causes post-flowering drought and reduces the grain yield considerably. Germination, seedling, flowering and grain formation stages are critical for irrigation and getting higher yield (Dastane, 1974). Water stress at an early stage reduces the amount of leaf area at flowering (Fischer and Hagan, 1965). Stress at critical stages limit the elongation of stalk and significantly reduces LAI. The period of 40 to 85 days after sowing - when flowering and grain formation stages are very sensitive to moisture stress – is very crucial (Oizumi *et al.*, 1965).

The expression of drought tolerance is dependent on the stage of development when stress occurs. This developmental interaction complicates the characterization and study of drought tolerance. In sorghum, developmentally specific patterns of drought tolerance have been identified and symptoms of susceptibility during each stage have been characterized (Rosenow and Clark, 1981). Susceptibility to drought can occur during the early vegetative seedling stage, during the period of panicle development prior to flowering and during the post-flowering stage of grain development. Susceptibility during the post-flowering stage is characterized by reduced seed size and grain yield, premature plant and leaf senescence, and increased stalk lodging.

One trait reported to be associated with post-flowering drought tolerance is 'staygreen'. Stay green is characterized as resistance to premature leaf and stalk death induced by post-flowering drought (Tuinstra *et al.*, 1997). Resistance to premature leaf and stalk death is thought to increase the potential period of grain development thereby stabilizing the expression of seed weight (Duncan *et al.*, 1981; Rosenow and Clark, 1981). Non-senescing lines may also be more resistant to charcoal rot and pathogen-induced lodging (Jordan *et al.*, 1984; Mughogho and Pande, 1984).

Sorghum lines with high levels of staygreen have been identified and are being used in a number of breeding programs. Genetic studies of staygreen have generally indicated a complex pattern of inheritance and, both dominant and recessive expressions have been reported. These studies also indicated that, the expression of staygreen is strongly influenced by the environment. Tenkouano *et al.* (1993) have proposed that inheritance of staygreen from the B35 genetic background may be less complex than previously thought. These studies point towards the fact that, staygreen was controlled by a single dominant factor with some epistatic interactions in certain genetic backgrounds. Seed weight is strongly influenced by post-flowering drought. Terminal post-flowering drought results in an abbreviated period of grain development and therefore reduces seed size. Variability in rate and duration of grain development could explain some differences in post-flowering drought tolerance. Genotypes with a high rate and reduced duration of grain filling may be more tolerant under terminal post-flowering drought stress conditions than lines with a low rate and prolonged duration of grain development (Sayed and Gadallah, 1983). In essence, this mechanism provides an opportunity to escape the effects of late season drought.

Chapter 3
Soil Management and Sowing

3.1 Soils

Sorghum is mainly grown on low potential soils which are usually not suitable for the production of other important crops. The crop is more tolerant of alkaline salts than other grain crops and can therefore be successfully cultivated on soils with a pH between 5.5 and 8.5. Soils with a clay percentage of between 10 per cent and 30 per cent are optimal for sorghum production. The most predominant soils in sorghum growing areas are Vertisols, Inceptisols, Entisols and Alfisols in Asia; Vertisols, Alfisols and Mollisols in North and Central America; Mollisols, Alfisols, Oxisols, and Ultisols in Southern America; Vertisols in Australia; and Vertisols, Alfisols, Entisols and Inceptisols in Africa (Myers and Asher, 1982; Clark, 1982a, d). Oxisols, Ultisols, and some Entisols, Alfisols and Inceptisols are acidic in reaction while Mollisols, Vertisols and some Inceptisols are alkaline. Soils with clay loam or loam texture, having good water retention capacity are best suited for sorghum cultivation. In India, rainy season sorghum is grown in Vertisols, Vertic soil types (Entisols, Inceptisols), and to a certain extent in Alfisols. Relative distribution of soil resources in production zones of sorghum is given in Tables 3.1 and 3.2. Post-rainy sorghum is largely confined to Vertisols (Tandon and Kanwar, 1984). Alfisols are light textured and shallow with poor in nitrogen and phosphorus content and rich in non-exchangeable potassium. These soils are mostly present in Andhra Pradesh and Karnataka and suited for *kharif* sorghum. Crust formation on surface is a serious problem in these soils. Black soils are predominant in the states of Andhra Pradesh, Tamil Nadu, Karnataka, Maharashtra, Gujarat and Madhya Pradesh. These soils are clayey (40 per cent to 70 per cent clay) with varying depths from shallow to deep and suitable for both rainy and post-rainy season sorghum cultivation. In general, stored available soil moisture of about 90 to 100 mm is required to sustain a *rabi* sorghum crop. The amount of moisture stored in the soil depends on its depth and the rainfall received during rainy season (Table 3.3). If winter showers are received, a good crop can be harvested on soils with less moisture storage capacity.

Table 3.1: Relative Distribution of Soil Resources in Production Zones of *kharif* Sorghum (Murthy *et al.*, 2007)

Primary Zone		Secondary Zone		Tertiary Zone	
Soil Type	Area (Per cent)	Soil Type	Area (Per cent)	Soil Type	Area (Per cent)
Entisols	45.6	Vertisols	38.0	Entisols	29.1
Alfisols	36.2	Entisols	27.5	Alfisols	25.7
Vertisols	9.3	Inceptisols	13.3	Inceptisols	20.7
Inceptisols	5.5	Alfisols	12.2	Vertisols	19.3
Aridisols	3.3	Aridisols	8.2	Aridisols	6.6

Table 3.2: Relative Distribution of Soil Resources in Production Zones of *Rabi* Sorghum (Murthy *et al.*, 2007)

Primary Zone		Secondary Zone		Tertiary Zone	
Soil Type	Area (Per cent)	Soil Type	Area (Per cent)	Soil Type	Area (Per cent)
Entisols	60.1	Vertisols	56.8	Alfisols	40.5
Vertisols	36.8	Entisols	38.0	Vertisols	30.7
Inceptisols	2.3	Alfisols	3.9	Entisols	21.6
Alfisols	0.8	Inceptisols	1.3	Aridisols	3.3
Inceptisols	2.5				

Table 3.3: Available soil moisture in different soil types

Sl.No.	Soil Type	Soil Depth (cm)	Available Soil Moisture (mm)
1.	Very shallow	7.5	15–20
2.	Shallow	22.5	30–35
3.	Medium deep	45.0	60–65
4.	Medium deep	60.0	80–90
5.	Deep	90.0	140–150
6.	Very deep	120.0	160–180

Sorghum is not tolerant of acid soils but is reported to be moderately tolerant to salinity (Francois *et al.*, 1984; Uleri and Ernst, 1997). It can be grown on soils with a wide range of pH, varying from 5.0-8.5 (Doggett, 1970), however the optimum pH range is 6.2 to 7.8 (Cothren *et al.*, 2000). Sorghum is most sensitive to salinity during the vegetative stage and least sensitive during maturity (Maas *et al.*, 1986). Nutrient requirements for grain sorghum are similar to corn, and in a growing season, a sorghum grain crop yielding 6.3 metric tons ha^{-1} will use around 38, 19, and 10 kg ha^{-1} of nitrogen, phosphorus, and potassium, respectively (Kramer and Ross, 1970; Whitney, 1998). Fertilizer amendments should be added based on, soil test results and plant requirements, during planting or shortly thereafter for the most efficient utilization by the crop (Cothren *et al.*, 2000).

Crop management practices for grain sorghum production vary widely depending on the production region. In low rainfall areas, in the semi-arid tropics, the main focus is on conserving soil moisture to help the crop reach its full yield potential. Cultivar selection is extremely important and they should be chosen from the latest maturity group that can be reliably grown in the region to help increase yield potential (Kramer and Ross, 1970; Martin *et al.*, 2006; Roozeboom and Fjell, 1998). Other important characteristics to consider when cultivar lodging, insect and disease resistance, cold tolerance, as well as the intended end-use of the grain where test weight, seed colour, or feed values may be important (Cothren *et al.*, 2000; Kramer and Ross, 1970; Roozeboom and Fjell, 1998).

3.2 Soil Management Practices

After harvest, lots of sorghum stubbles are left in/on the soil. Decomposition of these stubbles prior to planting the next crop is usually desirable. These residues/ stalks should be incorporated after harvest as soon as possible. Proper decomposition of residues before planting next crop reduces the problems with tillage and other planting operations. The early decomposition also makes plant nutrients found in residues available for the subsequent crop. Un-decomposed stubbles may lead to N-immobilization due to high C:N ratio and N- deficiency may occur early in the growth of subsequent crop.

A C:N ratio greater than 20 indicates that, soil microorganisms feeding on the stubble will require some N from the soil in addition to the N in stubble for decomposition to occur. The C:N ratio in grain sorghum ranges from 40:1 to 80:1. Nitrogen may be applied to the stubbles to speed up the decomposition and prevent the temporary N-deficiency. The amount of N applied usually ranges between 4.5 to 6.8 kg per 450 kg of stubbles produced (Bennett *et al.*, 1990).

Leaving crop residues on the soil surface is the most cost-effective method of reducing soil erosion. Covering 20 per cent of the surface with crop residues can reduce soil erosion caused by rainfall and runoff water by 50 per cent as compared to residue free condition (Shelton *et al.*, 1995). Stubbles also control wind erosion and assists in soil moisture conservation. A proper preparation of the seed bed is essential for uniform seedling emergence and early establishment of sorghum. It also improves soil aeration and moisture retention, and helps in weed control. Deep ploughing once with mould board plough, during off-season–especially during summer months–is very essential in controlling perennial weeds and insect-pests. In red soils, deep ploughing mixes bottom clay with top layers and thus improves moisture holding capacity and wetting depth. Deep tillage also conserves soil moisture by providing more opportunity time for water to infiltrate into the soil. Vijayalaxmi, (1987) reported 39 per cent increase in sorghum grain yield due to off season tillage. After receipt of pre-monsoon showers, the deep ploughed lands need to be cultivated twice with disc harrow followed by rotovator once to, break the clods, control perennial weeds and incorporate crop residues.

3.3 Time of Sowing

Due to slow initial growth rate, sorghum is highly vulnerable to insect-pests, diseases and weeds at seedling stage. Therefore, it is very important that its sowing time should be so adjusted that the crop passes through its life cycle at the most optimum environmental conditions for growth and developments. Temperature and soil moisture are the two most critical factors in deciding the proper planting date. Sorghum will not germinate readily at soil temperatures below $10°C$ (Anda and Printer, 1994). If adequate soil moisture at sowing is not available, it is recommended to either irrigate or delay planting until moisture becomes available. In tropical climates, the onset of monsoon, rainfall pattern, cultivar duration and seedling pests make the planting time an important factor (Dogett, 1988). In India, sorghum is grown during *kharif* and *rabi* seasons. Under rainfed conditions, *kharif* sorghum should be sown at the onset of monsoon. It generally coincides with last week of June to first week of July in different parts of the country. Progressive delay of 7, 14 and 21 days after the first monsoon rain cause substantial yield reductions (Singh, 1980). Under irrigated conditions, 4th week of June to 1st week of July for Uttar Pradesh and Delhi, 3rd to 4th week of June for Madhya Pradesh and 1st week of June for Tamil Nadu have been found optimum (Singh, 1980). Timely planted crop escapes the damage due to seedling pest 'shootfly' and midge. Pre-monsoon dry sowing, a week before the onset of monsoon, has also been reported beneficial (Rana *et al.*, 1999). Field experiments conducted under AICSIP at Parbhani, Dharwad, Indore, Surat, and Udaipur revealed that at Dharwad and Udaipur, sowing on 30th June produced maximum grain yield. Delayed sowing resulted in lower grain yield due to severe attack of shoot fly. At Indore, though delay in sowing from 15 June to 30th June reduced the grain yield, in all the genotypes, it was CSV 17 that was more affected. In Surat, however, there was no yield loss up to 30th June sowing irrespective of the cultivars (Table 3.4).

Rabi sorghum is completely rainfed and is grown on receding soil moisture. The productivity of *rabi* sorghum mainly depends upon soil moisture reserve or rains received in the month of September-October. Therefore, the crop should be managed in such a way that there is efficient utilization of available soil moisture. The recommended planting date for *rabi* sorghum is mainly based on soil moisture availability and the soil temperature at a 5 cm depth. Soil moisture content largely depends on rainfall pattern of the preceding *kharif* season and soil types. In general, the optimum sowing time varies from 3rd week of September to first week of October. Planting too early invites heavy infestation of shoot fly whereas delay in planting results in yield reduction due to considerable moisture loss through evaporation from the fallow soil surface. This leads to severe moisture stress at grain filling stage. With early planting, the crop covers the soil earlier in the season, thereby reducing water loss due to evaporation. Early planted crops take the greatest advantage of the rains received during late September/October months. The planting time can be conveniently adjusted if supplemental irrigations are available.

Rao *et al.* (1973) observed that seeding during late August to early September increased the yields of improved hybrids and varieties markedly as compared to local variety M 35-1. Singh (1980) reported first week of September for Rahuri; third week of September for Mohol, Solapur, Bijapur and Bellari; fourth week of September

Table 3.4: Interaction Effect of Dates of Planting and Sorghum Cultivars on Grain Yield of *Kharif* Sorghum (AICSIP, 2013)

Treatments	Dates of Planting				
	15 June	30 June	15 July	30 July	Mean
Dharwad					
Cultivars					
CSV17	–	5080	3691	0	2924
CSV23	–	6556	5846	0	4134
CSH16	–	6840	6006	0	4282
CSH23	–	6593	6543	0	4379
Mean		6267	5522		
CD (P = 0.05) Dates of planting (D) = 216	Cultivars (C) = 250	D x C = 353			
Udaipur					
CSV17	–	4751	4273	1696	3573
CSV23	–	4959	4963	993	3638
CSH16	–	6101	5627	908	4212
CSH23	–	5659	4799	861	3773
Mean		5367	4915	1114	
CD (P = 0.05) Dates of planting (D) = 331	Cultivars (C) = 382	D x C = 662			
Indore					
CSV17	2055	1227	679	450	1103
CSV23	5599	4684	890	795	2992
CSH16	5901	5156	999	857	3228
CSH23	4579	3914	915	701	2527
Mean	4533	3745	871	701	
CD (P = 0.05) Dates of planting (D) = 234	Cultivars (C) = 234	D x C = 468			
Surat					
CSV17	3430	3535	2946	2462	3093
CSV23	3388	3514	2988	2546	3109
CSH16	4061	4125	3325	2736	3562
CSH23	3998	4125	3241	2609	3493
Mean	3719	3825	3125	2588	
CD (P = 0.05) Dates of planting (D) = 275	Cultivars (C) = 275	D x C = 549			

for Hyderabad and first fortnight of November for Podalkur areas as the most optimum sowing time for *rabi* sorghum. Field experiments conducted under AICSIP at Parbhani, Rahuri, and Tandur revealed that, on location mean basis, sowing of *rabi* sorghum during 3rd week of September recorded the maximum grain yield (4102 kg/ha) followed by first week of September (3560 kg/ha) and first week of Oct (3474 kg/ha), both dates were at par with each other. Among the genotypes, Phule Revati produced the maximum yield at all the locations. At Parbhani, sowing during first week of October gave maximum grain yield, whereas at Tandur, first week to 1st week of October was better. At Rahuri, sowing during 3rd week of September was better. The interaction effect between dates of planting and genotypes was significant at Rahuri and Tandur. Phule Vasudha and Phule Revati showed consistent performance in terms of grain yield from 1st week of September to 3rd week of October at Tandur. Reduction in grain yield due to early and delayed sowing varied in different genotypes and locations. Irrespective of the genotypes, the percentage of reduction due to delayed sowing varied from 30.9 per cent at Tandur, to 44.5 per cent at Parbhani and 67.7 per cent at Rahuri (Table 3.5).

3.4 Seed Rate and Sowing Depth

In *kharif* sorghum, a density of 1.80 lakh plants per hectare (18 plants m^{-2}) is the optimum plant population to attain maximum yield. A seed rate of 8-10 kg/ha depending on the boldness of seed is recommended. In *rabi* season, under receding soil moisture conditions, a population of 1.35 lakh plants per hectare is optimum. However, under irrigated or assured soil moisture conditions, higher plant population of 1.85 lakhs/ha is recommended. Seed should be treated with azotobactor/azospirilum @ 250 g/10 kg seed before sowing. Sorghum is very sensitive to seeding depth. Depth of planting greatly affect emergence rate. The planting depth ranges from 2.5 to 7.5 cm depending up on soil moisture conditions. Planting depths should be deep if soil moisture conditions at planting are dry and shallow if sufficient moisture for germination is available in the top 2 cm of the soil (Anda and Pinter, 1994; Cothren *et al.*, 2000; Kramer and Ross, 1970). Seeds should be sown at a depth of 3-4 cm for better seedling emergence. Planting too deep – *i.e.* > 4 cm - may cause poor seedling emergence and vigour. Seeding too shallow – *i.e.*<1.5 cm - may cause poor rooting and therefore lodging of the mature crop. Planting depth is also determined by soil type. On heavy soils, planting depth should not be more than 2.5 cm, while on light soils; the depth can be upto 5 cm.

3.5 Row Spacing and Method of Sowing

Row spacing depends on the implements to be used in inter-cultivation for weed control after planting and moisture availability (Doggett, 1970; Kramer and Ross, 1970). Moisture availability is a key consideration in deciding row spacing and plant population. Standard row spacing for grain sorghum is 45 cm but wider rows may be more appropriate if moisture is expected to be limited (Bond *et al.*, 1964). Narrow rows are recommended if adequate moisture will be available during the growing season. Plant to plant distance should be 12-15 cm. The production practices that improve plant-available water, at reproductive growth stages may improve the ratio of grain yield to crop water use (WUE). Routley *et al.* (2003) has shown that sorghum

Table 3.5: Interaction Effect of Dates of Planting and Sorghum Cultivars on Grain Yield of *Rabi* Sorghum (AICSIP, 2013)

Treatments	Dates of Planting (D)					
	1ˢᵗ Week of September	3ʳᵈ Week of September	1ˢᵗ Week of October	3ʳᵈ Week of October	1ˢᵗ Week of November	Mean
PARBHANI						
Cultivars (C)						
CSH 15R	2468	3394	3584	2104	1763	2663
CSV 22	3009	3274	3449	2645	2130	2902
Phule Anuradha	2058	2670	2963	1766	1214	2134
Phule Vasudha	2999	3521	3874	2811	2323	3106
Phule Revati	3016	3470	3891	2866	2418	3132
Mean	2710	3266	3552	2439	1970	
CD (P = 0.05)	Dates of planting (D) = 167	Cultivars (C) = 167	D x C = 374 (NS)			
RAHURI						
CSH 15R	4298	4834	3493	1950	1618	3239
CSV 22	4713	5709	3693	2447	2020	3717
Phule Anuradha	3411	3910	2820	2074	1694	2782
Pphule Vasudha	4671	6583	4250	2241	1861	3921
Phule Revati	5727	7461	4202	2373	2003	4353
Mean	4564	5699	3692	2217	1839	
CD (P = 0.05)	Dates of planting (D) = 457	Cultivars (C) = 457	D x C = 1021 (Sig)			
TANDUR						
CSH 15R	3298	3207	2971	2603	1797	2775
CSV 22	3590	3565	3190	2984	2205	3107
Phule Anuradha	2988	2883	2759	2010	1604	2449
Pphule Vasudha	3380	3327	3308	3081	2976	3214
Phule Revati	3769	3721	3666	3396	3184	3547
Mean	3405	3340	3179	2815	2353	
CD (P = 0.05)	Dates of planting (D) = 195	Cultivars (C) = 195	D x C = 435 (Sig)			

roots grow in all directions at rates of 15 to 40 mm day⁻¹, depending on the growth stage. If the mean rate of root growth is 25 mm day⁻¹, this would imply that narrow-spaced sorghum will reach and exhaust all the available water early in the growing period, if there was no replenishment by rainfall. Conceivably, under low rainfall wider-spaced sorghum would use water stored in the inter-row soil regions to meet its needs during the reproductive stage and hence sustain high yields under dry conditions. Sojka *et al.* (1988) showed a contrasting effect of row spacing on water use efficiency of sorghum. Skip-row planting has been shown to conserve soil water for later use by the crop to improve water use and grain yield (McLean *et al.*, 2003; Routley *et al.*, 2003; Akwasi *et al.*, 2011). The method of skipping one row after 2 or 3 rows, produced a grain yield, which was at par with solid planting. However, skipping one row after planting 3 rows resulted in 18.9 per cent increase in grain yield and 25 per cent saving in seed of *rabi* sorghum (Radder *et al.*, 1993) (Table 3.6). Bandaru *et al.* (2006) reported that planting grain sorghum in clumps, in water stressed environments increased grain yield. Wide row spacing with high seeding rates and planting in clumps with three to six plants per hill reduced tiller formation, dry matter yield, and early water use with the benefit of saving soil water in the skipped area for use by plants during flowering and grain fill stages (Thomas *et al.*, 1980; Bandaru *et al.*, 2006).

Table 3.6: Effect of Skip-row Planting on Grain Yield of *Rabi* Sorghum (Radder *et al.*, 1993)

	Grain Yield (kg/ha)			
	1983-84	*1984-85*	*1985-86*	*Mean*
Planting Method				
Planting 3 rows and skipping 1 row	2066	1586	1462	1671
Planting 2 rows and skipping 1 row	1906	1148	1536	1530
Normal planting	1595	1128	1441	1405
CD (P = 0.05)	NS	NS	NS	–
Seed rate				
100 per cent of recommended	1904	1296	1520	1573
75 per cent of recommended	2018	1213	1475	1569
CD (P = 0.05)	NS	NS	NS	–

3.6 Thinning

Maintaining optimum plant population (thinning) is a very important operation in sorghum cultivation. Plant to plant population in a row should be kept 12-15 cm by thinning out extra plants at two stages. First thinning should be done 10-15 days after emergence and second when, the crop is 25-30 days old. All the diseased and insect-infested plants should be removed while thinning. Clegg and Marranville (1972) reported that thinning should be performed as early as possible, preferably before plants reach 7.5 cm in height. Yield was reduced when thinning was delayed until plants were, 15.0 cm to 23.0 cm in height.

Chapter 4
Varietal Improvement

The real development of hybrids in sorghum became feasible with the discovery of genetic male sterility (ms_2) by Stephen (1937) and the subsequent discovery of cytoplasmic male sterility msc_1 (Stephens and Holland, 1954, Doggett, 1988). An early hybrid in US was 'RS 610', a cross of combine Kafir 60A (male sterile) with combine 7078, which offered a substantial yield increase over the varieties. In India, while sorghum research was being carried out during pre-independence years, organized sorghum research was initiated in 1962 with the establishment of Accelerated Sorghum and Millet Improvement Project (ASMIP) and later on All India Coordinated Sorghum Improvement Project (AICSIP) in 1969 with 18 main centres spread over 13 State Agricultural Universities in 11 major sorghum growing states. First commercial sorghum hybrid 'CSH 1' was released in 1964 for all India cultivation using the parental line bred in USA and supplied by the Rockefeller Foundation. Indian sorghum breeding since then steadily gained competence and moved to the vanguard. In 1970, AICSIP was shifted from New Delhi to IARI Regional Station Hyderabad. In 1972 the International Crops Research Institute for Semi-Arid Tropics (ICRISAT) was established in Hyderabad, further spurring sorghum improvement research. National Research Centre for Sorghum was established in 1987 at Hyderabad by upgrading IARI Regional Station.

With the release of CSH 1 - the first commercial hybrid - in 1964, sorghum became the second crop after maize in developing high yielding hybrids using cytoplasmic genetic male sterility system. Since CSH 1, 30 more hybrids were added hither to centrally release for *kharif* season. A few more hybrids adapted to specific regions were released at State levels. Hybrids, CSH 1 to CSH 30 (Table 4.1), are a standing testimony of success of Indian sorghum breeding not only in terms of yield enhancement, but also in terms of diversification of parental lines and progressive advances in the incorporation of acceptable levels of resistance against major pests and diseases. The hybrids played a major role in pushing up productivity and production, particularly in the case of *kharif* sorghum. Among the *kharif* hybrids, the

Table 4.1: Performance of Released Hybrids and Varieties of Sorghum

Cultivars	Year of Release	Grain Yield (t/ha)	Stover Yield (t/ha)	Duration (Days)	Adoptation (Season)
(A) HYBRIDS					
CSH 1	1964	2.5-3.0	5.5-6.5	95-100	*Kharif*-low rainfall and light soils
CSH 2	1965	3.0-3.5	7.0-7.5	120-125	Mid-late *Kharif*, assured rainfall areas of Karnataka
CSH 3	1970	3.5-3.8	7.0-7.5	115-120	*Kharif*, assured rainfall tracts of Maharastra, Telangana region of Andhra Pradesh (AP), Tamil Nadu (TN), Malwa plateau of Madhya Pradesh (MP) and Bundelkhand region of Uttar Pradesh (UP)
CSH 4	1973	3.5-3.8	7.0-7.5	110-115	*Kharif*
CSH 5	1975	3.8-4.0	8.5-9.0	110-115	All *kharif* areas and late-kharif tracts of AP, summer irrigated areas in TN and Karnataka. Ideally suited for intercropping and ratooning.
CSH 6	1977	3.0-3.5	7.5-8.0	95-100	*Kharif* and late-kharif- low rainfall and light soils, suitable for intercropping and rationing.
CSH 7R	1977	2.5 – 3.0	5.0-6.0	110-115	Entire Deccan *rabi* tracts of Maharashtra, Karnataka, AP and also suitable for Gujarat
CSH 8R	1977	2.5 – 3.0	3.5-3.7	110-115	Entire Deccan *rabi* tracts of Maharashtra, Karnataka and AP
CSH 9	1981	3.8-4.0	8.5-9.5	105-110	All *kharif* sorghum growing areas except humid areas of Karnataka and TN
CSH 10	1984	3.5-3.8	12-14	105-110	*Kharif*, Karnataka
CSH 11	1986	3.8-4.0	10-12	105-110	All *kharif* sorghum growing areas
CSH 12R	1986	2.5-2.8	4.0-5.0	115-120	*Rabi*-Entire Deccan *rabi* tracts of Maharashtra, Karnataka and AP
CSH 13	1991	3.8-4.0 (*Kharif*) 3.2-3.5 (*Rabi*)	14-15 (*Kharif*) 5.0-5.5 (*Rabi*)	110-115	*Kharif* and *Rabi*- All sorghum growing areas
CSH 14	1992	3.8-4.0	8.0-9.0	100-105	All *kharif* sorghum growing areas, medium to heavy soils, low rainfall areas
CSH 15R	1995	3.0-3.5	5.5-6.0	110-115	*Rabi*-Maharastra, South Karnataka and north-west A.P
CSH 16	1997	4.0-4.5	9.0-10.0	110-115	All the *kharif* sorghum growing areas
CSH 17	1998	4.0-4.2	9-10	105-110	*Kharif*- Rajasthan, Tamilnadu, Maharashtra

Contd...

Table 4.1–*Contd...*

Cultivars	Year of Release	Grain Yield (t/ha)	Stover Yield (t/ha)	Duration (Days)	Adoption (Season)
CSH 18	1999	4.0-4.5	12.0 – 14.0	110-115	All *kharif* sorghum growing areas
CSH 19R	2000	2.5-3.0	5.5-6.0	115-120	All *rabi* sorghum growing areas of the country
CSH 23	2005	4.0-4.2	8.5-9.0	105-110	All *kharif* sorghum growing areas
CSH 25	2007	4.0-4.5	12.5-13.0	110-115	*Kharif*, Sorghum growing area of Maharashtra
CSH 27	2011	3.9-4.0	13.0-14.0	105-108	All *kharif* sorghum growing areas
CSH 30	2012	4.3-4.4	12-14	105-110	*Kharif* sorghum growing areas of Maharashtra, Gujarat, Karnataka and AP
(B) VARIETIES					
CSV 1 (Swarna)	1968	3.0-3.5	8.0-9.0	95-100	*Kharif* sorghum growing areas of Maharashtra, Gujarat, Karnataka and AP
CSV 2	1974	3.0-3.5	8.0-9.0	105-110	*Kharif* tracts of Maharashtra (Vidarbha and Marathwada), MP and adjoining areas of Rajasthan, Bundelkhand and north Telangana of AP
CSV 3	1974	3.5-4.0	8.5-9.5	105-110	All *kharif* sorghum growing areas
CSV 4	1974	3.0-3.58	8.0-9.0	105-110	All *kharif* sorghum growing areas, humid areas due to ability to tolerate grain mold.
CSV 5	1974	3.0-3.5	8.0-9.0	110-115	All *kharif*, early *rabi* and summer seasons. Suited for humid areas of TN, Karnataka and Maharashtra
CSV 6	1974	3.2-3.5	8.0-9.0	115-120	All *kharif* sorghum growing areas
CSV 7R	1974	2.0-2.5	6.5-7.5	120-125	All *rabi* sorghum growing areas of Maharashtra, Karnataka and AP. Suitable for early planting.
CSV 8R	1979	2.5-3.0	7.0-7.5	115-120	All *rabi* sorghum growing areas of Maharashtra, Karnataka and AP. Suitable for early planting.
CSV 9	1983	3.0-3.5	8.5-9.0	110-115	All *kharif* sorghum growing areas
CSV 10	1985	3.0-3.5	8.5-9.2	110-115	All *kharif* sorghum growing areas. Most suitable for Maharashtra, Karnataka, Rajasthan and AP
CSV 11	1985	3.0-3.58	9.5-10.0	110-115	All *kharif* sorghum growing areas

Contd...

Table 4.1—Contd...

Cultivars	Year of Release	Grain Yield (t/ha)	Stover Yield (t/ha)	Duration (Days)	Adoptation (Season)
CSV 12	1985	2.5-3.0	5.0-6.0	95-100	*Kharif*, Karnataka, TN and AP
CSV 13	1986	3.0-3.5	9.5-10.0	110-115	All *kharif* sorghum growing areas
CSV 14R	1992	2.2-2.5	5.0-5.5	110-115	All *rabi* sorghum growing areas
CSV 15	1996	3.5-3.8	11.5-12.5	110-115	All *kharif* sorghum growing areas
CSV 17	2002	2.5-3.2	6.5-7.0	95-100	*Kharif*, low rainfall and drought-prone areas of the country
CSV 18	2005	3.5-3.8	8.5-9.0	120-125	*Rabi* sorghum growing areas of Maharashtra, Karnataka and AP
CSV 20	2006	3.1-3.2	13.0-13.5	105-110	All *kharif* sorghum growing areas
CSV 23	2007	2.5-3.0	14.0-15.0	110-115	All *kharif* sorghum growing areas
CSV 26	2011	1.0-1.1	4.0-4.5	110-115	*Rabi* tract of Deccan, Maharashtra, Karnataka and AP
CSV 27	2011	2.8-3.0	16.0-17.0	115-120	All *kharif* sorghum growing areas, dual purpose
CSV 29	2012	2.5-2.8	6.5-7.0	118-120	*Rabi* tract of Deccan, Maharashtra, Karnataka and AP
M35-1	1969	2.0-2.5	6.0-6.5	115-120	*Rabi* tract of Deccan, Maharashtra, Karnataka and AP
Swati	1985	2.0-2.5	5.0-5.5	120-125	All *rabi* sorghum growing areas
CSV 216 (Phule Yashoda)	2000	2.0-2.5	7.5-8.0	120-125	All *rabi* sorghum growing areas
Phule Maulee	1999	1.5-2.0	4.5-5.0	110-115	Suitable for rabi season under shallow to medium soils of Maharashtra
Phule Uttara	2003	1.0-1.2	40-0-4.5	110-115	*Rabi*, Maharashtra, suitable for *Hurda* (green tender grains)
Phule Vasudha	2007	3.0-3.5	7.0-7.5	115-120	*Rabi*, Maharashtra
Phule Chitra	2006	2.0-2.5	5.5-6.5	110-115	*Rabi*, Maharashtra
Selection-3	1994	0.5-0.6	1.5-1.8	90-100	*Rabi*, Maharashtra
Parbhani Moti	2004	3.2-3.5	6.0-6.5	120-125	*Rabi*, Maharashtra
Pratap Jowar	2002	3.5-4.0	11.5-12.0	90-95	*Kharif*, Rajasthan
JJ 1041	1997	3.2-3.5	12.5-13.0	110-115	*Kharif*, Madhya Pradesh

Table 4.2: Recommended Hybrids and Varieties of Sorghum for different States

States	Areas of Adaptation/ Soil Types	Hybrids	Varieties
(A) *Kharif* season			
Maharashtra	Light soils	CSH 1, CSH 6, CSH 14	-
	Medium to heavy soils	CSH 9, CSH 10, CSH 11, CSH 13, CSH 16, CSH 18, CSH 23, CSH 25	CSV 10, CSV 11, CSV 13, CSV 15, PVK 400, PVK 801 and SPV 462
Karnataka	Low rainfall areas	CSH 1, CSH 6, CSH 14	SB 1066, DSV 1
	Assured rainfall areas	CSH 5, CSH 10, CSH 13, CSH 16 and CSH 25	CSV 10, CSV 11, CSV 13, CSV 15 and SPV 462
Andhra Pradesh	Low rainfall areas	CSH 6, CSH 14	CSV 10, CSV 11
	Normal rainfall areas	CSH 5, CSH 9, CSH 10, CSH 11, CSH 13, CSH 16, CSH 18, CSH 23 and CSH 25	SPV 462, CSV 10, CSV 11, CSV 13, CSV 15, CSV 17, CSV 20
	Late *kharif* (*Maghi*)	CSH 5, CSH 9, and CSH 13	Moti
Madhya Pradesh	Entire state	CSH 5, CSH 9, CSH 10, CSH 11, CSH 13 and CSH 16, CSH 18 and CSH 23	CSV 10, CSV 11, CSV 13, CSV15, CSV 17, CSV 20, SPV 462, and Jawahar Jowar 1041
Tamil Nadu	Madurai District	CSH 1, CSH 14	CSV 11, CSV 15
	Entire state	CSH 5, CSH 6, CSH 11 and CSH 13	Co 24, Co 25, Co 26, CSV 15, CSV 13, and CSV 17
Gujarat	South Gujarat	CSH 5, CSH 9, CSH 11 and CSH 13	CSV 10, SPV 462, CSV13, CSV 15, GJ 35, GJ 36, GJ 37, GJ 39, GJ 40, GJ 41
	North Gujarat and Saurashtra	CSH 6, CSH 10, SPH 468	CSV 10, SPV 462, CSV 15 CSV 13, GJ 37, GJ 38, 39 and GJ 40
Rajasthan	Medium to heavy soils	CSH 1, CSH 5, CSH 6, CSH 9, CSH 10, CSH 11, CSH 13, CSH 14, CSH 16 and CSH 23	CSV 10, CSV 13, CSV 15, CSV 17, CSV 20, CSV 23 and Pratap Jowar 1430
Uttar Pradesh	Entire state	CSH 9, CSH 10, CSH 11, CSH 14, CSH 13 and CSH 16	Bundela, CSV 10, CSV 11, SPV 462, CSV 13 and CSV 15, CSV 17, and CSV 20

Contd...

Table 4.2–*Contd...*

States	Soil Type	Area of Adaptation	Hybrids	Varieties
(B) *Rabi* season				
Maharashtra	Deep soil	Rainfed	CSH 15RCSH 19R	Phule Yashoda Phule Vasudha, Parbhani Moti, PKV Kranti, M 35-1,CSV 22
	Medium soil	Rainfed	—	Phule Chitra, Phule Maulee, M 35-1
	Shallow soil	Rainfed	—	Phule Anuradha, Phule Maulee, Sel. 3
	Medium-Deep soil	Irrigated	—	Phule Yashoda,Phule Vasudha, Parbhani Moti, PKV Kranti, CSV 18
	Medium-Deep soil	Rainfed	—	Phule Uttara (Hurda purpose)
Karnataka	Shallow soils	Rainfed	DSH 4	M 35-1, DSV 4
	Medium-Deep soils	Protective irrigations		DSV 5
	Deep soils	Irrigated	CSH 15 R	DSV 5, Phule Yashoda, CSV 18, CSV 22
Andhra Pradesh		Early *rabi* (Rayalseema region)	CSH 15 R	CSV 14R
		Normal *rabi*	CSH 15 R	M 35-1, CSV 14 R, CSV 216R, CSV 18, CSV 22
		Telangana region	CSH 14 R	CSV 22
		Coastal Andhra (Rice-fallows)	CSH 16, CSH 25, Mahalaxmi 296	—

role played and being played by CSH 1, CSH 5, CSH 6, CSH 9, CSH 14 and CSH 16 needs special mention. While CSH 5 and CSH 6 had a yield potential of 3.4 t/ha, this potential was raised to 4.0 t/ha in CSH 9 and more than 4.1 t/ha in CSH 16, CSH 23 and CSH 25, with distinctly superior quality grain, and fodder (stover).

Breeding could also identify high yielding varieties CSV 1 to CSV 29 and many more varieties were also released in various states. Some of these varieties are dual-purpose type. By and large, varieties encountered less acceptability among farmers in *kharif*. Better preference was received by dual-purpose varieties such as CSV 10, CSV 13, SPV 462 and CSV 15 in some restricted pockets. A major advantage of varieties over hybrids was their relative better grain quality and multiple resistance or tolerance against major pests and diseases. The dual-purpose varieties CSV 15, CSV 20, CSV 23 and CSV 27 could establish higher grain and fodder yield potential than our potential hybrids released earlier.

Improvement of *rabi* sorghum did not receive as much emphasis and effort as the *kharif* sorghum until the nineties. Six hybrids and five varieties were hitherto centrally

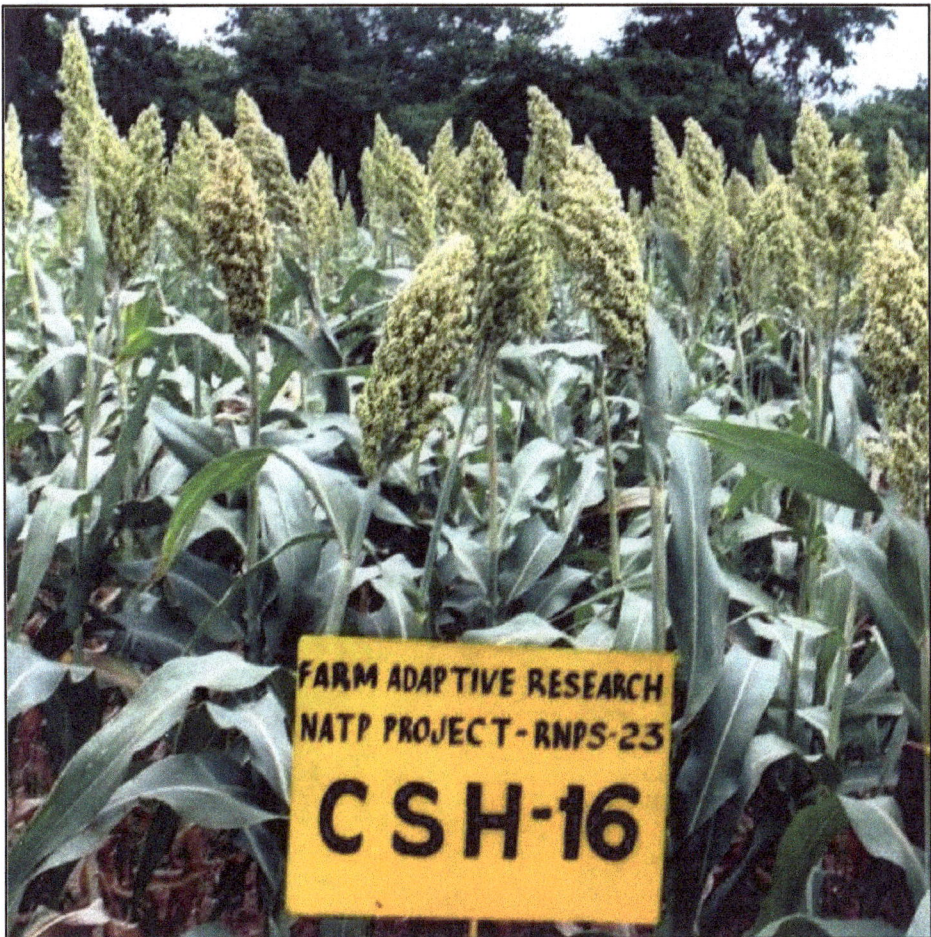

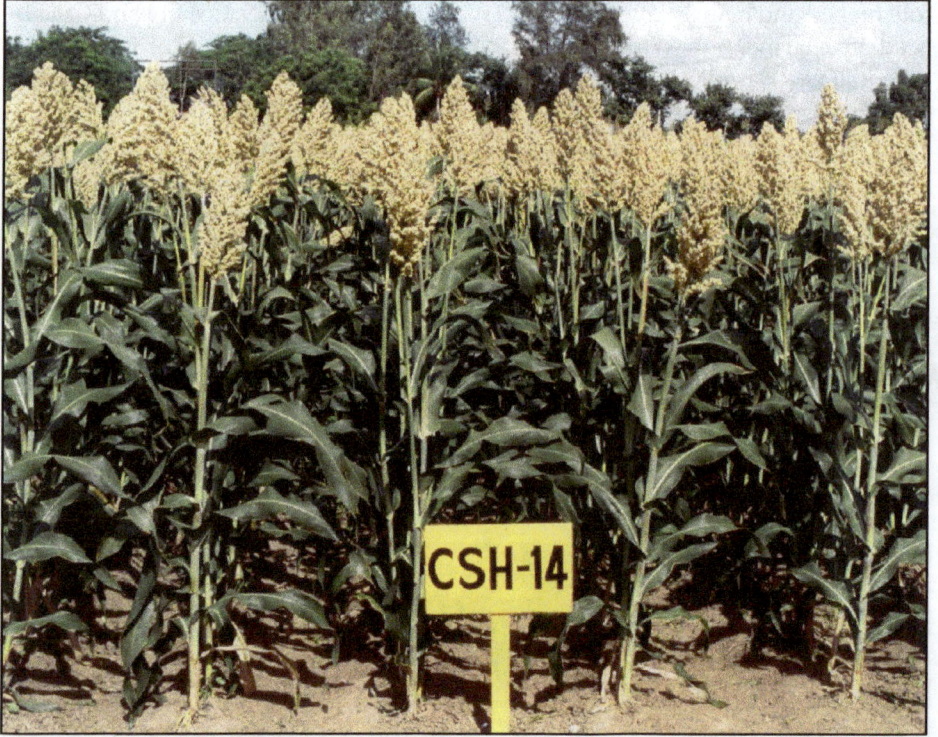

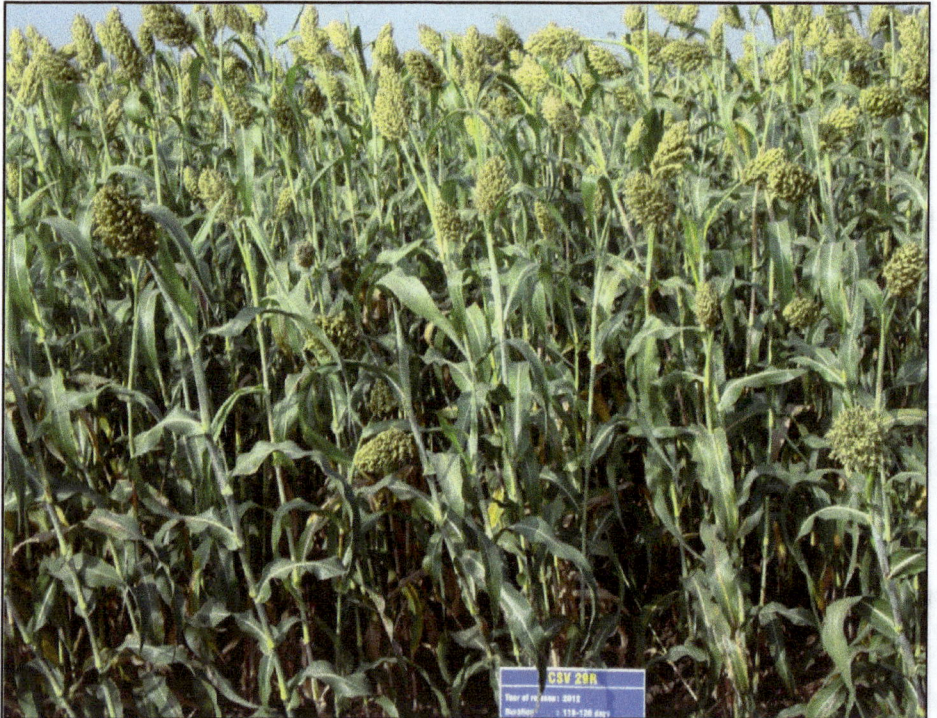

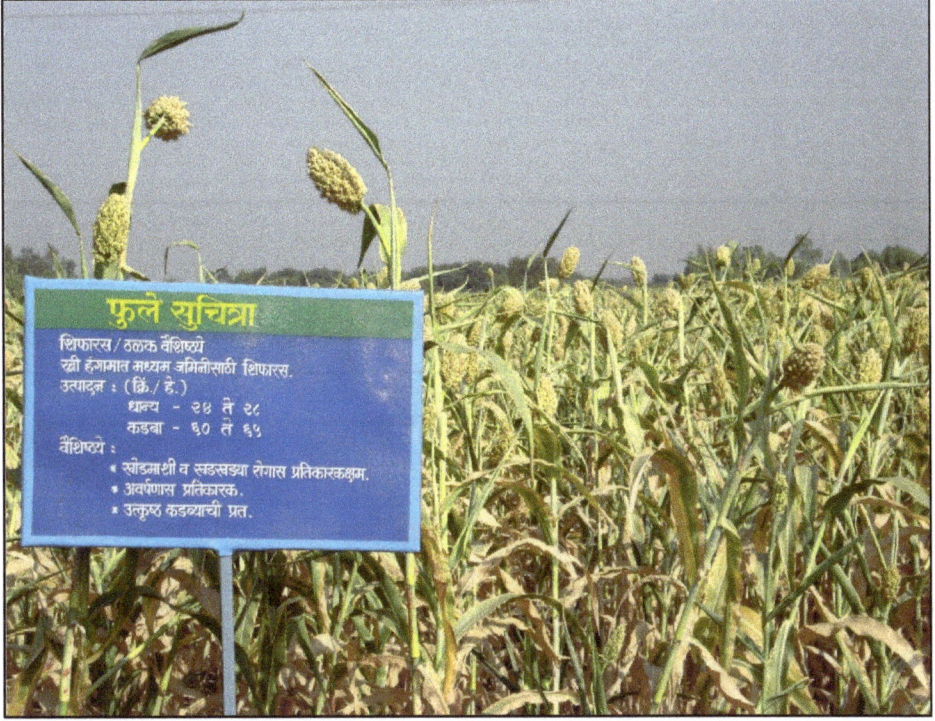

released for *rabi*. The first *rabi* sorghum hybrid CSH 7R and the latest hybrid CSH 19R were released keeping in view the importance of fodder. The *rabi* varieties CSV 8R, CSV 14R, CSV 18 and Swathi, were better received than the hybrids CSH 7R and CSH 8R. However, the recently developed hybrids CSH 15R and CSH 19R are more productive, but the acceptability among farmers is not high as they do not want to invest on hybrid seeds during *rabi* (dry season) without irrigation. A list of hybrids and varieties released and recommended for different states is given in Table 4.2.

Chapter 5
Sorghum-Based Cropping Systems

Cultivation of two or more crops simultaneously on the same field for higher yield and increased economic returns is important in the present context of agricultural scenario. The per capita availability of cultivable land has been shrinking due to increasing demographic pressures. Intercropping system improves cropping intensity as two or more crops occupy the land simultaneously. Intercropping can be defined as 'the growing of two or more crops on the same piece of land at the same time'. While intercropping has been traditionally practiced in India (Ayyangar and Ayyer, 1942) and found advantageous in comparison to sole cropping, agronomic research were initiated to determine the advantages in terms of the production stability, resource-use efficiency, risk reduction, protein production and higher monetary values.

When two or more crops are growing together, each must have adequate space to maximize cooperation, and minimize competition between them. To accomplish this, four things need to be considered:

1. Spatial arrangement,
2. Plant density,
3. Maturity dates of the crops being grown, and
4. Plant architecture.

5.1 Spatial Arrangements

There are at least four basic spatial arrangements used in intercropping.

☆ *Row Intercropping*: Growing two or more crops at the same time with at least one crop planted in rows.

☆ *Strip Intercropping*: Growing two or more crops together in strips wide enough to permit separate crop production using machines but close enough for the crops to interact.

☆ *Mixed Intercropping*: Growing two or more crops together in no distinct row arrangement.

☆ *Relay Intercropping*: Planting a second crop into a standing crop at a time when the standing crop is at its reproductive stage but before harvesting.

5.2 Benefits from Intercropping

1. Efficient Resource Utilization and Improved Yields

The main advantage of intercropping is the more efficient utilization of the available resources and the increased productivity compared to that of each sole crop of the mixture. When two or more crops with different rooting systems, different pattern of nutrient and water demand, and different above ground habit are planted together, growth resources such as nutrients, moisture and solar radiation are used more efficiently. Therefore, the combined yields of two crops grown as intercrops can be higher than the yields of the individual crops grown as pure stand.

2. Improved Soil Health

Intercropping of legumes with sorghum increases N_2-fixation and organic carbon in soil. Bandopadhyay and De (1986 a, b) reported that sorghum derived a part of N from the soil pool enriched by concurrently grown legumes in mixture. They ascribed it to the delaying of senescence of sorghum leaves due to continuous availability of nitrogen. Among different legumes, groundnut fixes the highest amount of atmospheric N (52 kg N/ha) followed by cowpea (32 kg N/ha) and greengram (30 days after sowing (Bandopadhyay, 1992). Sorghum + pigeonpea intercropping system improved soil N status (40 kg N/ha) at ICRISAT - Hyderbad, probably because of heavy leaf fall that occurs in pigeonpea before harvest (Willey, 1988).

3. Improved Fodder Quality

Intercropping of fodder legumes like cowpea, clusterbean, etc with sorghum provides nutritious fodder to supplement feed and also improves soil fertility of sorghum fields.

4. Reduced Incidence of Pests

Inclusion of legumes in sorghum based intercropping systems helps in reducing the incidence of insects and diseases. Intercropping of greengram, cowpea, blackgram and soybean with sorghum (paired row system), reduced the infestation of shoot fly in blackgram, whitefly in cowpea, yellow mosaic and podborer in greengram (Natarajan, *et al.*, 1991). Similarly, the incidence of charcoal rot in sorghum was reduced with sorghum + pigeonpea intercropping system as compared to sole crop of sorghum (Khune *et al.*, 1980).

5. Reduced Incidence of Weeds

Intercropping gives better control of weeds than sole cropping. Weed control can be improved where the intercrop situation provides a community of plants that are in total more competitive than the individual crops. (*see weed management chapter for details*).

6. Increased Biodiversity and Stability

Intercropping is the way to increase the diversity of the farming system. This means more stability, resulting in risk spreading and reduced pests and disease incidence.

7. Mitigates Adverse Effect of Climate Change

Intercropping of legumes helps in increasing carbon sequestration, soil organic matter, conserves soil moisture and maintains soil temperature and thus, reduces the adverse effect of increasing CO_2 and temperature in the atmosphere on sorghum yield.

5.3 Indices for Evaluation Productivity and Efficiency in Intercropping Systems

1. Relative Yield Total (RYT)

Relative yield total introduced by de Wit and Van den Bergh (1965) is the most important index of biological advantages in intercropping systems. The index is based on relating the yield of each crop in an intercrop treatment mixture to the yield of that crop grown as a sole crop. It is calculated as the sum of the intercropped yields divided by yields of sole crops.

2. Land Equivalent Ratio (LER)

The efficiency of intercropping systems are most often assessed in terms of their 'land equivalent ratio' (Willey, 1979), which is defined as the relative land area that would be required as sole crops to produce the yields achieved in intercropping. LER also indicates the relative yield advantage of intercropping. LER of more than 1 indicates yield advantage, equal to 1 indicates no grain or no gain or no loss and less than 1 indicates yield loss. It can be used both for replacement and additives series of intercropping. An LER value of 1.2 indicates that intercropping outyields sole cropping by 20 per cent. LER can be calculated as:

$$LER = La + Lb = \frac{Yab}{Yaa} + \frac{Yba}{Ybb}$$

where,

La and Lb are the LERs for the individual crops of the system

Yab = Intercrop yield of crop 'a'

Yba = Intercrop yield of crop 'b'

Yaa = Pure stand crop yield of 'a'

Ybb = Pure stand crop yield of 'b'

3. Income Equivalent Ratio (IER)

The ratio of the area needed under sole cropping to produce the same gross income as is obtained from 1 ha of intercropping at the same management level. The IER is the conversion of the LER into economic terms.

4. Area × Time Equivalency Ratio (LTER)

Area × time equivalency ratio was proposed by Hiebsch and Mc Collum (1987) as modification of LER. This takes into account the duration of the crop, and permits an evaluation of the crop on a yield per day basis.

$$ATER = \frac{(Ryc \times tc) \times (Ryp \times tp)}{T}$$

where,

Ryc = Relative yield of crop c (main crop)

Ryp = Relative yield of crop p (intercrop)

tc = Growth duration (days) for crop 'c'

tp = Growth duration (days) for crop 'p'

T = Growth duration (days) for the whole system

Competition Functions

1. Relative Crowding Coefficient (RCC)

The 'relative crowding coefficient' was proposed by de Wit (1960) relative crowding coefficient (K) can be calculated by the following formula:

$$Kab = \frac{Yab}{Yaa - Yab} - \frac{Zba}{Zab}$$

where,

Yab = Intercrop yield of crop 'a'

Yaa = Pure stand yield of crop 'a'

Zba and Zab are sown proportions of crop 'a' and 'b' in an intercropping system

2. Aggressivity (A)

Aggressively gives a simple measure how much the relative yield increase in crop *a*, is greater than that of crop *b* in an intercropping system. It is an index of dominanance. An aggressivity value Zero indicates that the component species are equally impective. A positive sign indicates the dominant species and a negative sign the dominated. The aggressivity (A) was proposed by McGilchrist (1965) and can be calculated by the following formula:

$$Aab = \frac{Yab}{Yaa \times Zab} - \frac{Yba}{Ybb \times Zba}$$

3. Competitive Ratio (CR)

Competitive ratio indicates the number of times a particular component crop is more competitive than the other. Relative species competition is often evaluated using competitive ratios (Putnam *et al.*, 1984). The competitive ratio as proposed by Willey *et al.* (1980) can be calculated by the following formula:

$$CRa = \frac{Yab}{Yaa \times Zab} \div \frac{Yba}{Ybb \times Zba}$$

If CRa < 1, there is a positive benefit and the crop can be grown in association; if CRa > 1, there is a negative benefit. The reverse is true for CRb.

5.4 Sorghum-Based Intercropping Systems

Traditionally sorghum was often mixed/intercropped with various crops in the semi-arid tropics of India. The traditional mixtures with sorghum were primarily developed as an insurance against total crop failure due to adverse weather conditions. With the development of high yielding sorghum cultivars from 1964 onwards, new vistas for the agronomists were opened for re-evaluating the cropping systems *viz.*, mixed-cropping, intercropping, multiple cropping and ratoon cropping to optimize production as well as security.

5.4.1 *Kharif* Sorghum-Based Intercropping Systems

Sorghum is mostly grown as intercrop with various oilseeds and pulses. In most of the agro-ecological regions of the country, sorghum + legume intercropping systems have been found more stable than sole crops. At IARI, New Delhi, Singh (1979) observed 8-34 per cent increase in sorghum grain yield due to intercropping of cowpea (fodder and grain), greengram, blackgram, groundnut and soybean.

Sorghum + Pigeonpea

Sorghum + pigeonpea is the most common intercropping system followed by the farmers in semi-arid tropics of India. This system provides greater stability of yield than sole cropping. In assured rainfall areas and medium to heavy soils, intercropping of sorghum with pigeonpea (2:1 or 2:2 or 3:2) not only produces higher yields per unit area and time but also improves soil health and provides nutritional security to rural poors of the semi-arid tropics. Sorghum+ pigeonpea intercropping at 2:1 or 2:2 row ratios was found to be promising (Rao *et al.*, 2003). The slow initial growth of pigeonpea does not provide any competition to sorghum crop for natural resources and being a leguminous crop, it helps in improving the soil fertility by fixing atmospheric nitrogen and heavy leaf fall. When the sorghum is harvested after 110-120 days, the pigeonpea grows vigorously utilizing the space left by the sorghum crop. Intercropping of sorghum also reduces the incidence of wilt disease in pigeonpea.

The sorghum genotypes vary in their growth behaviour, canopy development and duration. This may affect the growth and development of the pigeonpea crop grown in intercropping system. Intercropping of sorghum 'CSH 16' with pigeonpea (2:1) has been tested at different locations (like Coimbatore, Palem, Dharwad and Indore) of the country and found to be beneficial over sole cropping. This system gave the highest sorghum equivalent yield (6536 kg/ha) and benefit: cost ratio (3.83), besides improving soil health and nutrition of people living in rural areas (Table 5.1).

Sorghum + Soybean

In assured rainfall areas, soybean has tremendous scope for its inclusion in intercropping with *kharif* sorghum. Sorghum area in Maharashtra and Madhya

Table 5.1: Sorghum Equivalent Yield and Benefit : Cost (B: C) Ratio in Sorghum + Pigeonpea Intercropping System as Influenced by Sorghum Genotypes (Mean of 4 locations: Coimbatore, Palem, Dharwad, Indore)

Cropping System	Sorghum Equivalent Yield (kg/ha)	B:C Ratio
CSH16 + Pigeonpea(PP) (2:1)	6536	3.83
CSH23 + PP (2:1)	5895	3.35
CSV15 + PP (2:1)	6441	3.62
SPV1616 + PP (2:1)	6172	3.50
Local + PP (2:1)	6413	3.47
CSH16 sole	2749	2.54
CSH23 sole	2385	2.26
CSV15 sole	2486	2.43
SPV1616 sole	2553	2.44
Local sole	2550	2.533
CD (P = 0.05)	556	0.37

Table 5.2: Grain Yield of Sorghum and Soybean as Influenced by Row Proportions (Mean of Akola and Indore locations over 3 years)

Treatment	Yield (t/ha)			Monetary Return (Rs/ha)
	Sorghum	Soybean	Sorghum Equivalent	
Sorghum + soybean (1:2)	2.27	1.02	5.34	22,120
Sorghum + soybean (2:1)	3.41	0.50	4.92	21,913
Sorghum + soybean (2:4)	2.08	0.90	4.79	20,154
Sorghum + soybean (3:3)	2.69	0.71	5.16	21,298
Sorghum + soybean (3:6)	1.96	0.91	4.69	19,805
Sole soybean	–	1.34	4.02	14,697
Sole sorghum	3.90	–	3.90	18,990
CD (P = 0.05)			0.58	2,107

Pradesh has largely been replaced by soybean, because of its market price, which is supported by a growth in its utilization and allied industry. Intercropping of sorghum with soybean could sustain sorghum production in these states. In alfisols of Coimbatore with low to medium rainfall areas, sorghum + soybean intercropping at 3:6 ratio gave higher grain yields and economic returns (Subbian and Selvaraju, 2000) indicating that soybean can very well withstand the shade effect of sorghum. In Vertisols with medium to high rainfall sorghum + soybean in alternate rows resulted in higher yields and net returns (Gode and Bobde, 1993). Results of the experiments conducted at Akola and Indore under AICSIP revealed that intercropping system is highly beneficial as compared to either of the sole cropping systems (Table 5.2). In

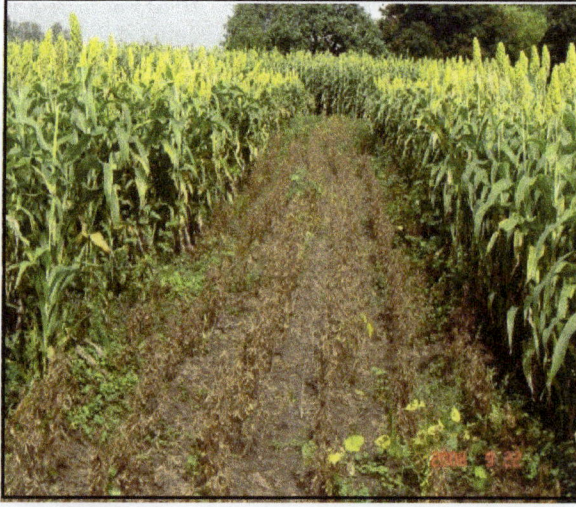

Sorghum + Soybean Intercropping (3 : 6)

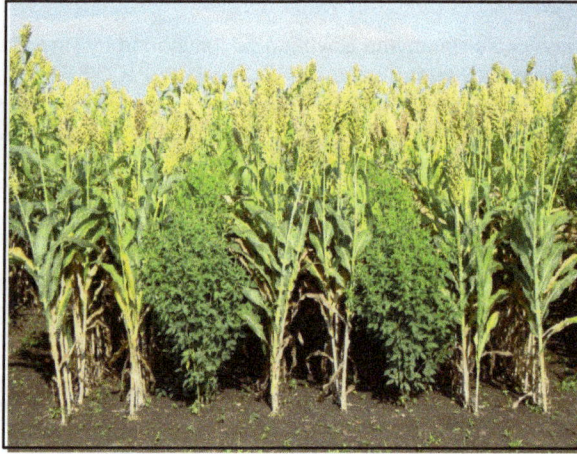

Sorghum + Pigeonpea (2 : 1 paired row) Intercropping (3 : 6)

Figure 5.1: Sorghum-based Intercropping Systems.

Malwa region of Madhya Pradesh sorghum genotypes JJ 1022, SPV 1616 and CSH 16 were most compatible with soybean intercropping (Table 5.3).

Sorghum + Groundnut

Groundnut being a leguminous and low profile canopy crop fits well with sorghum in intercropping system in semi-arid conditions. Results of the experiments conducted under AICSIP at Dharwad and Palem revealed that groundnut may be planted at 4 : 2 or 6 : 3 row ratios in order to get benefit of higher total productivity and gross returns (Table 5.4).

Table 5.3: Sorghum Equivalent Yield, Net Returns and Benefit : Cost (B : C) Ratio in Sorghum + Soybean Intercropping System as Influenced by Sorghum Genotypes at AICSIP, Indore (Madhya Pradesh)

Cropping System	Sorghum Equivalent Yield (kg/ha)	Net returns (Rs/ha)	B : C Ratio
CSH16 + soybean (2:4)	6337	56,274	5.33
CSH23 + soybean (2:4)	5369	46,959	4.62
CSV15 + soybean (2:4)	5993	55,244	5.25
SPV1616 + soybean (2:4)	6374	59,681	5.60
JJ 1022 (Local) + soybean (2:4)	6658	62,339	5.80
CSH16 sole	3305	29,472	3.02
CSH23 sole	2243	18,128	2.24
CSV15 sole	3498	33,651	3.31
SPV1616 sole	3382	34,172	3.34
Local (JJ 1022) sole	3421	33,465	3.29
Sole soybean	6835	49,152	5.12
CD (P = 0.05)	682	5,156	0.85

Table 5.4: Yield and Gross Monitory Returns in Sorghum+ Groundnut Intercropping System at AICSIP, Dharwad (Karnataka)

Treatment	Grain Yield (kg/ha)		Sorghum Equivalent Yield (kg/ha)	Gross Monitory Returns (Rs./ha)
	Sorghum	Groundnut		
Sorghum + Groundnut 1:2	3573	1667	8870	31057
Sorghum + Groundnut 2:1	3807	519	5180	23199
Sorghum + Groundnut 2:4	4724	1667	9946	35579
Sorghum + Groundnut 3:3	4701	827	7330	29212
Sorghum + Groundnut 3:6	3188	1358	7442	27263
Sorghum + Groundnut 6:3	4235	556	5999	25111
Sole sorghum	5541	–	5541	26348
Sole groundnut	–	1605	4012	13340
CD (P = 0.05)	541	159	675	2660

Sorghum + Short Duration Legumes

Intercropping of sorghum with short duration legumes like greengram, blackgram, cowpea etc. has been found more productive and profitable. In Alfisols of Southern Telangana region with low to medium rainfall, intercropping of sorghum with greengram/blackgram (1:1) with recommended row spacing for the crops has been found profitable inspite of adverse *kharif* season (Mastan and Goud, 1980-83). Sorghum + clusterbean intercropping system was found superior than other legumes in sandyloam soils of Hyderabad (Vishnumurthy and Vijayalakshmi, 1993) and

New Delhi (Singh and Balyan, 2000). Sorghum + cowpea (3:3 or 4:2) produced maximum net returns at Parbhani (Pawar and Shelke, 1992).

Rao *et al.* (2003) critically reviewed the research work done on different sorghum-based intercropping systems in rainfed regions of India and compiled the values of LER, equivalent yields and net returns (Table 5.5).

Table 5.5: Range of LER, Equivalent Yields, Net Returns and B : C Ratio Values in Sorghum- Based Intercropping Systems

Intercrops	Row Ratio	Range of Observations			
		LER	BCEY (t/ha)	Net Returns (Rs./ha)	B : C Ratio
Pigeonpea	2:1, 3:1, 4:2	1.19-1.51	1.56-6.90	2756-11312	–
Soybean	1:1, 2:2, 3:3, 3:6	1.16-1.57	3.30-5.28	11098-13220	3.28-3.93
Cowpea	1:1, 2:1, 2:2	1.60	–	–	1.87
Groundnut	1:1, 1:2, 2:2	–	–	6146-6181	–
Greengram	2:1, 1:4, 3:3	1.58	3.5-5.3	8672-11346	–

5.4.2 *Rabi* Sorghum-Based Intercropping Systems

As the moisture is a limiting factor during post-rainy sorghum production, intercropping is feasible only in deep soils. Sorghum + chickpea and sorghum+ safflower are the important intercropping systems in *rabi* sorghum growing regions of Maharashtra and Karnataka. Lomte *et al.* (1992) reported higher stability and profitability of *rabi* sorghum + safflower (6:3) at Parbhani.

Profitable Crop Sequences for *Rabi* Sorghum

Soybean - *rabi* sorghum has been found more productive and economically viable system under research trials. The profits from the different crop sequences are highlighted in Table 5.6.

Table 5.6: Profitable Crop Sequences for *Rabi* Sorghum (Patil *et al.*, 2013)

Kharif Crops	Yield (q/ha)	Yield of Rabi Sorghum (q/ha)		Profit (Rs./ha)
		Grain	Stover	
Greengram	10.19	18.77	35.51	41659
Blackgram	10.98	20.65	33.79	40720
Soybean	24.43	21.72	37.11	48361
Cowpea	8.91	18.12	32.53	32575
Pearl millet	27.25	19.57	32.92	36160

5.4.3 Forage Sorghum-Based Intercropping Systems

Sorghum is a major source of green and dry fodder for the cattle. Forage sorghums are generally cut at 50 per cent flowering with 8 per cent protein content and fed to the

Table 5.7: Productivity of Sorghum-Based Intercropping Systems (Mishra *et al.*, 1997)

Intercropping Systems	Fodder Yield of Sorghum (t/ha)	Total Fodder Yield (t/ha)	Total Dry Matter Yield (t/ha)	Crude Protein Yield (q/ha)	LER	Net Returns (Rs/ha)	B : C Ratio
Sole sorghum	29.8	29.8	6.84	4.31	–	4156	2.29
Sorghum + cowpea (1: 1)	15.9	36.0	6.98	7.72	1.15	5664	2.70
Sorghum + cowpea (1:2)	13.1	37.5	7.20	8.64	1.18	5944	2.72
Sorghum + cowpea (2; 2)	17.8	42.5	8.17	9.26	1.35	6804	2.77
Sorghum + horse gram (1:1)	20.4	27.1	5.58	4.53	1.11	3689	2.19
Sorghum + horsegram (1:2)	19.5	27.5	5.47	4.62	1.16	3780	2.21
Sorghum + horse gram (2: 2)	22.1	28.3	5.96	4.67	1.13	3791	2.15

animals. Suitable incorporation of protein rich leguminous crops with sorghum would improve the fodder quality and subsequently the potential of animals. (Sankaranarayana *et al.*, 2005). Sorghum + cowpea intercropping (Table 5.7) has been observed as the most suitable cropping system for total biomass productivity, forage quality and improving soil health. This might be attributed to complementary effect of cowpea, which supplemented nitrogen to sorghum, as well as made better utilization of environmental resources (Mishra *et al.*, 1997). Singh and Sogani, (1968) obtained, significantly more 'total digestible nutrients' and starch equivalent yields with sorghum + cowpea (3:1) intercropping. Intercropping of sweet sorghum + field bean (2:1) produced significantly higher mixed green forage yield and crude protein, crude fiber and total ash followed by sorghum + cowpea (2:1) and sweet sorghum + horsegram (2: 1) ratio (Thippeswamy and Alagundagi, 2001). Clusterbean has also identified as an important intercrop with sorghum in arid and semi-arid ecosystems (Table 5.8).

Table 5.8: Intercropping of Cowpea and Clusterbean in Forage Sorghum (Ram and Singh, 2001)

Intercropping Systems	Green Fodder Yield (q/ha)	Dry Fodder Yield (q/ha)	Sorghum Green Fodder Equivalent Yield (q/ha)	Net Returns (Rs./ha)	B : C Ratio
Sole sorghum	382	96	382	6888	1.28
Sorghum + cowpea (1: 1)	452	110	577	12502	2.06
Sorghum + clusterbean	406	100	456	8426	1.34
LSD (P = 0.05)	28	7	33	1072	0.15

Chapter 6
Nutrient Management

Adequate supply and balance of mineral elements are required for proper growth and development of sorghum plant. Nutrient requirements vary with soil, climate and cultivar. Sorghum is generally grown under less favourable conditions and meager amounts of fertilizers are applied. Prior to 1950's relatively little or no fertilizer was used on sorghum. In a survey during 1968-71, sorghum accounted for 3.5 per cent of the total fertilizer used with overall nutrient consumption of 4 kg/ha N + P_2O_5 + K_2O (NCAER and FAI, 1974). However, with the development of improved sorghum cultivars and other improved production practices the average nutrient consumption reached to 5.5-22.7 kg/ha during 1978-80 (Tandon and Kanwar, 1984) and 47.5 kg/ha (29.2, 14.2 and 4.1 kg N + P_2O_5 + K_2O) in 2003-04 as against 60.2 kg/in maize, 119.1 kg/ha in paddy and 136.7 kg/ha in wheat (FAO, 2005). Development of better adapted, high yielding sorghum cultivars has increased the yield potential and the amounts of plant nutrients required by the crop. Consequently, the fertilizer application in sorghum has increased substantially. Policy interventions to reduce fertilizer cost and improve grain marketing efficiency will further enable smallholders to increase fertilizer use for substantial increases in sorghum production.

6.1 Nutrients Deficiency Symptoms

Sorghum is gown on diverse range of soils. This range is so wide that some soils are unusually low in certain nutrients or have excessive quantities of certain nutrients. Nutritional stress problems in soils are often related to the type of parent material and the soil-forming processes characteristic of that soil (Dudal, 1976; Clark 1982a, d). Acid soils (Oxisols, Ultisols and some Entisols, Alfisols and Inceptisols) are usually low in exchangeable bases. Acidity increases the solubility of iron, aluminium and manganese and hence, these elements may reach to the toxic levels. However, acid soils are deficient in phosphorus, calcium, magnesium, molybdenum and zinc (Clark 1982a). Alkaline soils (Mollisols, Vertisols and some Inceptisols) often contain fairly high concentration of salt in the soil profile. These soils are rich in calcium, magnesium and potassium but deficient in sulphur. The deficiency symptoms of iron, zinc and manganese are the most common in sorghum grown on alkaline soils (Tandon and Kanwar, 1984).

There is a widespread deficiency of nitrogen, phosphorus, iron and zinc under both rainfed and irrigated conditions. Nitrogen, phosphorus, potassium and magnesium are phloem-mobile elements. When a deficiency of these elements occurs, plants tend to withdraw these elements from older leaves and redistribute them to young and actively growing parts of the plant through phloem (Robson and Snowball, 1986). Hence, the first and most obvious symptoms of deficiency of these elements occur on lower, older leaves. Elements such as calcium, iron, manganese and boron are phloem-immobile elements and hence, are not redistributed to any great extent under deficiency conditions (Robson and Snowball, 1986). The first and most obvious symptoms of deficiency of these elements occur on young, actively growing parts of the plant, including root tips. The nutrient elements such as sulphur, zinc, copper and molybdenum often have variable mobility in the phloem (Robson and Snowball, 1986). Hence, for these elements, symptoms may appear on young or old growth depending on the species, nitrogen supply, etc. However, Grundon *et al.* (1987) reported that in grain sorghum, only sulphur and zinc exhibited variation in the location of visible symptoms of deficiency, and that too only when the deficiency was very severe and persisted for some period of time. The key deficiency symptoms of nutrient elements in sorghum are listed in Table 6.1.

Table 6.1: Visible Symptoms of Nutrients Deficiency in Sorghum

Nutrients	Deficiency Symptoms
Nitrogen	☆ Deficient plants appear pale green to pale yellow in colour, stunted growth, thin and spindly stem, and often show delayed flowering and maturity. ☆ Nitrogen is mobile in plants and under conditions of low soil supply; it is easily mobilized from older to younger leaves. Hence, the deficiency symptoms appear first on older leaves and then advance up the stem to younger leaves. ☆ The leaf blades progressively become pale green with pale yellow chlorosis and pale brown necrosis.
Phosphorus	☆ Phosphorus deficiency symptoms appear first on the older leaves with purple suffused pigmentation and progress upwards. ☆ Affected plants appear stunted with thin stems and dark green leaves. ☆ Under severe deficiency, plant growth is greatly reduced and dark green older leaves turn purple or purple-red in colour.
Potassium	☆ Potassium deficiency symptoms appear first on older leaves with marginal yellow chlorosis, and brown necrosis. ☆ Deficient plants lose stalk strength and are prone to lodging. ☆ The internodes are shortened and thin and the older leaves develop a marginal necrosis.
Magnesium	☆ Older leaves are pale green to yellow in colour with many brown lesions. The symptoms advance upwards to younger leaves. ☆ In case of severe deficiency, the whole plant appears pale green or pale yellow in colour.

Contd...

Table 6.1–Contd...

Nutrients	Deficiency Symptoms
Calcium	☆ Young leaves have torn or serrated leaf margins and leaf tips are deformed, missing or joined together. ☆ Under severe deficiency, the upper internodes may be very short and the young leaves are crowded together to give the appearance of 'rosette'.
Sulphur	☆ Sulphur is not easily mobilized from older to younger leaves; the deficiency symptoms appear first on younger ones. ☆ Young leaves have faint yellow interveinal chlorosis and turn pale green in colour while older leaves remain dark green.
Iron	☆ Sorghum is the best indicator plant for iron deficiency. ☆ Prominent pale yellow or white interveinal chlorosis, leaving the veins green and prominent on young leaves.
Zinc	☆ Young leaves with broad yellow or white bands between the margins and midvein in lower half leaf. In case of severe deficiency, the chlorosis extends towards the leaf tip and often turns nearly white or pale brown. ☆ Shortening of internodes resulting in stunted plants. ☆ Delayed flowering and maturity.
Boron	☆ Young leaves with transparent white interveinal lesions. ☆ Shortening of internodes and stunted plant growth. ☆ Short, erect and dark green leaves. ☆ In case of severe deficiency, apical meristem often dies and tillers develop.
Manganese	☆ Plants are pale green to yellow in colour with thin spindly stem. ☆ Young leaves with yellow interveinal chlorosis and red-brown interveinal lesions.
Copper	☆ The young leaves and the leaves which are still within the whorl turn pale green in colour. ☆ The whorl of the expanding leaves may remain tightly rolled and become bent to one side. ☆ Young leaves with brown twisted leaf tips. ☆ Stunted plant growth with thin stems and pale green foliage.

6.2 Nutrient-Use Efficiency (NUE)

In semi-arid tropis where sorghum is an important crop, inorganic fertilizer use is limited due to high cost, non–availability, and limited soil moisture availability. To reduce the impact of nutrient deficiency on sorghum production, the selection of genotypes that are superior in the utilization of available nutrients - either due to enhanced uptake capacity or because of more efficient use of the absorbed nutrients in grain production - can be a desirable option. Nutrient-use efficiency can be expressed in many ways. Prasad (2009) described 4 agronomic indices in relation to nutrient-use efficiency. These are: Agronomic Efficiency (*AE*), Recovery Efficiency (*RE*), Physiological Efficiency (*PE*), and Partial Factor Productivity of Fertilizers (*PFPf*).

Agronomic Efficiency

It is expressed as 'kg crop yield increase per kg nutrient applied' and calculated as:

$$AE = \frac{Yf - Yc}{Na}$$

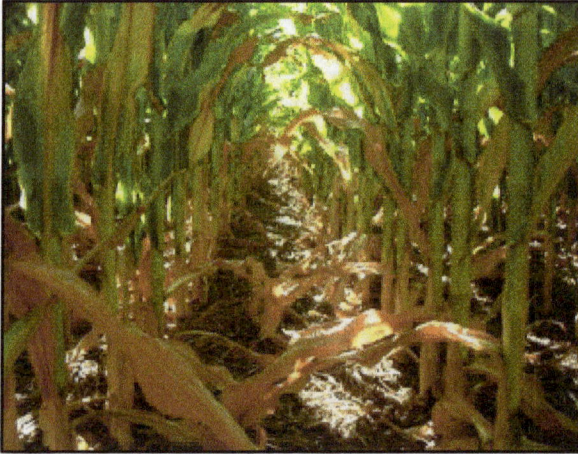

N Deficiency: Courtesy of the International Plant Nutrition Institute

P Deficiency: Courtesy of the International Plant Nutrition Institute

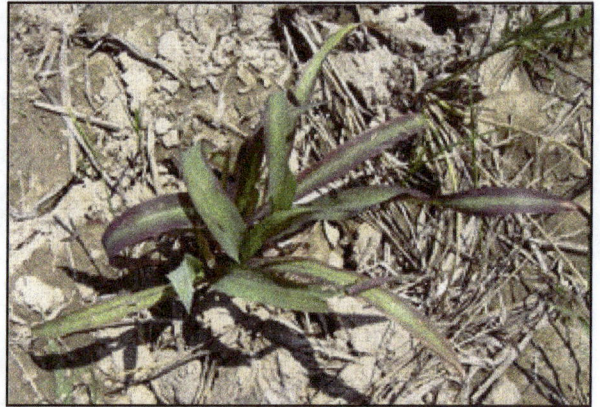

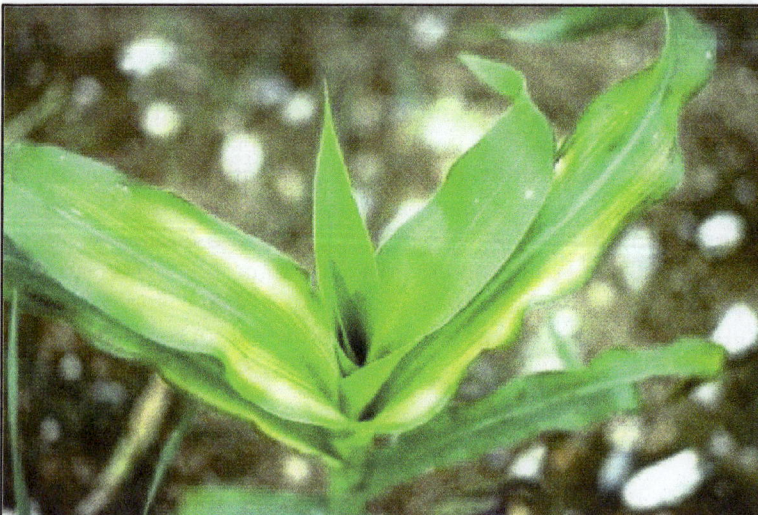

Zn Deficiency

Figure 6.1a: Nutrients Deficiency Symptoms in Sorghum.

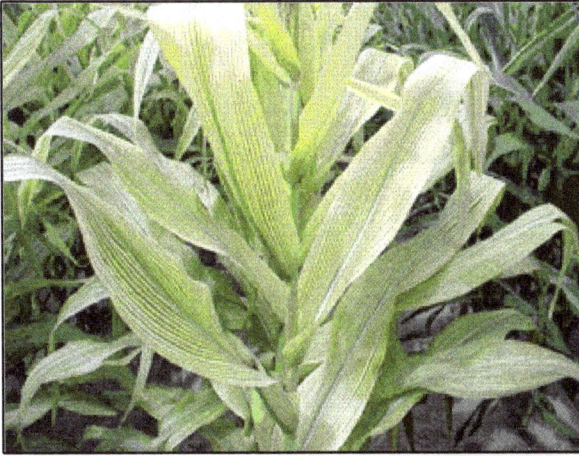

Fe Deficiency

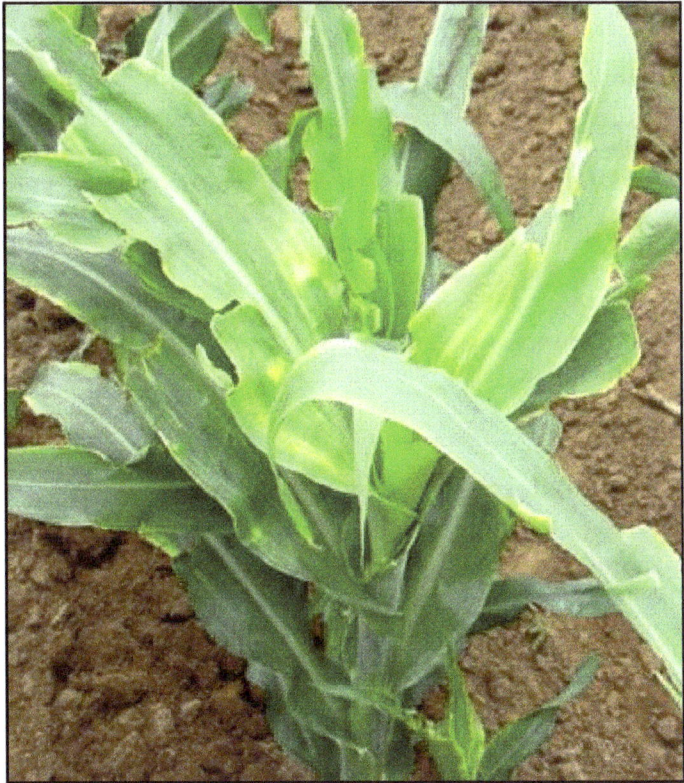

Ca Deficiency

Figure 6.1b: Nutrients Deficiency Symptoms in Sorghum.

Recovery Efficiency

It is expressed as 'kg nutrient taken per kg nutrient applied' or in other words 'per cent of nutrient taken by a crop'. Recovery Efficiency can be calculated as:

$$RE = \frac{NUf - NUc \times 100}{Na}$$

Physiological Efficiency

It is expressed as 'kg yield increase per kg nutrient taken up by a crop' and calculated as:

$$PE = \frac{Yf - Yc}{NUf - NUc}$$

Partial Factor Productivity of Fertilizers

The PFPf is expressed as 'kg crop yield per kg nutrient applied' and calculated as:

$$PFPf = \frac{Yf}{Na}$$

Here, *Yf* and *Yc* are the yields (kg/ha), in fertilized and control (no fertilizer) plots, respectively. *NUf* and *NUc* are the amounts of nutrients taken up by a crop in fertilized and control plots, respectively and *Na* refers to the amount of nutrient applied (kg/ha). *AE* is the same as "crop response ratio" or productivity index used by FAO (1989) and can be determined for a single nutrient (N, P, or K) or for a combination of nutrients (NP, NK, PK, or NPK), or for a fertilizer material *per se. PFPf* can also be determined for a single or a combination of nutrients or for a fertilizer *per se.* For calculating *PFPf*, 'no-fertilizer control' plot yield is not required. This gives a comparison of fertilizer use efficiency in different countries or in different regions of a country. The term is useful in comparing the advantages of fertilizer use in experiments on tillage, irrigation, weed control etc., where a 'no fertilizer control' is typically not provided.

Factors Affecting NUE in Sorghum

Production practices that lead to affecting crop yields will have impact on nutrient-use efficiency. Nutrient requirements and NUE in sorghum vary with soil, climate, cultivar and management practices.

Soil Factors

Sorghum is gown on diverse range of soils. This range is so wide that some soils are unusually low in certain nutrients or have excessive quantities of certain nutrients. Nutritional stress problems in soils are often related to the type of parent material and the soil-forming processes characteristic of that soil (Dudal 1976; Clark 1982a, d). Acid soils (Oxisols, Ultisols and some Entisols, Alfisols and Inceptisols) are usually low in exchangeable bases. Acidity increases the solubility of iron, aluminum and manganese and hence, these elements may reach to the toxic levels. However, acid soils are deficient in phosphorus, calcium, magnesium, molybdenum and zinc (Clark 1982a). Alkaline soils (Mollisols, Vertisols and some Inceptisols) often contain fairly high concentration of salt in the soil profile. These soils are rich in calcium, magnesium and potassium but deficient in sulphur. The deficiency symptoms of iron, zinc and manganese are the most common in sorghum grown on alkaline soils (Tandon and Kanwar 1984). The nutrient use efficiency in these soils is greatly influenced by the time and method of fertilizer application. High bulk density, poor soil structure and crust formation, low water holding capacity, water logging and poor soil aeration can also reduce NUE.

Climate and Weather Factors

Nutrient availability in soil and the ability of plants to absorb and utilize the nutrients and subsequent yields are greatly influenced by temperature, solar radiation, and rainfall during crop growth (Arkin and Taylor 1981; Baligar and Fageria 1997). The rate of nutrient release from organic and inorganic sources, and the uptake by roots and subsequent translocation and utilization in plant is influenced by soil temperature (Arkin and Taylor, 1981; Cooper, 1973). Solar radiation directly affects photosynthesis which in turn influences a plants' demand for nutrients (Baligar *et al.*, 2007). Higher rainfall and humid weather during the growing season favours weed growth and causes more attacks of insect-pests and diseases in sorghum. This reduces crop yields and nutrient-use efficiency.

Cultivars

In semi-arid tropics where sorghum is an important crop, inorganic fertilizer use is limited due to high cost and non-availability, and limited soil moisture availability. To reduce the impact of nutrient deficiency on sorghum production, the selection of genotypes that are superior in the utilization of available nutrients either due to enhanced uptake capacity or because of more efficient use of the absorbed nutrients in grain production can be a desirable option. Sorghum cultivars differ in growth, rooting pattern, maturity duration, etc. and hence the nutrient uptake pattern and the efficiency are also likely to differ. Exploiting these differences in nutrient demand and efficiency is a possible alternative for reducing the cost and reliance upon fertilizer. Gardner *et al.* (1994) demonstrated the genetic diversity for N use efficiency in grain sorghum and concluded that, the differences among sorghum cultivars for higher NUE mechanisms were associated with individual morphological, anatomical and biophysical traits like, larger canopies comprising of fewer but larger leaves with low N concentration, thicker leaves, larger leaf phloem transactional area, rapid solubilisation and remobilization of N from older to younger leaves, and lower 'dark respiration' rates. At low N levels (50 kg N ha^{-1}) the improved genotype had the highest nitrogen-use efficiency and the commercial hybrid had the lowest. However, at high levels of N (200 kg N ha^{-1}) the commercial hybrid showed the highest NUE (Bernal *et al.*, 2002). The 'nutrient-use' efficiency of rainy season grain sorghum was influenced by nutrient levels. Hybrid sorghum 'CSH 16' had maximum NUE (7.06 kg grain/kg NPK applied) with 150 per cent RDF (150 : 60 : 60 kg NPK/ha) (Figure 6.2) but sorghum variety 'SPV 462' recorded maximum NUE (7.22 kg grain/kg NPK applied) at 100 per cent RDF (80:40:40 kg/ha)(AICSIP 2010-11).

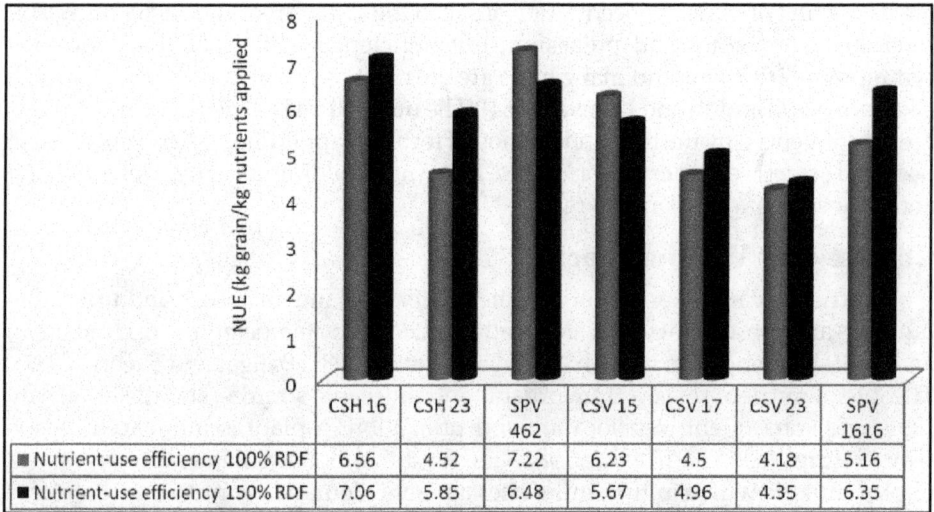

Figure 6.2: NUE of Grain Sorghum Cultivars.

	CSH 16	CSH 23	SPV 462	CSV 15	CSV 17	CSV 23	SPV 1616
■ Nutrient-use efficiency 100% RDF	6.56	4.52	7.22	6.23	4.5	4.18	5.16
■ Nutrient-use efficiency 150% RDF	7.06	5.85	6.48	5.67	4.96	4.35	6.35

Fertilizer Management

The 'nutrient-use' efficiency is affected by fertilizer dose, sources of nutrients, method and time of application, interaction of different nutrients, soil moisture, micorhyza and others. The availability and recovery efficiency are greatly influenced by addition of organic matter, liming, inclusion of legumes in sorghum-based cropping systems and others.

6.3 Nutrients Removal by Sorghum

Many factors are involved in determining the mineral requirement of sorghum (Maiti, 1996).

1. Amount of available and residual mineral elements in soil.
2. Physico-chemical properties of soil.
3. Availability of soil moisture.
4. Yield and end product desired.

Cultivars producing large amounts of biomass remove greater quantities of soil nutrients. Sorghum crop producing 5.5 t/ha grain removes a total of 335 kg nutrients (149 kg N + 61 kg P_2O_5 + 125 kg K_2O)/ha from soil. High yielding varieties remove 22 kg N, 9 kg P_2O_5 and 30 kg K_2O to produce 1.0 t of grain (Tandon and Kanwar, 1984). Sorghum crop yielding approximately 8 t of grain/ha removes about 250 kg N, 40 kg P_2O_5, 160 kg K_2O, 45 kg Mg, 40 kg S/ha from soil (Maiti, 1996). Nutrients removed by sorghum hybrid 'CSH 5' in Alfisols under rainfed conditions is given in Table 6.2 (Vijayalakshmi, 1979). Further studies revealed that sorghum grown in India removes on an average 22 kg N, 13.3 kg P_2O_5 and 34 kg K_2O to produce one tone of grains (Kaore, 2006).

Table 6.2: Nutrients Removal by Rainfed Hybrid Sorghum.

Nutrients	Grain Yield (t/ha)	Total Uptake by Grain and Stover
N	4.4	78 kg
P_2O_5	4.4	35 kg
K_2O	4.4	117 kg
Ca*	2.6	28 kg
Mg*	2.6	17 kg
Fe	4.4	705 g
Mn	4.4	447 g
Zn	4.4	132 g
Cu	4.4	37

*Vertisols (CSH 1) (Lakhdive and Gore, 1978)

Large quantities of N and P and some potassium are translocated from the other plant parts to the grain as it develops. Unless adequate nutrients are available during grain filling, this translocation may cause deficiencies in leaves and premature leaf loss that reduce leaf area duration and may decrease yields. Roy and Wright (1974) observed that, Nitrogen and P accumulation by whole plants increased almost linearly until maturity, but K accumulation was more rapid early in the season. Nitrogen, P, and K accumulation rates were higher during the 35th to 42nd day and 70th to 91st day which coincided with the peak vegetative growth period and the grain-filling stage, respectively. In unfertilized plants relatively higher translocation of N and P from the vegetative parts to the developing grain occurred. Little K was translocated. A much smaller percentage of total K was found in the head and more K was accumulated in the stem than N and P.

A grain crop of 8.5 t/ha contains (in the total aboveground plant) 207 kg of N, 39 kg of P and 241 kg of K (Vanderlip, 1972). Pal *et al.* (1982) reported that in early stage of crop growth, N and P accumulated slowly compared with the rapid accumulation of K. In later stages, uptake of K decreased relative to that of N and P.

6.4 Nitrogen

Nitrogen is one of the most abundant mineral nutrients required for sorghum growth. The level of nitrogen fertility has more influence on the growth and yield of grain sorghum than any other single plant nutrient. The amount of fertilizer N required will vary, depending on the yield potential of the cultivar and the amount of residual N available in the soil prior to planting. Preplant soil analysis can be very useful in estimating the nitrogen need of the crop. Only about 50 per cent of the N applied to soil is taken up and used by plants (Maiti, 1996). The reminder is left for microbial use, leaching and other reactions and processes occurring in the soil. Venkateswarlu (2004) indicated that sorghum belts in south India receives 6-12 kg N/ha from atmosphere depending on the level of precipitation. It has been estimated that 1.95-3.2 t soil/ha is lost annually due to wind and water erosion in sorghum belt (ICRISAT, 1986). This eroded soil carries away precious nutrients and reduces topsoil depth.

Alfisols, Vertisols and Red Lateritic soils where sorghum is prominently grown are prone to soil erosion (Sharda and Rattan Singh, 2003). Therefore, appropriate nutrient management strategies need to be adopted for improving soil health and productivity.

6.4.1 Nitrogen Concentration in Plant Tissues

Nitrogen accumulation in sorghum plants usually continues until maturity of the crop (Srivastava and Singh, 1971). The young plants accumulate relatively high concentration of N and the N content decreases in the various plant parts with age. Most of the plant N is absorbed during the vegetative stage and by early grain filling stages. Singh and Bains (1973) observed a continuous decline in N content in whole plant tissues until 75 days after planting followed by increased N content up to maturity. This late season increase in N content in whole plant after boot leaf stage was the result of the build-up of N in grains. The N content in plant tissues is influenced by the dose and time of fertilizer application, plant population, variety, irrigation and other management practice. There was a strong association between N content in whole plant at 30 and 60 days after sowing and grain yield (Hariprakash, 1979). Jones (1983) reported that the N concentration in sorghum grain ranged from 1.02 to 3.20 per cent (mean 1.67 per cent) and in stover 0.36 to 1.26 per cent (mean 0.80 per cent).

6.4.2 Nitrogen Uptake

The N-uptake curve is generally similar to sigmoidal growth curve in sorghum (Figure 6.3). Nitrogen accumulation rate by the whole plant was usually slower in the early growth stage, it became faster in the log phase of crop growth and again slowed down at maturity (Table 6.3) (Srivastava and Singh, 1971). Upon reaching the maximum accumulation in the vegetative plant parts, coinciding mostly with heading stage, nitrogen from vegetative parts starts getting translocated into the panicles (Singh and Bains, 1973). More N is translocated from leaves than from stem. Earheads contain the major portion of the N accumulated by the whole plant. Only 12-47 per cent of applied N is utilized by sorghum (Pal *et al.*, 1982). The recovery of N influenced by the rates and method of N application, soil types, variety, soil moisture and management practices. The results from a study with 15_N labeled urea at ICRISAT, 1982 and 1983 revealed that sorghum recovered 62.5 per cent of added N in the alfisol and 55.0 per cent in the vertisol. About 27.1 per cent of applied N was distributed in the alfisol profile and 38.6 per cent in the vertisol profile accounting to 89.6 per cent and 93.6 per cent N by the soil + crop system. In alfisols, crop recovery of N varied from 46.3 per cent to 51.1 per cent as N levels increased from 40 to 160 kg N/ha. At the highest N level tested, soil + crop system could account for 78.9 per cent of added N, as compared to 93.2 per cent at 40 kg N/ha. Although considerable fertilizer N was present in the soil profile after the harvest of rainy season sorghum, this residual N was of limited value either for safflower grown in the post-rainy season or for sorghum grown in the following rainy season (Moraghan *et al.*, 1983). The N response (kg grain/kg nitrogen applied) of rainfed sorghum to optimum or near optimum levels of N during rainy season varied from 21.7 kg in alfisols, 18.32 kg in vertisols11.9 kg in molisols and 20.15 kg in entisols (Tandon and Kanwar, 1984). A significant positive interaction between nitrogen and moisture has been well established in sorghum

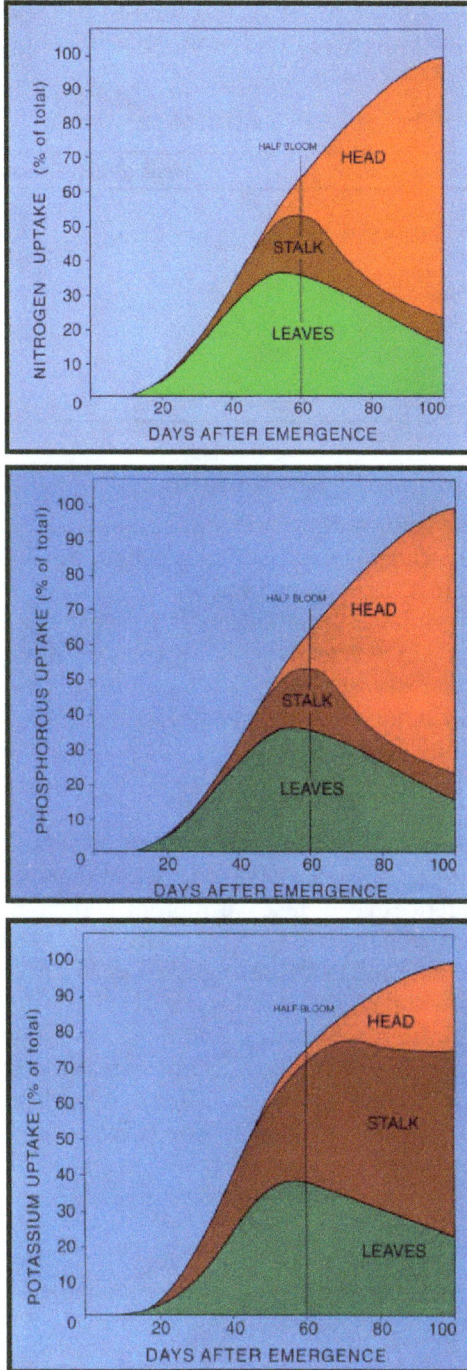

Figure 6.3: NPK Uptake Pattern in Grain Sorghum.

Source: R. L. Vanderlip, *How a Sorghum Plant Develops*, Kansas State University, January 1993.(*http://www.nasecoseeds.com/products/sorghum/47.html*)

and this interaction is stronger in an Alfisol than in a Vertisol (Kanwar, 1978). Nitrogen uptake was also improved by P and Fe fertilization in calcareous soils (Patil, 1979).

Table 6.3: N Accumulation Rates by Sorghum (CSH-1)

Growth Stages (Days after Sowing)	N Accumulation Rates (mg N/plant/day)
0-30	4.05-5.14
30-45	17.24-21.75
45-60	18.53-23.75
60-75	20.00-21.10
75-90	6.47-6.71
90-full maturity	0.40-2.10

6.4.3 Nitrogen × Moisture Interaction

Moisture availability, moisture use and nutrients supply to the plants are closely interacting factors influencing plant growth and yield production (Viets, 1972). There is a significant and positive correlation between fertilizer N and soil moisture for sorghum grain yield. The response was more in Alfosols than that of Vertisols (Kanwar, 1978). Water application in the Alfisols probably compensates for it comparatively shallow depth and low moisture storage, as compared with the Vertisol. With 58 or 120 kg N/ha, grain yield in non-irrigated Vertisol were similar to those in the Alfisol irrigated at 50 per cent moisture depletion (Tandon and Kanwar, 1984).

6.4.4 Nitrogen × Genotype Interaction

Sorghum genotypes greatly influence the nutrient accumulation in plants due to variation in rate of absorption, translocation and accumulation of nutrients in plant tissues. Genotypic difference in N uptake partitioning and NUE (unit dry matter per unit N in dry matter) has been reported for grain sorghum (Maraanville *et al.*, 2002). The varietal differences for N and P uptake might be due to additive gene action for N and non-additive for P (Krishna *et al.*, 1985). In general hybrids deplete greater amount of nutrients than that of varieties. Sorghum genotypes vary significantly for various root characteristics which may affect the nutrient uptake (Seetharama *et al.*, 1990). Long-term studies conducted in Vertisols indicated that sorghum absorbs mere 5 per cent of the total N during first 5 weeks followed by rapid N uptake. The crop accumulated 88 kg N/ha in 40-70 days, at the rate of about 3 kg N/ha/day (ICRISAT, 1984).

6.4.5 N × P Interaction

Long-term studies have indicated positive interaction between N and P in sorghum. The response to N may subside, if sufficient levels of P are not maintained on Vertisols and Alfisols. The positive N × P interactions have resulted in net advantage of 300-500 kg grains/ha (ICRISAT, 1984). N × P interactions may contribute up to 48-50 per cent of total response of sorghum to nutrient supply (Tiwari, 2006).

6.5 Phosphorus

Phosphorus is important in plant bioenergetics. As a component of ATP (Adenosine tri-phosphate), phosphorus is needed for the conversion of light energy to chemical energy during photosynthesis. There is widespread deficiency of phosphorus in soils of semi-arid tropics. It is estimated that only about 10 per cent of the P added to the soil is absorbed by plants and remaining 90 per cent become unavailable in the soil by adsorption or fixation by various soil fractions. Phosphorus accumulates extensively in the kernels (as phytin). A small fraction (16-22 per cent of total P uptake) of P is accumulated during early growth of the crop (42 days after sowing) owing to slower accumulation rate, whereas the major portion of the P is accumulated during later stages of crop growth (Srivastava, 1971; Roy and Wright, 1974).

Phosphorus uptake is enhanced by P fertilization. Excess P can interact with other nutrients (especially, Fe, Zn and Cu) and depress plant growth but causing deficiency of other plant nutrients. The response of phosphorus (kg grain/kg P_2O_5 applied) varies with soil types in order of Alfisols (17-32 kg) >Entisols (11-34 kg) >Vertisols (7-27 kg). In post-rainy crop, a response of 11 kg grain/kg P_2O_5 was obtained in Vertisols. Vertisols may require higher P application than other soils because of their high clay content and greater reactive surfaces/components (Rao and Das, 1982). On calcarious soils, P uptake by hybrid sorghum was highest when phosphatic fertilizers were applied on the surface, followed by 5 and 10 cm deep placement but the reverse was the case in non-calcareous soils (Venkatachalam, 1969). Apart from soil types, response to P is strongly affected by the yield potential of the cultivars, level of N applied, available soil P and favourable environment. Sorghum genotypes *viz.*, CSH 1, CSH 5 and CSV 3 were highly responsive to phosphorus (7.8 kg grain/kg P) compared to CSV 5 (3.5 kg grain/kg P) (Krishna, 2010). The residual response of P applied to sorghum on succeeding wheat crop is small and not consistent (Tandon and Kanwar, 1984). In general, 40-50 kg P_2O_5/ha is recommended for rainfed *kharif* sorghum and 20-30 kg/ha for *rabi* sorghum grown in medium and deep soils. In irrigated *rabi* sorghum, 40-50 kg P_2O_5/ha is recommended.

6.6 Potassium

Among the essential plant nutrients, potassium assumes greater significance since it is required in relatively larger quantities by plants. Besides increasing the yield, it largely improves the quality of the crop produce. Potassium regulates the opening and closing of stomata. Since stomata are important in water regulation, adequate potassium content in plants is associated with higher tolerance to drought and higher resistance to frost and salinity damage, and resistance to fungal diseases.

Potassium deficiency may not be a serious problem for sorghum in Indian soils. In general, black soils with higher clay and CEC showed high levels of exchangeable K and medium to high levels of non-exchangeable K content; Alluvial soils with higher contents of K rich mica with light texture, showed medium in exchangeable K and high in non exchangeable K content; and red and lateritic soils with kaolinite as a dominant clay mineral and light texture showed low in exchangeable as well as non-exchangeable K content (Srinivasarao *et al.*, 2011). However, recent studies indicated an application of 40-50 kg K_2O/ha in rainfed *kharif* and irrigated *rabi* sorghum.

Similar to N and P, K content in plant tissues also decreases as the crop advances from seedling stage (2.16-2.26 per cent in the leaves) to maturity (1.33 per cent in the leaves) and the ear heads contain less K than the leaves (Gopalkrishnan, 1960b). At harvest, the K content in grain declined from 0.41 per cent to 0.39 per cent and increased in stover from 1.24 to 1.29 per cent (Venkateswarlu, 1973). The potassium accumulated in sorghum plants rapidly during the early growth period and slowly at later stages (Roy and Wright, 1974). They further observed that 50-60 per cent of the total K uptake was completed before heading and around 68-78 per cent of total K was contained in the vegetative parts and 22-32 per cent in the heads.

6.7 Micronutrients

Among micronutrients, deficiency of zinc is more widespread in sorghum growing areas. Of the 2,51,660 soil samples analyzed for micronutrients, 49 per cent were deficient in Zn and 12 per cent in Fe content (Singh, 2001). Most Zn in sorghum is taken up by the early grain-fill stage. Next to Zn, iron nutrition to sorghum has importance in some soils. Sorghum is sensitive to iron stress and is less efficient in its absorption and translocation. Since Fe uptake decreases with increased $CaCO_3$ content of the soil, the problem of Fe deficiency is more on calcareous soils. Soils containing more than 1.2 ppm Zn and 3-5 ppm Fe (critical limit for sorghum) did not respond to Zn/Fe application (Tandon and Kanwar, 1984). Application of 20 ppm Fe as $FeSO_4$ increased the grain yield by 0.9 t/ha (Babaria and Patel, 1981). Koraddi *et al.* (1969) observed complete recovery from lime induced chlorosis and obtained higher sorghum yield with spraying of $FeSO_4$. Singh and Vyas (1970) reported 5.1 per cent and 13.9 per cent increase in grain yields application of manganese and zinc, respectively in Jodhpur. Joshi (1956) reported significant increase in yield of sorghum due to $CuSO_4$ application in Maharashtra. Kanwar and Randhawa, (1967) observed 35 per cent and 40 per cent increase in the yield of sorghum due to application of boron and boron (B) + manganese (Mn). Foliar application of $MnSO_4$ @ 10 kg/ha was found to increase the sorghum grain yield by 24-35 per cent (Gill and Abichandani, 1972). Experiments conducted under All India Coordinated Sorghum Improvement Project (AICSIP) revealed that deficiency of Zn and Fe can be corrected either through soil application of respective sulphate forms or through foliar application (Table 6.4).

An antagonistic relationship was reported with Fe and Cu, Zn and Mn, whereas Cu showed antagonism with Fe and Zn and synergism with Mn in sorghum shoot (Singh and Yadav, 1980)

6.8 Biofertilizers

A bio-fertilizer is a substance which contains living microorganisms which, when applied to seed, plant surfaces, or soil, colonizes the rhizosphere or the interior of the plant and promotes growth by increasing the supply or availability of primary nutrients to the host plant (Vessey, 2003). Biofertilizers add nutrients through Nitrogen fixation, solubilizing phosphorus, and stimulating plant growth through the synthesis of growth promoting substances. Biofertilizers can be expected to reduce

Table 6.4: Effect of Iron and Zinc on Grain and Dry Fodder Yield of Sorghum (AICSIP, 2011)

Treatment	Grain Yield (kg/ha)					
	Coimbatore	Parbhani	Akola	Dharwad	Surat	Mean
RDF + ZnSO$_4$ 25 kg (Soil appl.)	1833	2737	3178	2462	3045	2651
RDF + FeSO$_4$ 25 kg (Soil appl.)	1502	2312	3114	2862	3491	2656
RDF + 0.2 per cent ZnSO$_4$ Foliar spray at 15 and 30 DAS	1730	2328	2609	2289	2955	2382
RDF + 0.5 per cent FeSO$_4$ Foliar spray at 15 and 30 DAS	1553	2197	2525	2466	3024	2353
RDF + ZnSO$_4$ 15 kg (Soil appl.) + 0.20 per cent as foliar spray at 15 and 30 DAS	1936	2662	3136	2882	2826	2689
RDF + FeSO$_4$ 15 kg (Soil appl.) + 0.50 per cent asfoliar spray at 15 and 30 DAS	1562	2009	3093	2598	2971	2447
RDF + Soil application of 15 kg ZnSO$_4$ + 15 kg FeSO$_4$	1636	2793	4798	2953	3676	3171
RDF + Foliar application of 0.20 per cent ZnSO$_4$ + 0.50 per cent FeSO$_4$	1698	2036	2925	3184	3367	2642
RDF(80:40:40 kg NPK/ha) alone	1438	1847	2883	2939	2868	2395
Mean	1567	2252	3072	2509	3028	2486
C.D. (P = 0.05)	160	437	643	355	228	482
CV per cent	5.94	11.3	12.2	8.24	4.38	15.1

Source: (AICSIP 2010-11).

the use of chemical fertilizers and pesticides. Through the use of biofertilizers, healthy plants can be grown while enhancing the sustainability and health of soil. Biofertilisers form an important component in the integrated nutrient management. A number of biofertilisers *viz.*, Azotobactor, Azospirillum, vermicompost, etc., are now commercially available for cereals.

Field research on using microorganisms on increasing nutrient-use efficiency was started during 1970's. Various strains of microorganisms like *Azotobactor, Azospirillum, Phosphobacterin* and *Mycorrhiza* were found promising. Senthil Kumar and Arockiasami (1995) reported that Arbuscular mycorrhizas (AM) inoculated sorghum seedlings contained 11.5 mg Zn/g dry root but non-mycorrhizal seedlings had 7.5 mg Zn/g dry root. Sorghum genotypes also vary with regards to AM mycorrhizal colonization in roots and P uptake (Seetharama *et al.*, 1988). The net advantage from AM symbiosis to sorghum seems to be 10-20 kg P/ha (Krishna *et al.*, 1985). Studies conducted at TNAU, Coimbatore revealed that fertilizer-N application could be reduced by inoculating with *Azospirillum* (TNAU, 2003). In sorghum-chickpea system, biofertilizer [*Azospirillum* and phosphate-solubilizing bacteria (PSB)] gave significantly higher grain and fodder yields (Gawai and Pawar, 2006).

6.9 General Nutrient Recommendations

In light soils with low rainfall, a fertilizer dose of 60 kg N, 30 kg P_2O_5 and 20 kg K_2O/ha is generally recommended, however for medium-deep soils and moderate to high rainfall areas 80 kg N, 40 kg P_2O_5 and 40 kg K_2O per ha is desired for high yielding *kharif* sorghum cultivars. For *rabi* sorghum, inorganic fertilizers should be applied based on soil types and moisture conditions (Table 6.5).

Table 6.5: Recommended Dose of Nutrients for *rabi* Sorghum

Area of Adaptation/Soil Type		Inorganic Fertilizer (kg/ha)		
		N	P_2O_5	K_2O
Rainfed	Shallow	25	–	–
	Medium	40	20	–
	Deep	60	30	–
Irrigated	Medium	80	40	40
	Deep	100	50	50

6.10 Method and Time of Fertilizer Application

Nitrogen (N) should be applied as close to planting as possible. Placement of urea or diammonium phosphate with or near the seed is not recommended due to the risk of seedling injury due to ammonia toxicity. Nitrogen utilization by sorghum plant is quite rapid after the plant reaches to five-leaf stage, with 65-70 per cent of the total N accumulated by the bloom stage of growth (Cothren *et al.*, 2000). Apparent N recover also markedly improves when N is applied in 2 or 3 splits in a high rainfall year (Venkateswarlu *et al.*, 1978). Sorghum yields are adversely affected if the dose of N at planting is either reduced to less than 50 per cent of the total dose or the top dressing is delayed beyond the flower primordia initiation stage (Tandon and Kanwar, 1984). Application of half amount of N at planting and half at 30 days after sowing produced significantly higher yields of hybrid sorghum (Lingegowda *et al.*, 1971; Sharma and Singh, 1974; Turkhede and Prasad, 1978). However, in light soils and in high rainfall areas, three splits of N fertilizer, 50 per cent at sowing, 25 per cent at floral primordial initiation and 25 per cent at flowering has been found beneficial (Choudhary, 1978). In heavy black soils of Maharashtra, Bodade (1964, 1966) concluded that the application of 50 per cent N through foliar application was as effective as the full dose of N through soil application. Choudhary (1978) recommended 2 equal splits of N for foliage application: first at floral primordial initiation and second at mid-bloom stage of crop. Narayana Reddy *et al.* (1972) reported 6 per cent concentration of urea solution as the best for foliar spray. It is generally recommended that all phosphatic and potassium fertilizers should be applied as basal, and deep-placed.

6.11 Integrated Nutrients Management (INM)

Importance of the use of organic sources of nutrients along with chemical fertilizers for maintaining soil health has been emphasized by Katyal (2000). The use of chemical fertilizer or biofertilizer has advantages and disadvantages in the context of nutrient supply, crop growth and environmental quality. The advantages need to be integrated in order to make optimum use of each of the fertilizers to achieve balanced nutrient management for crop growth (Jen-Hshuan Chen, 2006). Combined use of inorganic and organic manures improves physical and chemical properties of soils. Application of sorghum stubbles, sunhemp and glyricidia has recommended dose of fertilizer resulted in maximum response with only 50 per cent under rainfed condition. Application of 75 per cent recommended dose of fertilizer (RDF) + farmyard manure (FYM) + biofertilizer [*Azospirillum* and phosphate-solubilizing bacteria (PSB)] gave significantly higher plant height, dry mater, yield attributes and grain and fodder yields of sorghum, and was on a par with application of 100 per cent RDF through inorganics alone showing 25 per cent saving of nutrients (Gawai and Pawar, 2006, Patil *et al.*, 2008). Incorporation of FYM, wheat straw and glyricidia leaves for 25 or 50 per cent N substitution in conjunction with balanced dose of NPK fertilizers increased infiltration rate, water stable aggregates and organic matter, the values of which ranged from 0.88 to 0.92 cm h^{-1}, 0.82 to 0.96 mm and 1.10 to 1.27 per cent, respectively; whereas bulk density decreased from 1.32 to 1.22 Mg m^{-3}. The soil reaction and electrical conductivity remained unaffected while the organic carbon content increased appreciably and ranged from 0.68 to 0.74 per cent. The available N, P$_2$O$_5$ and K$_2$O status improved after harvest of both the crops due to integrated nutrient management by the application of 50 per cent recommended dose of fertilizers and 50 per cent N equivalent with FYM to sorghum in *kharif* and recommended dose of fertilizers to wheat in *rabi* than the continuous application of recommended dose of fertilizers to both the crops (Bhonde and Bhakare, 2008). Crop residue recycling is a vital aspect of sorghum cultivation as it reduces run-off induced soil and nutrient loss (Dhruvanarayan and Rambabu, 1983). Among the residues, prunings from *Leaucaena* and *Glyricidia* enhance carbon sequestration better than cereals residue. Integration of vermicompost at 2 t/ha + 50 per cent RDF was found on a par with RDF in sorghum – chickpea/field pea/lentil system (AICSIP, 2007). Minimum tillage with 80:40:40 kg NPK/ha or conventional tillage with 60:30:30 kg NPK/ha, of which 75 per cent through inorganic + PSB + *Azospirillum* + *Dhaincha* incorporation/mulching at 30 DAS were found promising (Mishra *et al.*, 2012).

Chapter 7
Water Management

Water is a limiting factor in crop production in many areas. One should match an appropriate crop and genotype with available soil moisture. There is no advantage in planting a high yielding crop if the water is not available to support the high biomass yield. Sorghums are known for their ability to extract soil moisture and tolerate drought better than most other grain crops due to their well developed and finely branched root system. It also has a small leaf area per plant, which limits transpiration. The leaves fold up more efficiently during warm, dry conditions than that of maize. It has an effective transpiration ratio of 1:310, as the plant uses only 310 parts of water to produce one part of dry matter (Lima, 1998), compared to a ratio of 1:370 for maize (Chapman and Carter, 1976). The epidermis of the leaf is corky and covered with a waxy layer, which protects the plant form desiccation. The stomata close rapidly to limit water loss. During dry periods, sorghum has the ability to remain in a virtually dormant stage and resume growth as soon as conditions become favourable. Even though the main stem can die, side shoots can develop and form seed when the water supply improves.

In semi-arid regions, plant-available water is often the most limiting factor for crop growth and yield potential, in dry land agriculture. Grain sorghum is known for its drought tolerance and is well adapted to semi-arid dry land conditions. Water deficit during the early reproductive and grain filling stages of growth is a common cause of low grain yield and inefficient water use. Water supply at reproductive growth stages of grain sorghum has more impact on total grain yield than at the vegetative or ripening stages (Ockerby *et al.*, 2001; Maman *et al.*, 2003). Water stress during boot and flower stages can reduce grain yield by 85 per cent (Crawford *et al.*, 1993).

7.1 Water Requirement and Water-Use Efficiency

Sorghum is grown primarily in semi-arid and arid regions in the world with limited or no irrigation. Water requirement of sorghum varies from 350 to 700 mm depending on the season, crop duration, soil, nutrition and other environmental conditions. For optimum yields on good soil, short-growth, average-growth, and long-growth varieties requires 500 to 600 mm, 650 to 800 mm, and 950 to 1100 mm of well distributed rainfall, respectively. Raheja (1961) reported that sorghum crop requires about 610 mm water for optimum yield, whereas Chandramohan (1970) stated that 488 mm water was adequate for sorghum under Tamil Nadu conditions. Water requirement of main and ratoon sorghum was assessed at 520 and 293 mm, respectively when irrigation was scheduled at 50 per cent available soil moisture (Subbarayalu, 1982). Higher grain yield of 4.92 t/ha was obtained by applying 45 kg N/ha with a water requirement of 425 mm (Sharma and Neto, 1986). The water requirement for pure sorghum was lesser than sorghum + groundnut intercropping systems respectively (Shinde and Umrani, 1988).

Water use efficiency (WUE) is a measure of yield per unit of water consumed. Water use and WUE vary by site conditions. The FAO document on China states that for sorghum, maize and wheat, the transpiration ratio is 141, 170, and 241 kg/kg plant material, respectively (Turhollow *et al.*, 2010). For grain sorghum grown in the North Plains of Texas over the 6-year period of 1998 to 2003, water consumption was 1060 and 842 kg water/kg grain for dryland and irrigated production, respectively (New, 2004). Roots of mature sorghum plant can extract soil moisture from up to 2 m of soil depth, although higher yields are obtained when moisture is available in the top 76 cm of soil (Cothren *et al.*, 2000). Water availability to plants largely depend on soil texture (Table 7.1).

Table 7.1: Soil Texture and Available Water Capacity (Klocke and Hergert, 1990)

Soil Texture	Available Water Capacity (cm/m)
Course sand	2.1 - 6.2
Fine sand	6.2 - 8.3
Loamy sand	9.2 - 10.0
Sandy loam	10.4 - 11.7
Fine sandy loam	12.5 - 16.7
Silty loam	16.7 - 20.8
Silty clay loam	15.0 - 16.7
Silty clay	12.5 - 14.2
Clay	10.0 - 12.5

Kharif sorghum is mainly grown under rainfed conditions. Very often rainfed sorghum crop experiences soil moisture stress when rains fail during the monsoon season. However, the post-rainy season sorghum is grown on residual soil moisture with limited irrigation facilities. It is often argued that under the driest conditions millet is preferred over sorghum and maize (corn) as it produces more, under semi-arid conditions it is sorghum which is preferred over millet, and with ample moisture, corn performs best. Singh and Singh (1995) reported that maize and sorghum performed best at unstressed conditions. Just because a crop has a higher WUE does not mean it has a higher biomass yield. Different crops draw different amounts of water from different parts of the soil profile. Sorghum draws water from more of the soil profile than corn. The Table 7.2 below clearly shows that, under unstressed conditions, maize has a higher WUE than sorghum, but yields are same. Farré and Faci (2004) also reported that sorghum extracted more water from the deeper soil layers whereas maize from the upper soil layers.

Table 7.2: Biomass Production, Evapotranspiration, and Water Use Efficiency for Corn, Sorghum, and Millet in Northern India in 1979 and 1980 (Singh and Singh, 1995)

Irrigation Level	Dry Biomass (Mg/ha)			Evapotranspiration (mm)			Water Use Efficiency (Dry biomass kg/ha/mm)		
	Maize	Sorghum	Millets	Maize	Sorghum	Millets	Maize	Sorghum	Millets
Unstressed	9.0	9.0	8.3	567	582	568	15.9	15.4	14.6
Mildly stresses	5.2	7.1	5.9	403	432	429	12.8	16.4	13.8
Moderately stresses	4.7	6.1	5.4	342	329	331	13.7	18.5	16.3
Severely stressed	3.0	4.1	4.0	276	288	224	11.0	14.4	17.9

7.2 Water Use by Sorghum Plant

Knowledge of the growth stages of sorghum is necessary for better understanding of its moisture use pattern. For optimum 'plant stand' establishment, a good 'seed-to-soil' contact at sowing, adequate soil moisture and optimum soil temperature are necessary. Although sorghum takes less amount of water during germination and at seedling stage, but it is critical and thus sufficient moisture is required. During seedling stage more amount of moisture is lost through evaporation than by transpiration. Soil moisture conservation practices such as compartmental bunding, tide ridging, green manuring and mulching, narrow row spacing, proper planting time and suitable cultivar for early canopy development and timely weed control are very important. During early stage of growth, the root zone of sorghum is not much deeper and therefore, deeper soil moisture might not be critical at this stage.

The rapid growth starts about 25 days after seedling emergence, when 6-7 leaves are visible. Remaining leaves emerge with in next 30-35 days and maximum leaf area is attained. As the leaves develop and full canopy is formed at boot stage, the water use by sorghum reaches its peak stage (Figure 7.1). Therefore, the adequate soil moisture is required, 2 weeks prior to boot leaf stage through the boot stage for better seed set and higher productivity. With the start of soft dough stage, moisture requirements decline rapidly.

7.3 Critical Stages for Irrigation in Sorghum

Germination, seedling, flowering and grain formation stages were critical for irrigation and getting higher yield (Dastane, 1974). Water stress at early stage reduces the amount of leaf area at flowering (Fischer and Hagan, 1965). Stress at critical stages limits the elongation of stalk and significantly reduced LAI (Oizumi, *et al.*, 1965). The period of 40 to 85 days after sowing when flowering and grain formation stages are very sensitive to moisture stress (Figure 7.1).

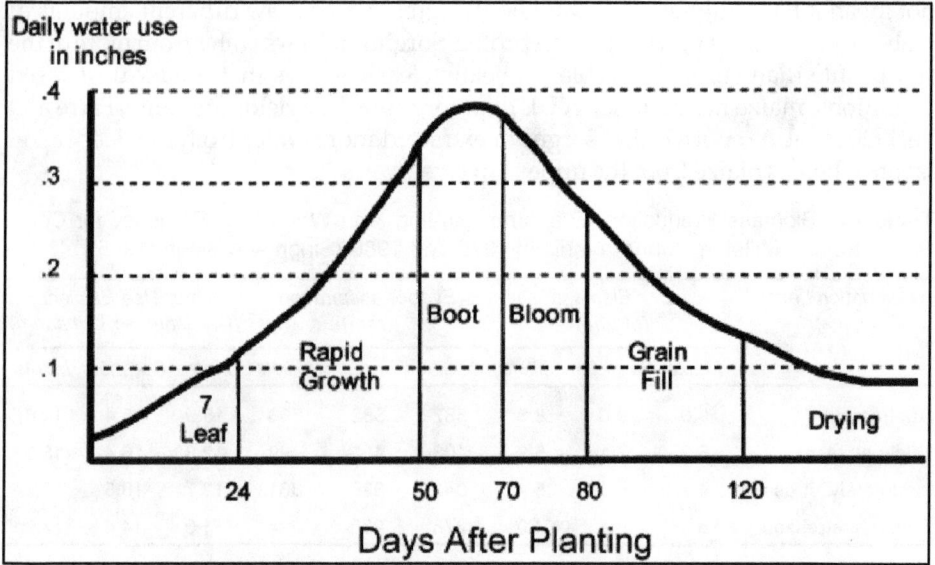

Figure 7.1: Daily Water Use (in inches) by Sorghum during Entire Growing Season.
Source: http://sanangelo.tamu.edu/agronomy/sorghum/gsprod.htm.

The critical growth stages of sorghum in relation to water requirement are:

1. Initiation of grand growth stage 20-25 DAS
2. Flag-leaf stage or boot stage 50-55 DAS
3. Flowering stage 70-75 DAS
4. Grain-filling stage 90-100 DAS

In case water is available for providing irrigation at all four stages, it would be advantageous. In case of limited water availability, it should be given at the flower primordial initiation stage (30-35 DAS) followed by flowering stage.

7.4 Irrigation Scheduling

Various approaches based on transpiration ratio, soil moisture depletion, phenological stages, etc., have been developed for scheduling irrigation in sorghum. Dastane *et al*. (1970) reported that one irrigation at 25 per cent available soil moisture (ASM) in upper 30 cm soil layer in heavy clay soil was adequate for *kharif* sorghum. However, in *rabi* sorghum irrigation at 50 per cent ASM was found better (Hukkeri *et al*., 1977). Irrigation scheduled at 0.60 IW/CPE ratio was found better than that of 0.80 and 1.0 IW/CPE ratio in terms of grain production (Kandasamy and Subramanian, 1980). In sorghum + cowpea/blackgram intercropping system, irrigating at 25 per cent ASM was found optimum for higher yields of both main as well as intercrops (Vasimalai, *et al*., 1981). Done *et al*. (1984) determined an optimum irrigation interval of 12-18 days for higher grain yield of sorghum. Seedling, pre-flowering and grain formation stages coinciding with 2 to 4, 12 to 14 and 17 weeks after sowing respectively were critical for water demand (Balasubramanian, *et al.*, 1966). Irrigations scheduled at seedling, vegetative, flowering and grain formation stages were as effective as irrigating at 50 per cent ASM (Palaniappan *et al.*, 1977). One irrigation applied at pre-boot stage produced as much grain yield as that of 2 irrigations at pre-boot and boot stages or 4 irrigations at pre-boot, boot, flowering and milky stages in *rabi* sorghum under black soil conditions at Rahuri, Maharashtra (Dhonde *et al.*, 1986). Field experiments conducted at Solapur and Tandur revealed that 3 irrigations each at 35, 55 and 75 days after sowing gave the maximum grain (3663 kg/ha) at both the locations (Table). In case of only one irrigation, it should be applied either at 55 DAS. In case of 2 irrigations, it should be applied at 55 and 75 DAS (AICSIP, 2012) (Table 7.3).

Table 7.3. Effect of number of irrigations and stages on grain and Stover yields (AICSIP, 2012).

Treatments	Grain Yield (kg/ha)			Stover Yield (kg/ha)		
	Solapur	Tandur	Mean	Solapur	Tandur	Mean
One irrigation at 35 DAS (Flower primodia initiation stage)	1517	1949	1733	7387	3540	5463
One irrigation at 55 DAS (flag-leaf or boot stage)	1646	2254	1950	4198	3878	4038
Two irrigations each at 35 and 55 DAS	2277	2569	2423	6626	4240	5433
Three irrigations each at 35, 55 and 75 (flowering stage) DAS	3951	3375	3663	5597	4417	5007
Two irrigations each at 35 and 75 DAS	1580	2811	2196	8107	4209	6158
Two irrigation each at 55 and 75 DAS	3195	3079	3137	4403	4026	4214
Control (rainfed)	1158	1147	1153	5206	2889	4048
CD (P = 0.05)	1093	338	827	657	2584	

7.5 Soil Moisture Conservation Practices in *Kharif* Grain Sorghum

Kharif sorghum cultivation is primarily rain dependent. The crop faces frequent drought spells during its growth and reproductive periods. Early withdrawal of monsoon by mid-September, often causes post-flowering drought and reduces the grain yield considerably. Therefore, the moisture conservation practices like mulching crop residues between the rows or opening furrows at 3 weeks after sowing have been found beneficial in conserving soil moisture and increasing grain yield (AICSIP, 2009) (Table 7.4).

Table 7.4: Grain and Stover Yields of *Kharif* Grain Sorghum as Influenced by Moisture Conservation Practices.

Moisture Conservation Practices	Grain Yield (t/ha)					Stover Yield (t/ha)				
	Parbhani	Akola	Dharward	Udaipur	Mean	Parbhani	Akola	Dharward	Udaipur	Mean
Flat-bed sowing (45cm)	1620	4377	3463	3489	3237	8.47	10.54	11.25	11.45	10.43
Sowing at 45cm and opening furrows 3 weeks after sowing (WAS)	1898	4704	3701	4048	3597	8.5	1081	11.88	12.86	11.01
Paired planting at 30:60cm and opening furrows at 3 WAS	1798	4236	3871	4059	3491	8.49	10.03	12.84	13.08	11.11
Paired planting at 30:60cm and intercropping of green gram/cowpea	1574	4142	3502	3669	3222	8.3	10.19	11.46	11.62	10.39
CD (P = 0.05)	174	443	163	283	238	0.48	1.01	0.88	0.8	NS

7.6 Soil-Moisture Conservation Practices for *Rabi* Sorghum

The productivity of *rabi* sorghum is dependent on the quantity of rains received during rainy season, water holding capacity of soil, moisture conservation practices, use of high yielding cultivars and nutrient management technologies based on soil types. Occurrence of terminal drought is a major concern. Of the several factors responsible for increasing the productivity of *rabi* sorghum, *in-situ* moisture conservation contributes 35 per cent and therefore, every effort should be taken during preceding rainy season to conserve every drop of water.

Compartmental Bunding

The pioneering research work done at Hagari (Karnataka) during early 1940s indicated that, compartmental bunding enhanced the sorghum yields appreciably (Gopalkrishna Rao *et al.*, 1975). It involves making square or rectangular compartments on the field to retain rain water and to arrest soil erosion in medium deep black soils. After receipt of early rains in June and July, land is harrowed to remove the germinating weeds. Then the compartmental bunds (0.15-0.25 m height) are formed using bullock drawn bund former. The size of bunds varies from 3 m × 3 m to 4.5 m × 4.5 m depending on the slope. Radder *et al.* (1991) obtained higher grain and stover yields with compartmental bunding at 3m × 3m or 4.5m × 4.5m as compared to 9m × 9m and unbunded check (Table 7.5). The cost of is Rs. 150-300/ha. These bunds are retained till the sowing of *rabi* crop during second fortnight of September to first fort night of October. Compartmental bunds provide more opportunity time for water to infiltrate into the soil and help in conserving soil moisture.

Results of the experiments conducted under All India Coordinated Sorghum Improvement Project (AICSIP) revealed that compartmental bunding during *kharif* season conserved more soil moisture and produced higher grain yield over farmers' practice (Tables 7.5 to 7.7).

Table 7.5: Effect of Size of Compartmental Bunding on Grain and Stover Yields of *Rabi* Sorghum (Radder *et al.*, 1991)

Mean	Grain Yield (kg/ha)			Stover Yield (kg/ha)		
	1982-83	1983-84	Mean	1982-83	1983-84	Mean
Compartmenta bunding at						
3m x 3m	1793	1180	1487	3989	2900	3450
4.5m x 4.5m	1727	1140	1434	4158	2817	3488
6m x 6m	1616	1091	1354	3794	2687	3241
9m x 9m	1400	1022	1211	3493	2500	3001
Unbunded check	1063	848	956	3302	2332	2817
CD (P=0.05)	328	158	–	496	310	–

Ridge and Furrow Method

In this system, ridges and furrows are formed across the slope by bullock-drawn plough before monsoon. The height of ridges is around 20 cm and width of furrows

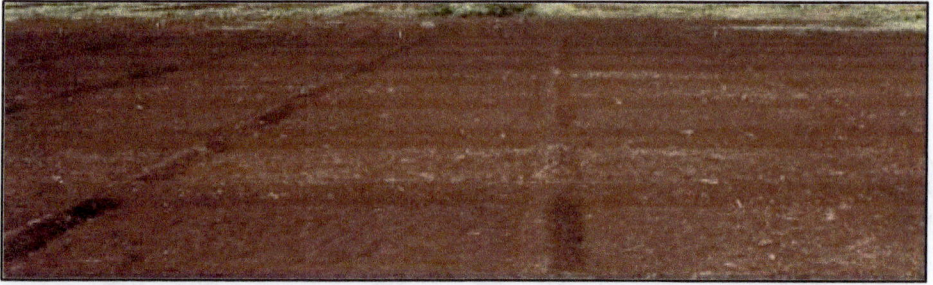

Field Layout of Compartmental Bunding.

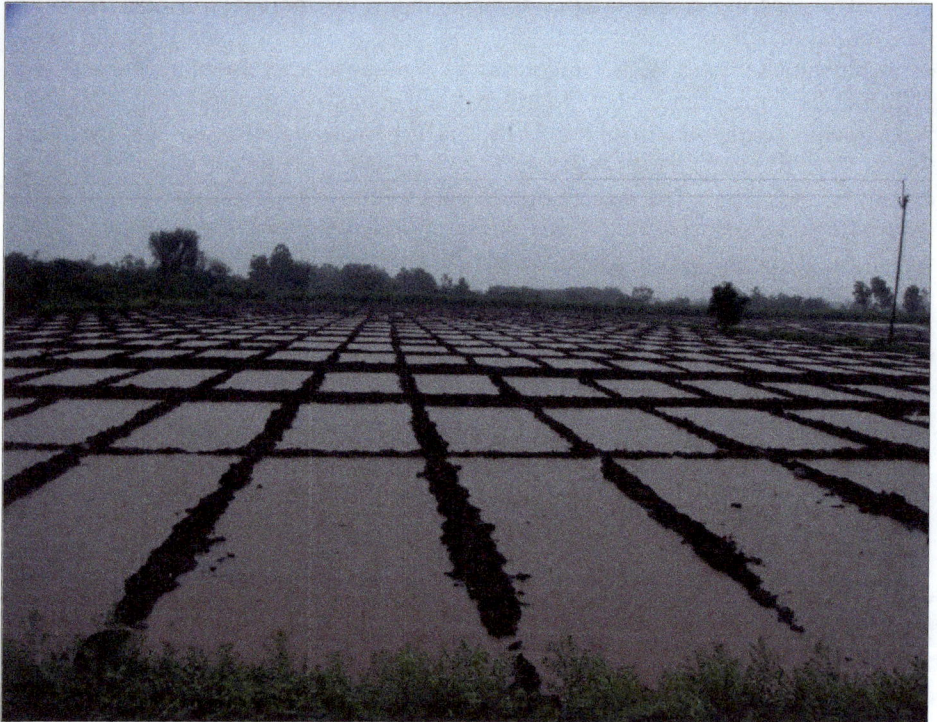

Rain water stored in compartments.

Figure 7.2: Compartmental Bunding.

is 45 cm. The rain water is stored in furrows and infiltrates into the soil and help in conserving soil moisture. Besides, opening of furrows in preceding (*kharif*) legumes (cowpea, mungbean, urdbean, soybean) after every 3rd or 4th row by 'Baliram Plough' conserves soil and moisture and improves drainage and increases the productivity of *rabi* sorghum.

Deep Ploughing

With mould board plough followed by 3-4 harrowing during summer (May-June) helps conserve rain water in deeper soil layers for a longer period.

Table 7.6: Effect of Moisture Conservation Practices on Grain Yield of *Rabi* Sorghum at different AICSIP Centres (Patil *et al.*, 2013)

Moisture Conservation Practices	Grain Yield (kg/ha)		
	Rahuri	Dharwad	Tandur
Compartmental bunding	3128	3039	3114
Ridge and furrow	2847	2994	2285
Green manuring with *dhaincha*	2856	3017	2879
Farmers' practice (flat sowing)	2625	2815	1845
CD (P = 0.05)	410	248	653

Table 7.7: Effect of Moisture Conservation Practices on Soil Moisture Content (AICSIP, 2012)

Moisture Conservation Practices	Soil Moisture Content (per cent)						
	At Sowing	At 35 DAS		At 55DAS		At 75 DAS	
	(0-15 cm Soil Depth)	0-15 cm	15-30 cm	0-15 cm	15-30 cm	0-15 cm	15-30 cm
Compartmental bunding	31.53	22.93	29.88	21.43	26.90	15.03	22.23
Ridge and furrow	29.05	19.80	28.10	18.33	24.78	14.93	20.10
Green manuring with *dhaincha*	30.93	22.18	28.70	20.73	26.05	14.33	21.35
Farmers' practice (flat sowing)	28.00	18.70	26.68	17.25	23.90	13.85	19.23
CD (P = 0.05)	0.94	0.70	1.06	0.65	1.00	0.92	1.59

Green Manuring

Whereever possible, green manuring crops like sunhemp or dhaincha should be grown during *kharif* fallow period and incorporated at 45 days after sowing (at 50 per cent flowering stage). This practice improves *rabi* sorghum productivity by conserving soil moisture in deeper layers, improving soil health and controlling weeds.

Table 7.8: Effect of *In-situ* Moisture Conservation Practices on Moisture Content, Grain Yield and Net Returns in *Rabi* Sorghum (Hiremath *et al.*, 2003)

In-situ Moisture Conservation Practices	Soil Moisture Content (cm) in 60 cm Profile at Flowering	Grain Yield (kg/ha)	Stover Yields (kg/ha)	Net Returns (/ha)	B:C Ratio
Flat bed	16.91	1405	2399	4,712	0.75
Compartmental bunding	17.35	2124	3282	9,491	1.45
Tied ridges	19.69	2210	3429	10,055	1.52
LSD (P = 0.05)	0.48	281	172	2,040	0.32

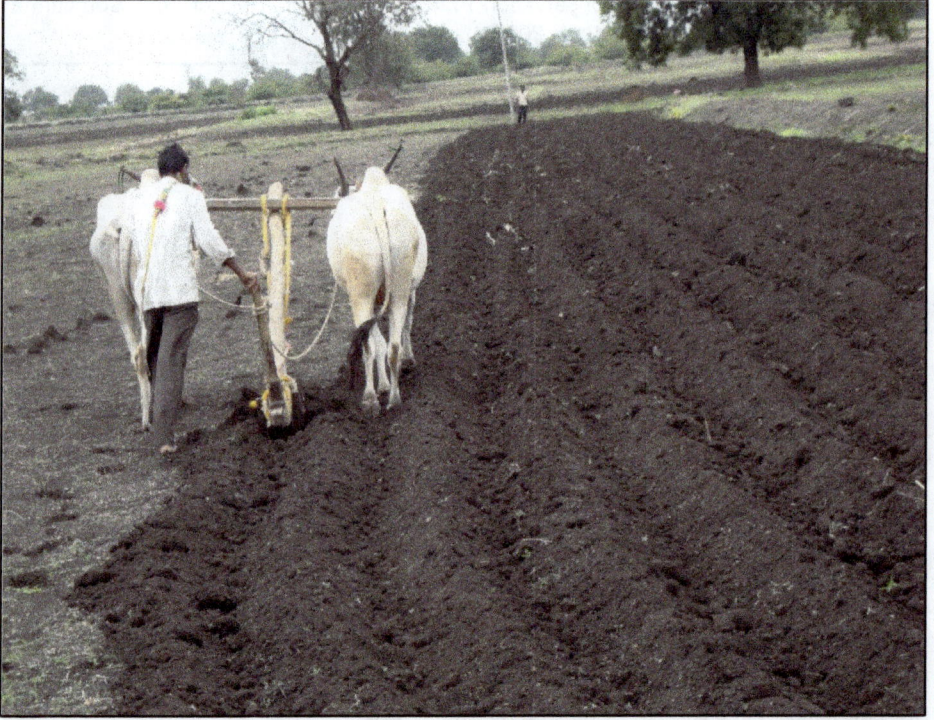

Opening of Ridges and Furrows

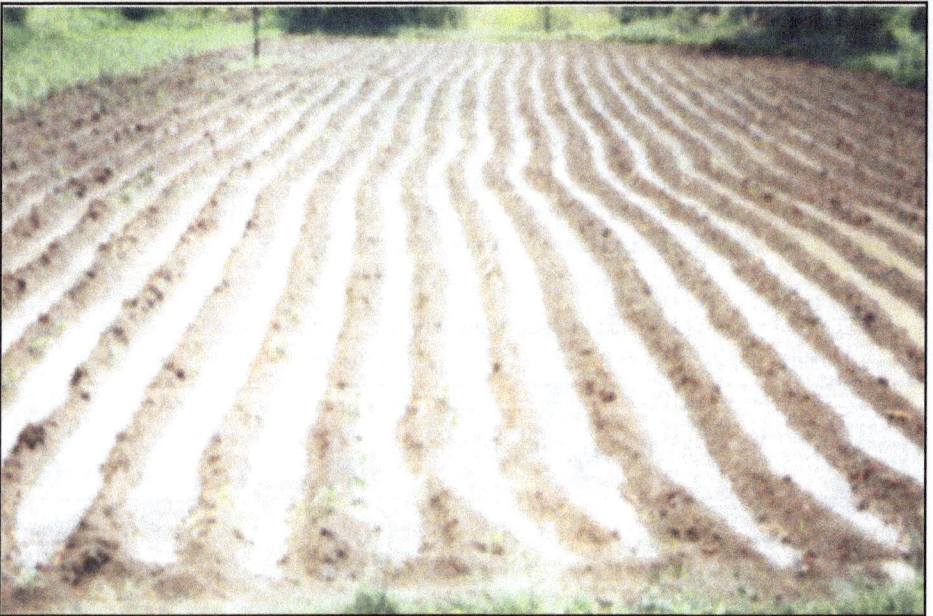

Rain Water Stored in Furrows

Figure 7.3: Ridge and Furrow.

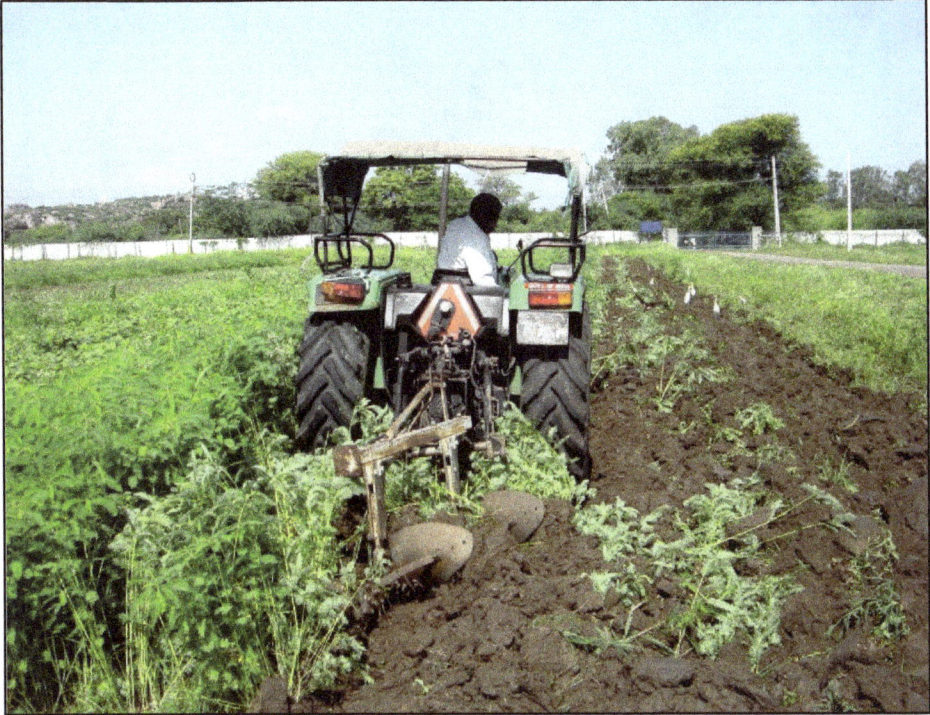

Figure 7.4: Incorporation of Dhaincha as Green Manure.

Moisture Conservation Practices after Sowing

Application of organic mulch (straw of preceding legume crops) in between rows after 3 weeks of sowing helps in conserving soil moisture by reducing evaporation.

In situ moisture conservation practices *viz.*, tied ridges and compartment bunding were found beneficial in conserving higher soil moisture, grain yield and net returns as compared to flat-bed method (Table 7.8).

Application of organic mulch (straw of preceding legume crops) in between rows after 3 weeks of sowing helps in conserving soil moisture by reducing evaporation. Spraying 2 per cent urea at the times of soil moisture stress experienced by crop also helps to overcome moisture stress.

Chapter 8
Weed Management

Weeds are a major deterrent in increasing the sorghum productivity. Grain sorghum seedlings are comparatively small and grow slowly for the first 20-25 days (Vanderlip, 1979) and consequently do not compete well with most weeds in the early stage of crop growth (Knezevic *et al.*, 1997), especially under adverse conditions. Planting sorghum in wider rows to facilitate inter-row cultivation and/or ditch furrow irrigation worsen the problems (Stahlman and Wicks, 2000). This is because the crop canopy forms slowly and provides little shading of weeds between rows until mid season; by then, most weeds are well established. Sorghum grown in rainy season is more heavily infested with weeds than grown in winter and spring seasons. Sorghum is mostly grown in rainfed areas where soil moisture and nutrients are limiting factors. Weeds compete with sorghum for light, soil moisture and nutrients (Smith *et al.*, 1990). Therefore, appropriate weed management would help to improve sorghum productivity and input use-efficiency. Burnside and Wicks (1969) discovered that weed competition had a greater effect on sorghum yield than crop row spacing or crop population. When improved agricultural technologies are adopted, efficient weed management becomes even more important, otherwise the weeds rather than the crops benefit from the costly inputs (Rao *et al.*, 1987).

8.1 Major Weed Flora

Sorghum is grown in both rainy and post-rainy seasons and under different cropping systems. Weeds are however a major problem in rainy season sorghum as the crop is sown soon after commencement of monsoon and the temperature is congenial. A mixed population of broad-leaved grasses and cyperaceous weeds grows with the sorghum crop under different agro-climatic conditions. Although typically, broad-leaved weeds are the major concern in grain sorghum, but annual grasses are also becoming a major matter of concern in some areas (Stahlman and Wicks, 2000). According to Holm *et al.* (1977), five of the world's major grass weeds *Echinochoa colona* (L.) Link. (jungle rice), *Echinochoa crus-galli* (L.) Beauv. (barnyard grass), *Eleusine indica* (L.) Gaertn. (goose grass), *Digitaria sanguinalis* (L.) Scop. (crab grass) and *Sorghum halepense* L. Pers. (johnson grass) infest grain sorghum. Among broad-leaved weeds, *Amaranthus palmeri* S. Wats (Palmer amaranth), *A. retroflexus* L. (Redroot pigweed), *Celosia argentea* L. (white cock's comb), *Trianthema portulacastrum* L. (horse weed), *Tribulus terrestris* L. (puncture vine), *Boerhaavia diffusa* L. (hog weed), *Acanthospermum hispidum* DC (Bristly starbur). *Striga asiatica* (L.) Kuntze. and *S. hermonthica* (Del.) Benth. (Witch weed) are the most common parasitic weeds worldwide.

The major weeds associated with sorghum in different sorghum growing regions of the country are classified as under (Table 8.1).

Table 8.1: Major Weeds of Sorghum

Scientific Name	English Name	Family
Grasses		
Cynodon dactylon Pers.	Bermuda grass	Poaceae
Brachiaria ramosa L.	Brown top millet	Poaceae
Digitaria sanguinalis (L.) Scop.	Crab grass	Poaceae
Dactyloctenium aegyptium L.	Crowfoot grass	Poaceae
Dinebra retroflexa Vahl.	Viper grass	Poaceae
Chloris barbata Sw.	Peacock plume grass	Poaceae
Eleusine indica (L.) Gaertn.	Goose grass	Poaceae
Echinochoa colona Link.	Jungle rice	Poaceae
Sorghum halepense (L.) Pers.	Johnson grass	Poaceae
Setaria glauca Beauv.	Yellow fox tail	Poaceae
Setaria viridis L.	Green foxtail	Poaceae
Panicum repens L.	Tarpedo grass	Poaceae
Paspalum paspaloides	Hilo grass, Sour grass	Poaceae
Broad-leaved		
Convolvulus arvensis L.	Field bind weed	Convolvulaceae
Acanthospermum hispidum DC.	Bristly starbur	Asteraceae
Achyranthes aspera L.	Prickly chaff flower	Amaranthaceae
Commelina benghalensis L.	Tropical spider wort	Commelinaceae
Ageratum conyzoides L.	Bill goat weed	Compositae
Amaranthus viridis L.	Pigweed	Amaranthaceae
Amaranthus palmeri S. Wats.	Palmer amaranth	Amaranthaceae
Amaranthus retroflexus L.	Redroot pigweed	Amaranthaceae
Boerhavia diffusa L.	Hog weed	Nyctaginaceae
Celosia argentea L.	White cock's comb	Amaranthaceae
Cleome viscosa L.	Cleome	Capparridaceae
Digera arvensis Forsk.	False amaranth	Amaranthaceae
Kochia scoparia (L.) Schrad.	Kochia	

Contd...

Table 8.1–*Contd...*

Scientific Name	English Name	Family
Portulaca oleracea L.	Common purslane	Portulacaceae
Euphorbia hirta L.	Pill pod spurge	Euphorbiaceae
Eclipta alba Hassk.	False daisy	Compositae
Corchorus acutangulus Lamk.	Jew's mallow	Tiliaceae
Ipomoea haderacea Jack.	Morning glory	Convolvulaceae
Portulaca oleracea L.	Purselane	Portulaceae
Salsola iberica Sennan and Pau	Russian thistle	
Trianthema portulacastrum L.	Horse purslane	Aizoaceae
Tridax procumbens L.	Coat buttons, tridax daisy	Compositae
Tribulus terrestris L.	Puncture vine	Zygophyllaceae
Xanthium strumarium L.	Common Cocklebur	Asclepiadaceae
Sedges		
Cyperus rotundus L.	Purple nut sedge	Cyperaceae
Parasitic		
Striga spp.	Witch weed	Scrophulaceae

8.2 Losses Due to Weeds

Weeds compete with sorghum for nutrients, soil moisture, sunlight and space when they are limiting, resulting in reduced yields, lower grain quality and increased production cost. The percentage of grain sorghum lost from weed competition exceeds that of most other grain crops (Stahlman and Wicks, 2000). Yield loss due to weeds ranges from 15 to 83 per cent depending on crop cultivars, nature and intensity of weeds, spacing, duration of weeds infestation and environmental conditions (Graham *et al.*, 1988; Okafor and Zitta, 1991; Mishra, 1997; Stahlman and Wicks, 2000). Competition from broadleaved weeds reduced grain sorghum yields more than grass species competition or mixture of broadleaved and grasses (Feltner *et al.*, 1969a). Tamado *et al.* (2002) observed that infestation of *Parthenium* in sorghum reduced its yield by 69-97 per cent depending upon its intensity. Moore and Murray (2002) reported that grain sorghum yields decreased 97 kg ha^{-1} for each increase of one *Amaranthus palmeri* plant per 15 m of row and decreased 392 kg ha^{-1} for each increase of 1 kg of dry matter of weed per 15 m of row. Grain yield was reduced by 3.10 kg ha^{-1} with every 1 g increase in weed dry weight m^{-2} (Sharma *et al.*, 2001). Uncontrolled weeds in sorghum removed 29.94-51.05, 5.03-11.58 and 48.74-74.34 kg ha^{-1} NPK, respectively from soil (Satao and Nalamwar, 1993). Weeds also act as an alternate host for insect-pests and diseases (Table 8.2). Weeds are an important plant resource for insects, although feeding by insects on weeds can have both positive and negative effects on crop productivity (Capinera, 2005).

Figure 8.1: Major Weeds of Sorghum.

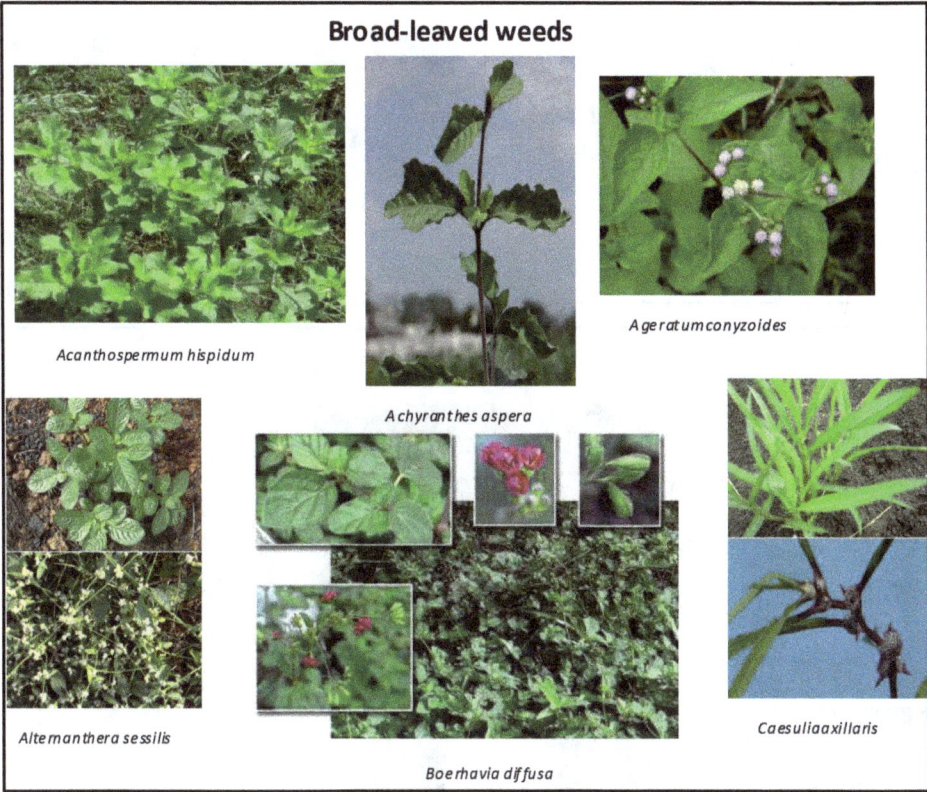

Broad-leaved weeds

Acanthospermum hispidum

Achyranthes aspera

Ageratum conyzoides

Alternanthera sessilis

Boerhavia diffusa

Caesulia axillaris

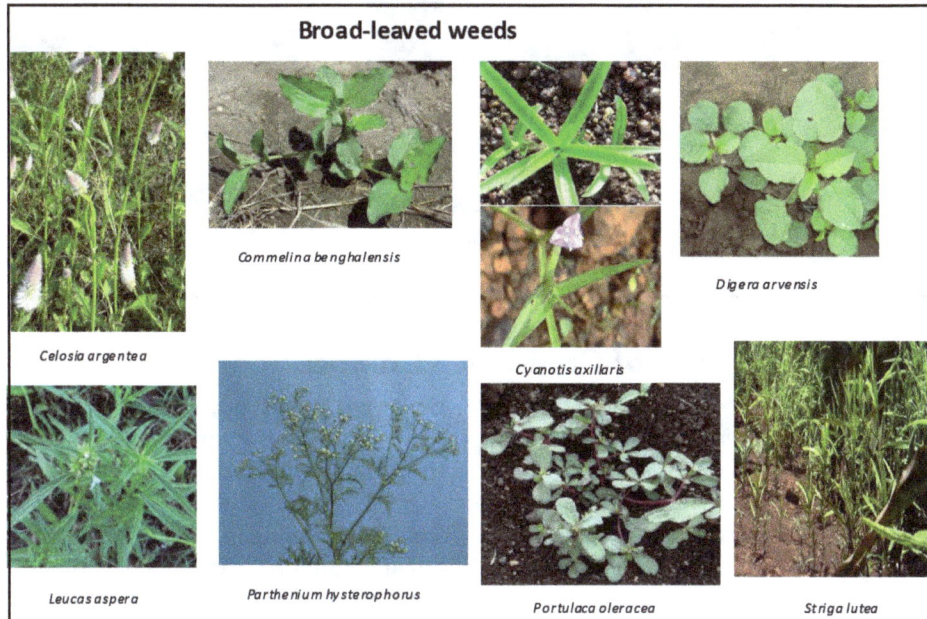

Broad-leaved weeds

Celosia argentea

Commelina benghalensis

Cyanotis axillaris

Digera arvensis

Leucas aspera

Parthenium hysterophorus

Portulaca oleracea

Striga lutea

Broad-leaved weeds

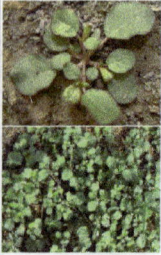

Tribulus terrestris

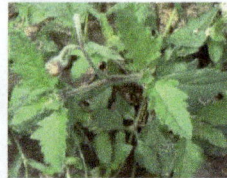

Tridax procumbens

Xanthium strumarium

Trianthema portulacastrum

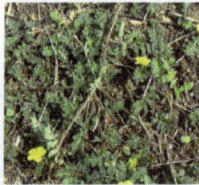

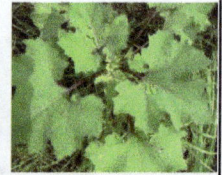

Grasses and sedges

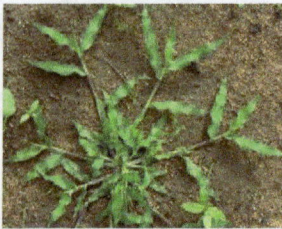

Brachiaria ramosa

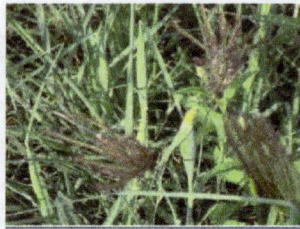

Chloris barbata

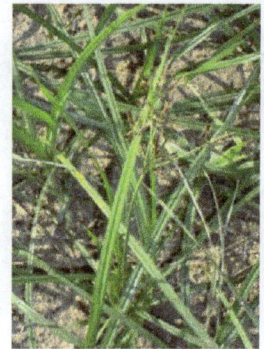

Cyperus rotundus

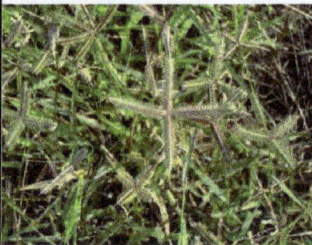

Dactyloctenium aegyptium

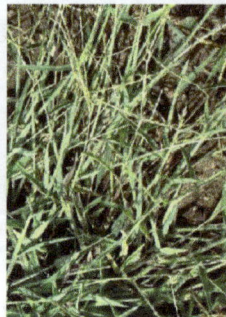

Digitaria sanguinalis

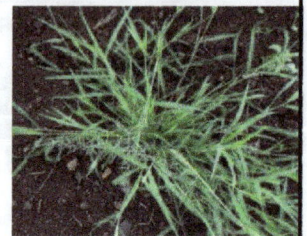

Dinebra retroflexa

8.3 Critical Period of Crop-Weed Competition

Emergence of weeds begins simultaneously with the crop, leading to severe competition between weeds and the crop right from the very early stage. In rainy season, weeds emerge in succession almost throughout the crop season. Removing weed competition any time during the growing season is not desired. Time of weed removal is as important as removal *per se*. 'Critical period' defines the maximum period of time in which weeds can be tolerated without affecting final crop yields (Zimdahl, 1980). This provides information on the active duration when the presence of weeds

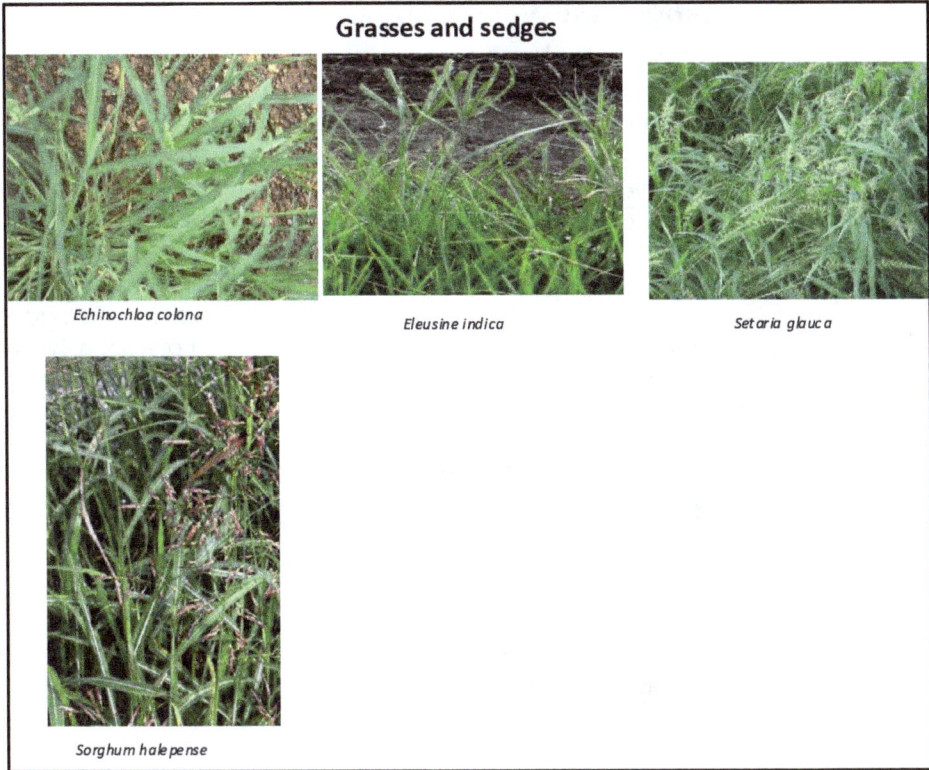

Grasses and sedges

Echinochloa colona

Eleusine indica

Setaria glauca

Sorghum halepense

make their deleterious effect on crops. In grain sorghum, 4-6 weeks after seedling emergence has been found as the 'critical period' (Kondap and Bathakal, 1981; Sundari and Kumar, 2002).

Table 8.2: Weeds as an Alternate Host for Insect-Pests and Diseases of Sorghum

Weed Species	Organisms	Disease/Insect-Pests	References
Cynodon dactylon	Sporisorium sorghi	Sorghum covered smut	Marley (1995)
Sorghum halepense	Colletotrichum graminicola	Sorghum anthracnose	Frederiksen (1984)
	Stenodiplosis sorghicola	Sorghum midge	Monaghan (1978); Bilbro (2008)
	Claviceps Africana	Ergot	Reed et al. (2000)
Brachiaria distachya, Panicum repens, Setaria intermedia, Cyperus rotundus	Shoot fly		Nwilene et al. (1998)

8.4 Climate Change and Weed Competition

Changes in temperature and carbon dioxide are likely to have significant influence on weed biology and vis-à-vis crop-weed interaction. Ziska (2001) observed that the vegetative growth, competition and potential yield of sorghum (C_4) could be reduced by co-occurring of common cocklebur (*Xanthium strumarium*: C_3) as the atmospheric CO_2 increases. Watling and Press (1997) investigated the effects of CO_2 concentrations (350 and 700 μmol/mol) in sorghum with and without *Striga* infestation. They observed that a high CO_2 concentration resulted in taller sorghum plants, and greater biomass, photosynthetic rates, water-use efficiencies and leaf areas. A high CO_2 concentration resulted in lower *Striga* biomass/host plant and a greater rate of photosynthesis. Parasite stomatal conductance was not responsive to CO_2 concentration. *Striga* emerged above ground and flowered earlier under the lower CO_2 concentration.

8.5 Methods of Weed Management

8.5.1 Cultural Management

Despite the great progress made in developing improved management practices in agriculture, manual and mechanical methods continue to be important weed management practices in many sorghum growing regions of the world. Cultural methods mainly complement the manual and mechanical methods. Cultural practices are manipulated in such a way that they become more favourable for crop growth and less to weeds. They are not only eco-friendly but also reduce the use of costly herbicides.

Plant Geometry and Plant Density

Planting density and pattern modify the crop canopy structure and in turn influence weed-smothering ability. Narrow row spacing will bring variation in microclimate, *viz.* light intensity, evaporation and temperature at soil surface.

Sorghum is normally planted at 45 cm × 15 cm under rainfed conditions; however, it can be reduced to 45 cm × 12 cm under irrigated condition. The establishment of a crop with a more uniform and dense plant distribution may result in better use of light, water and nutrients and lead to greater crop competitive ability. Increased shading at soil surface will smother weed growth. It is observed that narrow row spacing and high seeding rate enhanced grain sorghum's competitiveness with annual weeds (Limon-Ortega *et al.*, 1998). Burnside *et al.* (1964) showed that weed growth increased with row width, unless rows were inter-cultivated.

Competitive Cultivars

Sorghum hybrids differ in their tolerance to weed competition (Burnside and Wicks, 1972). A quick growing and early canopy-producing cultivar would be expected to be a better competitor against weeds than crops lacking these characters. Rapid germination and emergence and early root and shoot growth are the major traits for weed suppression (Guneyli *et al.*, 1969). Traore *et al.* (2003) suggested developing tall sorghum hybrids with high LAI for integrated weed management.

Long-season hybrids with considerable vegetative growth competed better with weeds than other hybrids (Burnside and Wicks, 1972). As the level of shading by crops increased, weed seed production decreased (Shetty *et al.*, 1982). Sorghum hybrid CSH 5 was superior to CSV 3 in terms of weed suppression and grain yield (Kondap and Bathakal, 1981).

Nutrient Management

Kondap *et al.* (1985) reported that increasing levels of nitrogen decreased the population of *Cyperus rotundus* and *Panicum emeciforme* in sorghum. This study revealed the possibility of saving 30-90 kg N ha^{-1} by adopting either chemical or manual weed control. Okafor and Zitta (1991) observed a reduction in grain yield due to weed competition by 51.0, 37.8 and 32.2 per cent at zero, 60 and 120 kg N ha^{-1}, respectively, indicating that yield reduction due to weeds decreased at higher N levels. However, increased weed growth with higher levels of N as compared to lower level in grain sorghum was observed by several workers.

8.5.2 Mechanical Management

Traditional methods of weed control in sorghum include hand tools such as the sickle, hand hoe or animal-drawn mechanical equipment which is also used for line sowing and inter row cultivation, *e.g.*, blade harrow (Rao *et al.*, 1987). The success of mechanical weeding depends upon the stage of weeds, crop geometry and climatic conditions. Hand weeding may also be used after mechanical inter row weeding to deal with weeds left in crop rows. Manual weeding by hand tools or inter-row cultivators is used between 3 and 6 weeks after sowing (depending upon the physical condition of soil during the rainy season). It has been observed that, when only depending on mechanical methods, two weeding are a must to provide season-long weed control in rainy season sorghum (Patil and Shah, 1979). If preceded by pre-plant incorporated or pre-emergence or early post-emergence herbicide application, one inter-row cultivation or hand weeding is sufficient to provide season long weed control. Hand hoeing twice at 18 and 35 days after sowing (DAS) before the first and second irrigation was the best weed control treatment in sorghum (Attalla, 2002). Hand hoeing twice at 4 and 8 weeks after sorghum emergence or a smother crop (cowpea) in combination with hand hoeing once, consistently suppresses *Parthenium* (Tamado and Milberg, 2004).

8.5.3 Use of Herbicides

In India, the use of herbicides has revolutionized weed management practices in crops like wheat, rice, soybean, etc. However, they are seldom used in rainfed crops like sorghum because of the following reasons.

☆ Sorghum is mostly grown in intercropping system with pulses and oilseeds and selective herbicides are often unavailable.

☆ Lack of adequate soil moisture in semi-arid regions reduces the efficacy of pre-emergence herbicides.

☆ Farmers fear that the use of herbicides leaves toxic residues in fodder, grain and soil.

☆ Use of weeds as a source of green fodder for animals in semi-arid regions.

☆ Farmers think that the herbicides are expensive as they do not include the cost of family labours for weeding.

☆ Illiteracy among resource-poor farmers of dry-land areas and unavailability of suitable herbicides.

However, weed control through selective herbicides as pre-plant incorporation, pre- or post-emergence has been effective in managing weed problems and has also led to increased sorghum production. In rainy season sorghum, timely weed management only through mechanical methods is many a time risky as the continuous rains do not permit the use of this method. Under such a situation herbicidal approach provides effective control of weeds.

Herbicides are a major component of weed management, especially in grain sorghum grown under no-till conditions as they improve weed control and production efficiency (Brown *et al.*, 2004). However, the margin of selectivity of herbicides on sorghum has been rather narrow especially on coarse textured and low organic matter soils (Burnside and Wicks, 1968). Sorghum hybrids also vary in their tolerance to herbicides and this may become a factor in selection of herbicide.

2,4-D was the first widely used herbicide in grain sorghum (Stahlman and Wicks, 2000). It is applied as 'post-emergence' for control of broad-leaved weeds. Time of its application is most important. Untimely application of 2,4-D leads to serious crop injury. Phillips (1970) observed that 2,4-D should be applied in grain sorghum when it attains a height of 10-30 cm. Yield reduction occurred when 2,4-D was applied to sorghum at 21 days after sowing-DAS (beginning of tillering, first tiller detectable) and at 30 DAS (beginning of stem elongation) (Turk and Tawah, 2002). Symptoms of 2,4-D injury include temporary stalk brittleness, stalk leaning, retarded and abnormal root development and leaf rolling, commonly known as "onion leafing" or "buggy whipping". Crop injury caused by 2,4-D drift to non target crops occurs due to high winds (Enrique *et al.*, 2005). Crops like cotton and soybean were damaged by 2, 4-D drift and volatilization (Chamberlain *et al.*, 1970). Application of 2, 4-D provided inconsistent control of *Parthenium*, possibly because of its reemergence from soil seed bank after control (Tamado and Milberg, 2004).

Triazine herbicides were introduced in early 1960s to provide selective weed control in grain sorghum. These herbicides provide good weed control in grain sorghum for a period of few to several weeks depending on the herbicide, rate of application, soil and climatic factors (Stahlman and Wicks, 2000). Atrazine is the most versatile herbicide for weed control in grain sorghum. It can be applied as 'pre-plant incorporated', 'pre-emergence' or 'post-emergence' for control of many broad-leaved and grassy weeds (Stahlman and Wicks, 2000). 'Pre-emergence' application of atrazine proved to be better than its 'post-emergence' application. However, simazine at 1.5-3.0 kg ha^{-1} as 'post-emergence' resulted in good weed control (Tanchev, 1989). Bromoxynil applied at 240, 360 and 480 g ha^{-1} (registered rate) and prosulfuron at 14.2 g ha^{-1} also provided excellent weed control (Enrique *et al.*, 2005).

Table 8.3: Mode of Action of Herbicides Used for Weed Control in Sorghum

Herbicide	Herbicide Family	Mode of Action
Atrazine, simazine, propazine, prometryn	Triazine	Inhibition of photosynthesis at photosystem II
Pendimethalin	Dinitroaniline	Microtubule assembly inhibition
2,4-D	Phenoxy-carboxylic acid	Action like indole acetic acid (synthetic auxins)
Fluroxypyr	Pyridine carboxylic acid	Action like indole acetic acid (synthetic auxins)
Metolachlor, Pretilachlor	Chloroacetamide	Inhibition of cell division
Flumioxazin	N-phenylphthalimide	Inhibition of protoporphyrinogen oxidase(PPO)
Bentazon	Benzothiadiazinone	Inhibition of photosynthesis at photosystem II
Bromoxynil	Nitrile	Inhibition of photosynthesis at photosystem II

Patil and Shah (1979) found that pre-emergence application of pendimethalin at 2.0 kg/ha had adverse effect on crop but its application at lower rate (1.0 kg ha^{-1}) did not reveal any phytotoxicity. Sarpe *et al*. (1997) reported that pre-emergence application of pendimethalin at 1.32-1.98 kg ha^{-1} combined with a post-emergence application of dicamba/2, 4-D (0.4 or 0.6 kg ha^{-1}) resulted in the best control of *Digitaria sanguinalis* and in the greatest crop yields.

Fluroxypyr at 150-300 g ha^{-1} gave excellent control of broadleaf weeds in grain sorghum (Webb and Feez, 1987). Dhanapal *et al*. (1989) reported that pre-emergence application of oxyfluorfen at 0.2-0.3 kg ha^{-1} was phytotoxic to sorghum. Flumioxazin at 0.07-0.11 kg ha^{-1} applied at 0-30 days after sowing provided excellent control of *Amaranthus turculatus* and *Parthenium hysterophorus* but provided variable control of *Panicum texanum* without any injury to sorghum (Grichar, 2006).

Herbicide Mixtures

In early 1990s, sulfonylurea herbicides, *viz*. halosulfuron and prosulfuron were introduced for selective control of broad-leaved weeds in grain sorghum. However, these herbicides did not control weed biotypes resistant to acetolactate synthase (ALS)-inhibiting herbicides. Halosulfuron and bentazone were the only herbicides for control of nutsedge in sorghum (Ackley *et al.*, 1996). Ramakrishna *et al*. (1991) reported that pre-emergence application of metolachlor at 1.0-1.25 kg ha^{-1} or combination of atrazine+metolachlor or sequential application of metolachlor and bentazon, atrazine at 0.75 kg ha^{-1} and metolachlor at 1.0 kg ha^{-1} as pre-emergence followed by one manual weeding at 30 days after sowing, yielded as good as repeated weedings.

Wu *et al*. (2004) reported that soil incorporation of atrazine mixed with metolachlor at sorghum planting provided effective seasonal control of barnyard grass (*E. colona*). Metsulfuron causes toxicity to sorghum. Brown *et al*. (2004) evaluated the efficacy and safening of metsulfuron applied with dicamba, 2,4-D, clopyralid and fluroxypyr with and without nonionic surfactants and found that 2,4-D and dicamba safened grain sorghum from metsulfuron injury. Differential hybrids responses to metsulfuron + 2,4-D was observed at 1 and 2 week after treatment. Atrazine + pendimethalin or trifluralin applied late-post emergence (when weeds and sorghum were 10-15 cm tall) resulted in 99 per cent control of tumble pigweed (*Amaranthus albus*) with less than 3 per cent sorghum stunting (Grichar *et al.*, 2005). Ishaya *et al.* (2007) observed that pretilachlor + dimethametryne at 2.5 kg ha^{-1} or cinosulfuron 0.05 kg ha^{-1} or piperophos + cinosulfuron 1.5 kg ha^{-1} effectively controlled weeds, increased crop vigour, plant height, reduced plant injury and produced higher grain yield of sorghum.

8.5.4 Weed Management in Sorghum-Based Intercropping Systems and Crop Rotations

Crop intensification in time and space influences the weed dynamics and calls for changes in the weed management strategies. Crop diversity may also lead to the greater competitive effect with weeds. It is generally believed that intensive cropping reduces weed problems. However, the weed problems in cropping systems largely depend upon the crops and management practices adopted. Besides, herbicide selectivity and residual toxicity are also critical in intensive cropping systems.

Intercropping

Intercropping of sorghum with legumes suppresses the weeds (Shetty and Rao, 1979; Solaimalai and Sivakumar, 2002; Mohandoss *et al.*, 2002). Kondap *et al.* (1990) observed that sorghum alone was a poor competitor of weeds, but intercropping it with cowpea reduced the weed growth markedly. In sorghum + legume (lab-lab/ cowpea/blackgram) intercropping system, Shetty and Rao (1981) reported that inclusion of intercrops minimized weed infestation and replaced one hand weeding without any detrimental effect on the yields of sorghum.

Although intercropping may reduce weed infestation and growth, there is still a need for some degree of weed management in most cases. Manual or mechanical weed control is the main method in intercropping systems. Most of the herbicides are crop specific and thus, it is difficult to find out chemicals that will give a broad-spectrum control without causing damage to the component crops. The results obtained by Rao and Shetty (1976) in sorghum + pigeonpea intercropping and by Moody (1978) in sorghum + cowpea intercropping showed that just one weeding would be sufficient to get as high an yield as in case of weed free check. Gworgwor and Lagoke (1992) concluded that hoeing is important for effective season-long weed control in sorghum + groundnut intercropping. Pre-emergence application of isoproturon 0.60 kg ha^{-1} + 1 hoeing at 30 DAS (Balasubramanian and Subramanian, 1989) or metolachlor at 0.75-1.50 kg ha^{-1} + 1 inter-row cultivation at 30-35 DAS (Kandasamy *et al.*, 1999) controlled the weeds effectively. Metolachlor was however, not effective against *Celosia argentea*. Singh and Singh (1999) reported that pendimethalin 1.0 kg ha^{-1} + 1 hand weeding (HW) at 30 DAS or 2 HW at 25 and 50 DAS provided effective control of weeds in pigeonpea + sorghum intercropping system.

In sorghum + cowpea intercropping system, pre-emergence application of isoproturon at 0.50-0.60 kg ha^{-1} (Kempuchetty and Sankaran, 1990), butachlor at 0.75-1.0 kg ha^{-1} + 1 HW at 40 DAS (Krishnasamy and Krishnasamy, 1996), and metolachlor at 1.0 kg ha^{-1} + hoeing at 40 DAS (Solaimalai and Sivakumar, 2002; Ponnuswami *et al.*, 2003) were safe and effective for both the crops, while pendimethalin 1.0 kg ha^{-1} was toxic for sorghum germination.

In sorghum + blackgram intercropping system, pre-emergence application of isoproturon at 0.50 kg ha^{-1}, followed by manual weeding (Ramamoorthy *et al.*, 1995), metolachlor at 1.0 kg ha^{-1} and hand hoeing on 40 DAS (Solaimalai and Muthusankaranarayanan, 2000), and metolachlor at 1.5 kg ha^{-1} (Sundari and Kathiresan, 2002) were effective in controlling weeds. Promising weed management practices in sorghum-based intercropping system have been summarized in Table 8.4.

Table 8.4: Weed Management Practices in Sorghum-Based Intercropping Systems (Mishra and Rao, 2011)

Intercropping System	Weed Management Practices
Sorghum + pigeonpea	Fluchloralin 0.50 kg/ha or metolachlor at 0.75 kg/ha or pendimethalin 0.50-0.75 kg/ha as pre-emergence + 1 hand weeding or inter-row cultivation at 25-30 days after sowing.
Sorghum + cowpea	Butachlor at 0.75-1.0 kg/ha or metolachlor at 1.0 kg/ha as pre-emergence + 1 hand weeding at 30-35 days after sowing.
Sorghum + groundnut	One hoeing at 25-30 days after sowing.
Sorghum + blackgram/ greengram	Metolachlor at 1.0 kg/ha as pre-emergence followed by one hand hoeing at 40 DAS.

Sequence Cropping/Double Cropping Systems

Weed management in sequential cropping is slightly different from those in intercropping systems. Continuous presence of crop cover, residual toxicity of herbicides applied to the previous crops on succeeding crops and changing weed flora with the season, all need a different approach in weed management practices. In sorghum-cotton cropping sequence, pre-emergence application of atrazine 0.25 kg ha^{-1} in sorghum and pendimethalin 1.0 kg ha^{-1} in cotton was effective for control of broad-leaved weeds. Atrazine applied as pre-emergence at 0.50 kg ha^{-1} gave effective weed control in sorghum but the establishment of legumes such as greengram and groundnut which followed sorghum was poor. The following cotton was not affected (Palaniappan and Ramaswamy, 1976). In sorghum-safflower sequence, Giri and Bhosle (1997) observed that pre-emergence application of atrazine at 0.75 kg ha^{-1} alone or atrazine at 0.50 kg ha^{-1} combined with weeding and hoeing 6 weeks after sowing were as effective as 2 weeding and hoeing at 3 and 6 weeks after sowing in controlling weeds without any phytotoxic effect on succeeding safflower.

8.5.5 Integrated Weed Management

Considering the diversity of weed problem, no single method of weed control, whether manual, mechanical or chemical could reach the desired level of efficiency under all situations. The most promising single approach to weed control in cropland combines manual, cultural and mechanical methods with herbicides. Herbicides are being used as a supplement, at as low a rate as possible. On environmental grounds emphasis has been given to judicious combinations of cultural and chemical methods of weed control. In rainy season, because of the continuous rains many a times, early weed removal might not be possible. The use of pre-emergence herbicides, for removing early weed competition and supplementary hoeing or hand weeding for removing later emerging weeds, might form a package of weed control practices. It is observed that, a combination of, cultivation, narrow rows and 'pre-emergence' herbicides, controlled weeds more effectively than any single method (Zimdahl, 1980). Mohamed Ali and Sudhakar Rao (1987) reported that pre-emergence application of atrazine at 0.25 kg ha^{-1} + 1 HW at 30 DAS was better than atrazine 0.50 kg ha^{-1} alone. Similarly, 2,4-D at 1.0 kg ha^{-1} applied at 15 DAS + 1 HW at 30 DAS was better than 2,4-D at 2.0 kg ha^{-1} alone in reducing weed populations. Atrazine 1.0 kg ha^{-1} + 1 hand hoeing at 30 DAS recorded the highest weed control efficiency and grain yield (Satao *et al.*, 1995). Kalyansundaram and Kuppuswamy (1999) reported that tank mix application of butachlor at 0.75 kg ha^{-1} + atrazine 0.75 kg ha^{-1} followed by 1 HW at 45 DAS controlled the weeds effectively and produced the highest grain yield.

Upadhyay *et al.* (1981) stated that atrazine 0.50-1.0 kg ha^{-1} supplemented with 1 HW or 2,4-D Na salt at 6 weeks after sowing (WAS) was effective. Grichar *et al.* (2004) reported that twin-row spacing (2 rows spaced 20 cm apart on a single bed) and atrazine at 0.56-1.12 kg ha^{-1} gave higher control of *Panicum texanum* (*Texas panicum*) as compared to conventional row spacing (single rows spaced 91 cm apart on a bed) with herbicide. Smother cropping using cowpea or mungbean and pre-emergence application of metolachlor at 1.5 kg or pendimethalin at 1.0 kg ha^{-1} followed by manual weeding at 45 DAS produced as higher yield as weed-free treatment (Ramakrishna, 2003). Application of nitrogen at 80 kg/ha + inter-cultivation recorded the highest yield (Sharma *et al.*, 2000). Field experiments conducted under All India Coordinated Sorghum Improvement Project at six locations (Coimbatore, Udaipur, Dharwad, Parbhani, Indore, Surat) revealed that application of atrazine 0.25 kg/ha pre-emergence fb 2 HW/interculture at 30 and 45 DAS gave effective control of weeds, higher grain yields and benefits. Among herbicidal combinations, atrazine 0.25 kg/ha pre-emergence *fb* pendimethalin 0.50 kg/ha at 30 DAS (after first hand weeding as pre-emergence between rows- *Layby* application) was very effective (Table 8.5).

8.6 Allelopathy

Sorghum is a potential allelopathic crop and contains numerous water soluble allelochemicals, phytotoxic to many plant species (Cheema *et al.*, 2007). Sorghum cultivars differ considerably in their allelopathic potential. They can be selected for inclusion in cropping systems for suppression of weeds and the aquous leachetes obtained from mature herbage of the cultivars with higher allelopathic potential can be used as foliar sprays for weed suppression in field crops. It can be used as sorgaab (water extract of mature sorghum plants), sorghum mulch, sorghum soil incorporation or included in crop rotation. Sorgaab can be used as a natural weed inhibitor in maize (Cheema *et al.*, 2007). Sorgaab controlled up to 35-49 per cent weeds and increased wheat yield by 10-21 per cent. Matured sorghum chopped herbage (2-6 Mg ha^{-1}) incorporated in the soil at sowing controlled up to 40-50 per cent weeds and increased wheat yield by 15 per cent. Two foliar sprays of 10 per cent sorgaab at 30 and 60 days after sowing was the most economical method for controlling weeds with maximum net benefits and 535 per cent marginal rate of return (Cheema and Khaliq, 2000). Sorgoleone is a natural product isolated from root exudates of grain sorghum. Nimbal *et al.* (1996) reported that sorgoleone was phytotoxic to *Digitaria sanguinalis, Abutilon theophrasti* and *Echinichloa crus-galli*. They concluded that sorgoleone was a potent inhibitor of photosynthetic electron transport and acted similar to classical diuron-type herbicides at the same site in the PS II complex. Arif Mohmood and Cheema (2004) determined the effect of sorghum mulch on nutsedge (*Cyperus rotundus*) in maize and found that soil incorporation or surface application of 15 t sorghum mulch/ha reduced the nutsedge dry weight.

8.7 Weed Management in Forage Sorghum

Weed control is one of the most important factors in the production of nutritious fodder from forage sorghum. It has been observed that usually grain crops get priority over fodder crops with regards to weed control. Weeds usually cause greater loss in forage sorghum than insects-pests and diseases. Weeds generally grow faster than forage sorghum and compete for plant nutrients, space, light and moisture. Weeds culminate forage or dry-matter yield reduction to an extent of 15-54 per cent (Singh *et al.*, 1988; Raghuvanshi *et al.*, 1990).

Atrazine at 0.50-1.0 kg ha^{-1} as pre-emergence was found to be effective and economical in forage sorghum (Latchanna *et al.*, 1989; Thakur *et al.*, 1990). There was a saving of 60 kg N ha^{-1} due to effective weed control. Split application of atrazine 0.50 kg/ha as pre-emergence and 0.50 kg ha^{-1} at 20 DAS gave the best weed control in fodder sorghum (Singh and Bajpai, 1992). Balyan *et al.* (1993) observed that *Trianthema portulacastrum* and *Echinochloa colona* were the most problematic weeds in forage sorghum in Haryana (India). Atrazine at 0.50 kg ha^{-1} applied at 7 and 14 DAS and 2,4-D applied at 14 and 21 DAS resulted in the greatest control of weeds and resulted in higher yields of forage sorghum. Atrazine controlled both broadleaved weeds and grasses but was less effective against *E. colona, C. rotundus* and *Saccharum spontaneum*. Mukherjee *et al.* (2000) recorded the highest green forage yield with atrazine + one hand weeding. Herbicide mixture (atrazine at 200 g + metolachlor at 300 g L^{-1}) provided excellent control of broadleaf weeds in forage sorghum (Archangelo *et al.*, 2002).

8.8 Management of *Striga* spp. (a parasitic weed) in Sorghum

Striga is a major biotic constraint in the subsistence agriculture and causes considerable crop damage in the semi-arid tropics. *Striga* species on cereals continue to be more serious in many countries owing to continued loss of soil fertility (Parker, 2008). The weed threatens the lives of over 100 million people in Africa, seriously in 17 countries and moderately in 25 countries (Mboob, 1986). It caused significantly greater yield loss (65 per cent) compared to 32 per cent by non-parasitic weeds (Bebawi and Farah, 1981). Incidence of *Striga* alone caused 75 per cent reduction in grain yield of Sorghum (Rao, 1978). Crop losses of 10-90 per cent, with an average loss of 35

Table 8.5: Effect of Weed Control Methods on Weeds, Growth, Yield and Economics in *Kharif* Grain Sorghum (AICSIP, 2012)

Treatment	Weed Density (No./m²) at Harvest	Weed Dry Weight (g/m²) at Harvest	Grain Yield (kg/ha)	Net Returns (Rs./ha)	B:C Ratio
Atrazine 0.50 kg/ha as pre-em. *fb* 1 hand weeding (HW) at 30 DAS	44	77	3805	44174	2.74
Atrazine 0.25 kg/ha pre-em *fb* 2 HW at 30 and 45 DAS	20	29	4293	49912	2.86
Pendimethalin 0.50 kg/ha pre-em *fb* 1 HW at 30 DAS	38	68	3845	44200	2.75
Pendimethalin 0.50 kg/ha as pre-em *fb* 2,4-D 0.50 kg/ha at 25 DAS	40	72	3562	41077	2.71
Atrazine + pendimethalin each at 0.25 kg/ha as pre-em. (tank mixed)	47	82	3278	37014	2.58
Atrazine 0.25 + pendimethalin 0.50k/ha as pre-em. Tank mixed) *fb* 2,4-D 0.50 kg/ha as post- em.	34	64	3633	43967	2.86
Atrazine 0.25 kg/ha pre-em. *fb* 2,4-D 0.50 kg/ha as post-em.	43	71	3525	42707	2.84
Atrazine 0.25 kg/ha pre-em *fb* pendimethalin 0.50 kg/ha at 30 DAS (after first hand weeding as pre-emergence between rows- *Layby* application)	27	42	3646	45689	2.89
Weedy check	108	231	2118	19028	1.64
CD (P = 0.05)	34	73	533	15617	0.63

per cent in sorghum have been attributed to *Striga hermonthica* in Nigeria. The loss is estimated to be worth $250 million US annually (Parkinson *et al.*, 1986; Lagoke, 1987). *Striga* reduced the sorghum plant height by 50 per cent and shoot and root dry matter by 70 per cent and 50 per cent, respectively (Gworgwor *et al.*, 1991). In sub-Saharan Africa, *S. hermonthica* caused 70-100 per cent crop loss in sorghum, maize and pearl millet (Emechebe *et al.*, 2004).

8.8.1 Control Measures

Early removal of *Striga* (after its emergence), and thereafter at regularly weekly intervals, may help to improve crop yields. Gbehounou *et al.* (2004) observed reduced infestation of *Striga* in delayed sowing as compared to early sowing. However, the grain yield was reduced in delayed sowing. Therefore, transplanting after cultivation in a *Striga*-free nursery for 4-6 weeks, is a better alternative as it combines the respective beneficial effects of early sowing and the effects on *Striga* of delayed planting.

Intercropping of sorghum with groundnut significantly reduced *Striga* infestation in sorghum (Tenebe and Kamara, 2002). Jost (1997) found that *Striga* seed bank in soil decreased by 33 per cent after cotton and 34 per cent after soybean grown as

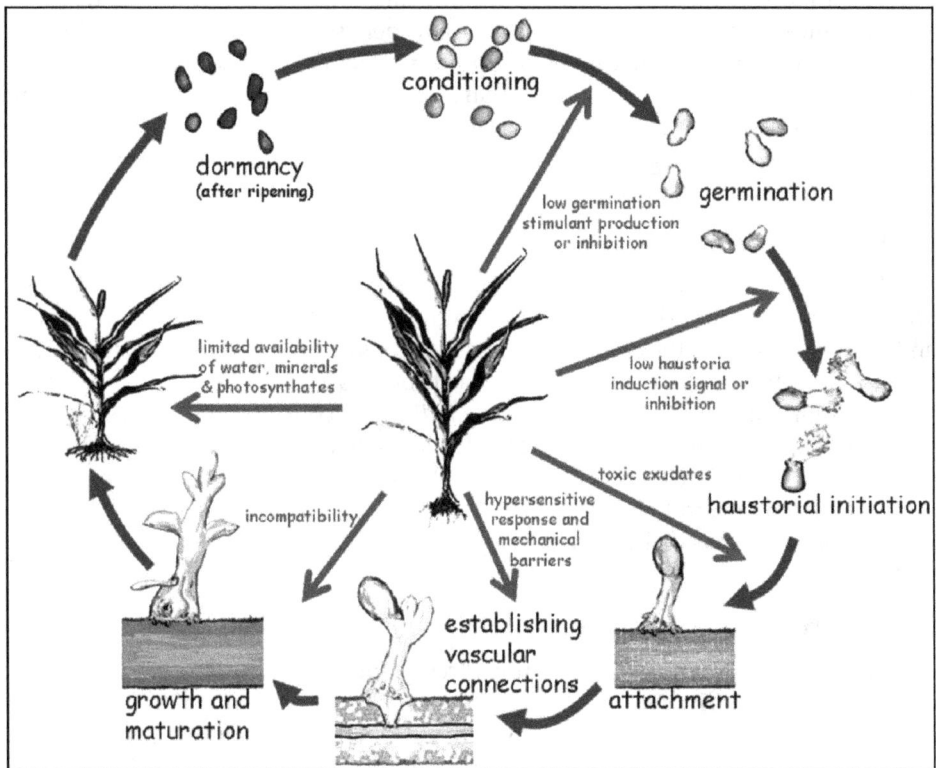

Figure 8.2: Life Cycle of *Striga*.

Source: http://www.falw.vu.nl/en/research/molecular-cell-biology/ecology-and-physiology-of-plants/student-projects/project-6-molecular-dissection-of-parasitic-plants.asp.

trap crops. One year trap cropping of cotton depleted more than 90 per cent of *Striga* seed bank in soil (Bekker *et al.*, 2003). Intercropping of sorghum with cowpea [(*Vigna unguiculata* (L.) Walp.], greengram [(*Vigna radiata* (L.) Wilczek], and Crotolaria (*Crotolaria ochroleuca* G. Don), significantly reduced the *Striga* population in sorghum Khan *et al.* (2007). Legume-cereal rotation was the most effective control option for *Striga* management (Emechebe *et al.*, 2004).

Lowest *Striga* population was observed in 10 per cent urea spraying at 45 DAS followed by 2 HW or atrazine 0.25 kg ha^{-1} + 2,4-D. Seed treatment with brine (NaCl) at 1.5 M significantly reduced the *Striga* emergence resulting in increased crop growth and grain yield of sorghum (Gworgwor *et al.*, 2002). A combination of nitrogen fertilizer between 50-100 kg/ha and some level of *Striga* tolerance in sorghum varieties is an ideal control package of *Striga* menace (Showemimo *et al.*, 2002). Pre-emergence application of chlorsulfuron at 4-6 g ha^{-1} was however damaging to sorghum crop. Hoffmann *et al.* (1997) showed that application of 2, 4-D at 30 DAS delayed the appearance of *Striga* and reduced the density of infestation in sorghum and maize.

Genetic control of *Striga* is effective, although sources of resistance are limited in most crops. Maiti *et al.* (1984) studied 10 sorghum cultivars for their mode of *Striga* parasitization and the factors conferring resistance. He observed that in resistant cultivars most of the *Striga* haustoria failed to penetrate beyond the endodermis, whereas in susceptible cultivars the hastoria penetrated the endodermis and became established. Resistant cultivars showed marked endodermal and pencyclic thickening and the deposition of silica in their endodermal cells, which were lacking in the susceptible cultivars. Sorghum variety ICSV 145 was found resistant to *Striga asiatica* (ICRISAT, 1988).

Biological Control of *Striga*

In a survey conducted by Gworgwor, *et al.* (1998) in sorghum fields in Nigeria, *Striga* plants were found to be attacked by an insect, *Smicroynx unbrinus* Hustache and up to 40 per cent of the plants produced fruit galls due to infestation This indicated that the insect has a great potential as a parasite of *Striga*. Marley *et al.* (2004) accessed the possibility of using neem (*Azadirachta indica*) for control of *Striga* in sorghum. They reported that neem seed powder reduced the emergence of *S. hermonthica* (1.7 per 3 m^2) as compared to control (30.3 per 3 m^2). They further, observed that integrated *Striga* management strategy involving *Fusarium oxysporum* (isolate PSM 197)-based mycoherbicide increased the profitability of sorghum production on *Striga*-infested soils.

8.9 Herbicide Tolerance

Sorghum is grown under moisture stress conditions with low inputs. Under moisture stress conditions, the efficacy of pre-plant and pre-emergence herbicides, especially on grassy weeds decreases (Tapia *et al.*, 1997). These weeds need to cultivated or treated with post-emergence herbicides. Therefore, herbicide tolerance through genetic enhancement is the viable option. Herbicide-tolerant crops make it possible to control weeds with non-selective herbicides. Miller and Bovey (1969) evaluated 40 varieties of sorghum representing 27 diverse groups for tolerance to herbicide propazine, norea, GS 14260, linuron and propachlor and observed that herbicide tolerance was most evident in caudatum, durra and conspicuum groups. Scifres and Bovey (1970) reported that, of seven sorghum varieties, 'Pioneer 820' seedlings were the most tolerant to picloram, 'Tophand' was the least tolerant and GA 615, RS 626 and RS 671 were intermediate.

ALS-inhibitor herbicides *viz.*, nicosulfuron and nimsulfuron are widely used to control broadleaf and grassy weeds in corn (*Zea mays*), but sorghum is susceptible to these herbicides. However, by transferring a major resistance gene from wild sorghum relative, researchers at Kansas State University (KSU), USA developed a grain sorghum that is resistant to several ALS-inhibiting herbicides as Steadfast (nicosulfuron + rimsulfuron), Accent (nicosulfuron), Resolve (rimsulfuron) and Ally (metsulfuron) (Tuinstra and Al-Khatib, 2007; Tuinstra *et al.*, 2009).

Herbicide tolerance through transgenic technology is not addressed worldwide because of the opinion of development of "Super Weed". It is understood that crops and related wild or weedy plants can and will exchange genes through pollen transfer, if provided with the opportunity, and have been doing so ever since there have been crops and weeds (Harlan, 1982). Hybridization occurs readily between grain sorghum and johnsongrass (*Sorghum halepense*) (Dogget, 1976). Transfer of herbicide tolerant gene to johnsongrass from cultivated sorghum is considered a threat during hybrid development due to their cross compatibility. Arriola and Ellstrand (1996) found that the rate of hybridization varied with distance between the two species but was as high as 2 per cent at a distance of 100 m. They concluded that under natural field conditions, crop-to-weed gene flow is much more likely to occur than is weed-to-crop gene flow. Thus the risk of transgene providing a particular trait, such as resistance to herbicide, escaping into wild relatives is relatively high. Therefore they added that, the risk associated with transformation and subsequent wide-scale commercial release of transgenic sorghum must be considered, when strategies are being developed to minimize the threat of transgene escape. Smeda *et al.* (2000) reported that resistance to fluazifop in *Sorghum halepense* was inherited by a single dominant gene and transfer of herbicide resistance from johnsongrass to sorghum can occur due to natural hybridization. Schmidt and Bothma (2006) also cautioned that presence of fully fertile crop wild relatives and the weedy relative of johnsongrass, which may form hybrids with crop sorghum. Based on the fact that gene flow takes place, there is strong evidence that introgression of genetically modified (GM) sorghum into crops and crop wild relatives will take place once GM-sorghum is deployed.

Chapter 9
Insect-Pest Management

Sorghum crop is attacked by number of insect-pests right from germination till maturity. A detailed account of various insect-pests infesting the crop at different growth stages is shown in the Figure 9.1.

Shoot Fly (*Atherigona socatta* Rondani)

Shoot fly is a major pest of sorghum. Plants up to 4 week age are more susceptible to this pest. Maggot feeds on the growing tips causing first wilting of leaf and later

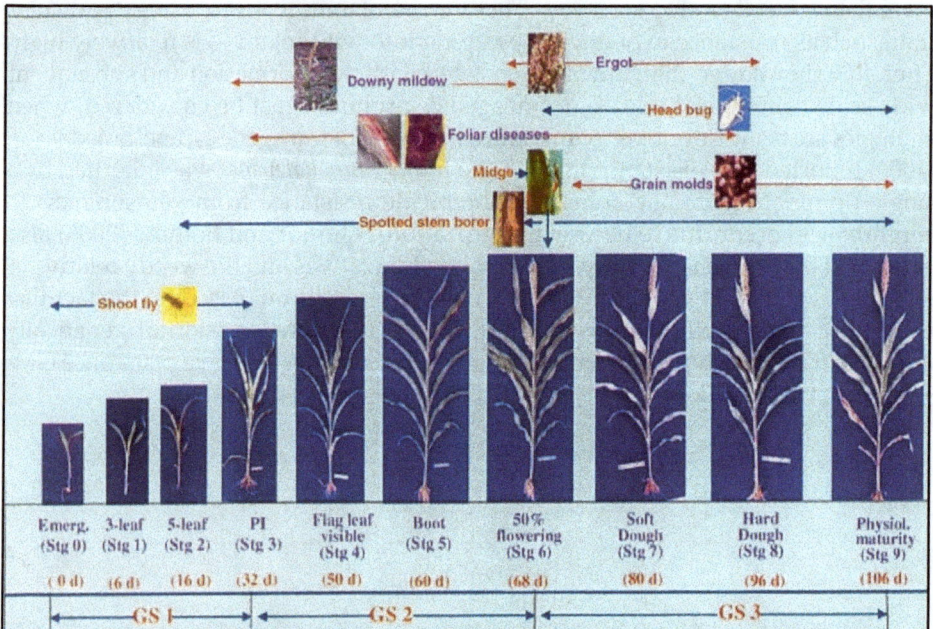

Figure 9.1: Insect-Pests Attacking Sorghum Crop at different Stages of Crop Growth.

drying of central leaf, giving a typical symptom of 'dead heart'. The damaged plants produce side tillers which again are infested increasing the population build up. Early planting with the onset of monsoon is effective in avoiding the infestation of shoot fly during *kharif*, however in *rabi*, planting during 15th September to first week of October is ideal to escape the shoot fly damage. Higher seed rate and removal and destroying the 'dead heart' seedlings are the other important management practices. Seed treatment with imidacloprid @14 ml or carbosulfan 25 SD @ 200 g/kg of seed has also been found effective. Carbofuron 3G or Phorate 10 G as soil application in furrows (20 kg/ha) before sowing also checks the pest incidence. In case soil application of phorate is not done, damage can be minimized by spraying seedling at 7 and 14 days stages with cypermethrin 2ml/liter water.

Stem Borer (*Chilo partellus* Swinhoe)

Stem borer attacks the plant throughout the growing season. Initially the larvae feed on the upper surface of whorl leaves leaving the lower surface intact. As the severity of the feeding increases, blend of punctures and scratches of epidermal feeding appears prominently. Sometimes 'dead heart' symptoms also develop in younger plants due to early attack. Subsequently, the larvae bore into the stem resulting in extensive stem tunneling. Effective control of the borer can be achieved by removing the stubbles immediately after the crop harvest. Application of carbaryl 4G or carbofuran 3G in the leaf whorls @ 8-12 kg/ha at 20 and 35 days after emergence is found effective. Biopesticides *viz., Bacillus thuringiensis* (1 g/litre), NSKE (5 per cent), nimbecidine (5ml/litre) and *Metarhizium anisopliae* (1g/litre) were also found effective in reducing stem borer damage by 5.1 to 24.4 per cent (Jose *et al.*, 2008).

Sorghum Midge (*Contarinia sorghicola* Conquillett)

Sorghum midge is one of the most destructive pests to grain sorghum. The insect damages the crop at the blooming stage. The female sorghum midge deposits a single egg between the glumes of a floret. Larvae destroy the seed, resulting in "blank" or shriveled seed coats that often appear discoloured. Heads with severe midge damage appear small and compressed with blank areas. The midge infestation can be prevented by removing the weed Johnson grass and other grasses which serve as alternate hosts. Spraying of carbaryl 50WP or dusting of carbaryl 10D at 90 per cent head emergence (prior to flower opening) can effectively check the midge infestation.

Shoot Bug (*Peregrinus maidis* Ashmead)

It is a sporadic pest of sorghum. Under favourable conditions, it produces several generations and cause heavy damage to sorghum. Both the adults and nymphs suck sap resulting in yellowing and drying up of the plant. Heavy infestation at vegetative stage may results in twisting of top leaves and may prevent the formation and emergence of panicles. Application of carbaryl 3G@ 8kg/ha in the leaf whorls can effectively check the incidence of the pest. Spraying 5 per cent Neem seed kernel suspension acts as a repellent and spraying 5 per cent extract of Vitex leaves also controls the nymphs and adults.

Headbug (*Calocoris angustatus* Lethierry)

The head bug infests on the panicle and feed mainly on the developing seeds and to lesser extent on other panicle parts. They cause economic damage by reducing the grain weight, seed quality and viability. Grain mold damage is also severe in bug affected panicles. Application of Carbaryl 50SP @ 3.0kg/ha as spray or Carbaryl 5D @ 20 kg/ha as dust to panicles once at pre-bloom and once at milk stage can effectively check the infestation.

Aphids

Aphids have piercing, sucking mouth parts that they use to suck juices from plant tissue, causing stunted plant growth. Aphids inject a toxin along with saliva into plant tissue, causing a yellowish spot to develop around the point of feeding. Such damaged tissue quickly results in a reddish color on the leaf surface. These reddish areas gradually enlarge as the aphid colonies on the underside of leaves increase in numbers. Eventually, feeding causes the leaves to start browning at the outer edges and ultimately to die. Attack during boot stage may result in poor panicle exertion. Spraying of metasystox 35 EC @ 1 litre/ha in 500 litre of water effectively controls aphids.

Mite (*Oligonynchus indicus*)

Mites suck up the plant sap from leaves, first from the under surface of the functional leaves and the infested area initially is pale yellow, however it later turns reddish or brownish on the upper surface of the leaf. Spraying of Kelthane 35 EC or Monocrtophos 35 EC or Dimethoate 35 EC @ 1 litre/ha in 500 litre water has been found effective.

Management of Stored Grain Insect-Pests

The important sorghum storage pests may be classified as;

Internal Feeders

Rice weevil (*Sitophilus oryzae*), Lesser grain borer (*Rhizopertha dominica*), Angoumois grain moth (*Sitotroga cerealella*).

External Feeders

Khapra beetle (*Trogoderma granarium*), Red flour beetle (*Tribolium castaneum, T. confusom*), Saw toothed grain beetle (*Oryzaephilus surinamensis*), Rice moth (*Corcyra cephalonica*), Tropical warehouse moth (*Ephestia cautella*), Indian meal moth (*Plodia interpunctella*) and Grain mite (*Acarus siro*).

At harvest, sorghum grain contains 20-28 per cent moisture depending upon season and weather conditions (Babu and Prasad, 2011). High moisture content in grain during storage offers congenial environment for storage pest attacks. Sun drying and use of mechanical dryers can be opted to bring down the moisture content up to 10-12 per cent before grain storage. In fumigation of stored grains, either shed fumigation (entire store house or godown) or cover fumigation (only selected blocks or bags) is desirable depending upon the intensity of pest attack. Fumigation may be done with aluminium phosphide (3 tablets of 3 g each each per tonne of grain for cover fumigation and 21 tablets of 3 g each for 28 cubic meters for shed fumigation), or ethylene dibromide (EDB) (22 g per cubic meter for shed fumigation and 3 ml/100 kg grain for cover fumigation) and the period of fumigation should be 7 days.

Chapter 10

Diseases and their Control

There are more than a dozen of foliar and panicle diseases affecting productivity and quality of sorghum crop. In grain sorghum, grain mold, downy mildew, anthracnose and ergot are major diseases during *kharif* season whereas, root and stalk rot diseases like charcoal rot, and viral diseases are common during *rabi* season. Other diseases like leaf spot, pokkah boeng and smut occur sporadically and assume economic significance under specific environments depending on relative humidity and temperature during crop growth period. In forage sorghum, foliar diseases like leaf spot, sooty stripes, leaf blight, downy mildew, anthracnose and rust are more common. Leaf diseases destroy active leaf area required for photosynthesis, adversely affect sugar accumulation in stalk and thus, interfere with the quality and quantity of the fodder. Similarly in sweet sorghum, diseases adversely affect the stalk yield, sugar production and ethanol yield. The major diseases of sorghum are listed in Table 10.1.

Table 10.1: Sorghum Diseases, Identification Keys and their Control Measures (Das, 2011)

Disease	Casual Organism	Field Identification Key	Control Measures
Foliar diseases			
Anthracnose	Colletotrichum sublineolum	Small circular lesions on the mid-rib speckled with black dots.	Use of clean seed, destroying plant refuses, crop rotation, removal of host weed plants like Sudan grass and Johnson grass.
Downy mildew	Peronosclerospora sorghi	Appearance of vivid green and white stripes on leaves and white patches of oospores. Whole leaves may become chlorotic and plants usually fail to exert panicles.	Deep ploughing before planting to destroy oospores. Rouging of infected plants, Seed dressing with Metalaxyl/Ridomil 25 @1 g ai/kg seed.
Sorghum stripe virus	Maize stripe virus-sorghum isolate	Chlorotic stripes and yellowish bands on the leaf. Stunted growth of the infected plant, which generally fails to produce earhead.	Practice of clean cultivation, removal of weeds from the bunds, and control of insect vector by spraying suitable insecticide.
Leaf blight	Bipolaris turcica	Lesions with dark margins but without distinct haloes	Use of clean seed and destroying plant refuse. Use of resistant genotypes.
Rust	Puccinia purpurea	Ruptured pustules releasing red to brown powdery masses from leaf	Use of clean seed, crop rotation, destroying of plant refuses, Spraying of Dithane M 45 @ 0.2 per cent thrice with 10 days intervals, starting at 30 days crop stage.
Sooty stripe	Ramulispora sorghi	Small, circular reddish brown spot on leaf with distinct yellow haloes.	Use of clean seed and destroying plant refuse. Use of resistant genotypes.
Zonate leaf spot	Gleocercospora sorghi	Circular lesions with concentric banding formed out of fungal growth.	Use of clean seed, crop rotation, destroying of plant refuses.
Grey leaf spot	Cercospora sorghi	Oval to rectangular lesions limited by the veins	Use of clean seed and destroying plant refuse. Use of resistant genotypes.
Stalk rot complex (Charcoal rot)	Macrophomina phaseolina, Fusarium moniliforme	Soft basal internodes, lodging, black sclerotia inside the disintegrated stalk, breaking of stalk, on upper side of the 3rd or 4th internodes.	Soil moisture conservation, maintaining optimum plant population, straw mulching and mixed cropping, use of early maturing cultivars and seed treatment with fluorescent Pseudomonas (10⁷cfu/ml) reduce the incidence.

Contd...

Table 10.1–Contd...

Disease	Casual Organism	Field Identification Key	Control Measures
Panicle diseases			
Grain mold	A complex of several fungi. Major being *Fusarium moniliforme* and *Curvularia lunata*	The infected grains are soft, powdery, with moldy growth of pink, white or black in colour.	Avoiding cultivars that are likely to mature in heavy rains. Harvesting of panicles at physiological maturity and artificial drying in community dryer. Spraying of fungicides (Captan 0.30 per cent, Tilt 0.20 per cent) or bioagents (Fluorescent Pseudomonas 10^7 cfu/ml) on panicles reduces mold incidence and improves seed quality.
Ergot/Sugary disease	*Sphacelia sorghi*	Droplet of sticky liquid exudes from the florets	Ensuring synchrony of flowering (A and R lines) in seed production plots. Early sowing, removal of collateral host from the field bunds. Mechanical removal of sclerotia from seeds. Two spray of 'Tilt' 25 per cent EC @ 0.2 per cent starting from flowering with 10 days interval
Smut			
Loose smut	*Sporisorium cruenta*	Individual grains replaced by small cream to brown sacs that ruptures soon after head emergence	Use of clean seed free from smut sori to reduce the field incidence. Removal and destruction of smutted panicles from the field. Seed dressing with sulphur @ 4g/kg or thirum 75 @ 3g/kg seed to control seed-borne infections in loose and covered smuts.
Covered smut	*S. sorghi*	Individual grains replaced by small sacs that persists up to threshing	
Head smut	*S. reilianum*	Panicle partially or completely converted in to a large whitish sac	
Long smut	*Tolyposporium ehrenbergii*	Few individual grains replaced by long white-cream fungal sacs	

Chapter 11

Genetics of Nutritionally Important Traits in Sorghum

In general, the nutritional quality of grain as human food is somewhat lower than other cereals. However, sorghum supplies important minerals, vitamins, protein, and micronutrients essential for optimal health, growth, and development. Starch content in the whole grain is about 70 per cent. Crude protein content is about 11 per cent (flour weight basis, 12 per cent moisture). Lysine is the limiting amino acid in sorghum than the normal maize and is about 2.0 per cent of total protein or about 0.25 per cent of flour weight (Axtell and Ejeta 1990), due in part, to sorghum's approximately 10 to 15 per cent higher prolamin content (Hamaker *et al.*, 1995) and lower amounts of high lysine containing non-prolamin proteins. Two sources of high lysine sorghum exist.

Protein Content

Although sorghum is the major source of protein for millions of people in the developing countries, its low nutritional quality makes it less competitive as a food and feed crop. Grain nutritional traits selection programs, for high protein or lysine are not successful in sorghum. Heritabilities of fodder digestibility, high protein and less fiber content are reasonably high and it is possible to breed for high grain yield and high fodder quality. Landraces of sorghum exhibit higher protein content than improved varieties. Protein content was higher in landraces like Dood Moghra (12.42 per cent), Yennigar Jola (11.55 per cent) and SPV 1155 (11.37 per cent).

To increase the efficiency of screening and selection of sorghum for increased levels of protein digestibility, turbidity assay is a significant achievement for sorghum nutritional quality research. Continuous research for improved nutritional quality at Purdue University has enabled the development of a sorghum mutant line – 'P-

851171'. This sorghum mutant line has a mutation that alters the protein bodies from the less digestible normal smooth and spherical shape to a folded and irregular shape that is comparable to maize in digestibility. 'P-851171' was developed from crosses between a high-lysine opaque mutant - 'P-721Q' - and a high yielding agronomically elite line. The 'P721' opaque mutant (designated 'P721Q') resulted in a 60 per cent increase in lysine content. The high lysine lines show high digestibility as well (Mohan 1975). The first is a naturally occurring Ethiopian mutant identified by Singh and Axtell (1973) from the world sorghum collection, with lysine levels of 3.1 per cent and a total crude protein content of 15-17 per cent (Axtell *et al.*, 1974). On a flour weight basis, the lysine content is 0.5 per cent. The second high lysine gene mutation was induced in sorghum by chemical mutagenesis by Axtell and colleagues (Mohan 1975, Axtell and Ejeta 1990).

The lysine concentration in P721 opaque mutant is controlled by a single gene that is simply inherited as a partially dominant factor. The study conducted to determine the inheritance of high protein digestibility and high lysine concentration in P-851171 suggested a one-gene partial dominance model for both high protein digestibility and high lysine concentration consistent with prior results for high lysine concentration. The map distance between hpd and opaque was estimated to be 42.7 cM suggesting that the two traits are unlinked. Results of QTL analysis indicated that both hpd and opaque loci were each associated with a SSR marker, Txp113, in linkage group A (Muthama 2001).

Starch Content

Starch is the major component of grain sorghum, constituting 70 per cent of dry grain weight (Hoseney *et al.*, 1981). Many important physicochemical, thermal, and rheological properties of starch are influenced by the ratio of amylose and amylopectin, the two major polymers in the starch granule, and by the structure of amylopectin. Most sorghum starch contains 70-80 per cent branched amylopectin and 21-28 per cent amylose. However, waxy or glutinous sorghum contains 100 per cent amylopectin. Hence amylose content of sorghum grain depends on the dose of a recessive gene (*wx*). The endosperm of waxy sorghum contains three recessive waxy genes (*wxwxwx*), that of heterowaxy sorghum contains at least one recessive gene (*WxWxwx* or *Wxwxwx*), and that of normal sorghum contains no recessive gene (*WxWxWx*) (Sang *et al.*, 2008).

Genetic studies revealed that the landraces were good general combiners for higher protein content, low starch and high soluble/free sugars content. Rao *et al.* (1982) also observed that positive 'general combining ability' (GCA) effect for protein content was accompanied by negative GCA effect for starch content. Correlation studies indicated that for improvement of protein content in terms of quantity, the starch content must decrease or compensate at biochemical level in the grain, during grain development stage (Deshpande *et al.*, 2003).

Tannins

Polyphenolic compounds, also known as tannins, present in the grain of some sorghum cultivars substantially reduce the big-availability of protein and other nutrients, which indirectly has a major negative effect on the nutritional quality of grain sorghum. However recently, they have been shown to promote human health because of their high antioxidant capacity and ability to fight obesity through reduced digestion. Tannins are present only in sorghums with a pigmented testa layer. The presence of the testa layer is controlled by *B1_B2_* genes. When *B1_B2_* is dominant, a pigmented testa is present.

Fe and Zn Content

Biofortification of sorghum by increasing mineral micronutrients [especially iron (Fe) and zinc (Zn)] in grain is of widespread interest (Pfeiffer and McClafferty 2007). Grain Fe and Zn in sorghum like in other crops are quantitatively inherited with continuous variation. Expression of grain Zn content in sorghum is governed predominantly by additive gene effects, and suggested high effectiveness of progeny selection in pedigree selection or population breeding to develop lines with increased levels of grain Zn contents. Low predictability ratio for Fe indicated that the expression of grain Fe content in sorghum is governed predominantly by non-additive gene effects in combination with additive gene effects, suggesting a scope for heterosis breeding to develop lines with increased levels of grain Fe content in addition to progeny selection (Ashok Kumar *et al.*, 2013).

Mineral Content

The mineral elements N, Mg, Si, P, S, CI, K, Ca, Mn, Fe, Cu, and Zn were studied in 49 experimental hybrids of forage sorghum. 'General combining ability' (GCA) effects exceeded specific combining ability (SCA) effects for all elements except P, CI, and Fe in females, and Sand CI in males. The GCA and SCA effects in females were low for both Fe and Cu (Gorz *et al.*, 1987).

Molecular Approaches for Identification of Genes Controlling Grain Quality Traits

Association analysis of 300 accessions between 333 SNPs in candidate genes and/or loci and grain quality traits resulted in eight significant marker–trait associations. A SNP in starch synthase *IIa* (*SSIIa*) gene was associated with kernel hardness (KH) with a likelihood ratio-based R^2 (R_{LR}^2) value of 0.08, a SNP in starch synthase (*SSIIb*) gene was associated with starch content with an R_{LR}^2 value of 0.10, and a SNP in loci *pSB1120* was associated with starch content with an R_{LR}^2 value of 0.09 (Sukumaran *et al.*, 2012).

A chromosomal segment located on LG F was found to play a major role in grain quality (Rami *et al.*, 1998). In a RIL, four QTLs for flouriness, dehulling yield, amylose content and mold resistance during germination were detected to be very closely linked with each other. On the same linkage group, four important QTLs were detected on another RIL for flouriness, kernel friability, kernel hardness and amylose content (Deu *et al.*, 2000). These results are consistent with the close correlation found between amylose content and endosperm texture. The B2/b2 gene controlling the presence of a high-tannin testa layer in the grain has been phenotypically mapped in this region. This explains the visual quality criteria used by breeders (a quality grain has a vitreous and hard endosperm and has no testa). QTLs for kernel friability, kernel hardness, dehulling yield and protein content were detected on LG A for RIL249. This is consistent with the close correlations found between these traits; the *guinea* allele conferred a higher mechanical resistance to the kernel. Co-localizations of QTLs for protein content and kernel physical properties were also found in other segments of the genome: for example, QTLs for protein content and flouriness had a same map position on LG C. Major QTLs for amylose content, dehulling yield, and kernel texture are not linked to productivity traits, while they are co-located with major QTLs for the mold resistance during germination and the tannin content. No genetic obstacle was observed for recombination of genetic components of both productivity and grain quality in *caudatum × guinea* crosses (Deu *et al.*, 2000). Great number of QTLs are involved in the regulation of the quantity of storage proteins in the grain, especially albumins and prolamins and that several QTLs for albumin quantity have a same map position as QTLs for grain hardness, flouriness and dehulling yield (Rami, 1999).

Among the six genes involved in synthesis pathways of starch (Sh2, Bt2, SssI, Ae1, and Wx), SssI and Ae1 were associated with peak gelatinization temperature, a trait influenced by amylopectin amount. Sh2 was associated with amylose. Grain storage proteins (O_2) and Wx were associated with hardness and endosperm texture. No association was found between O_2 and protein content (Peng 2013).

Chapter 12
Biotechnology of Sorghum

The increase in yield and productivity cannot be sustained indefinitely by traditional approaches to crop improvement, as these approaches have several limitations (Vasil, 1994). In recent years Biotechnology has provided a powerful tool to supplement traditional methods through the use of molecular genetics in cloning and sequencing of genes leading to the analysis of the genome structure, evolution and expression. Improving sorghum through biotechnology is the latest technology that has been applied to this crop. Five basic tools of technology have been developed for sorghum improvement: (1) *in vitro* protocols for efficient plant regeneration; (2) molecular markers; (3) gene identification and cloning; (4) genetic engineering and gene transfer technology to integrate desirable traits into the sorghum genome; and (5) genomics and germplasm databases (Maqbool *et al.*, 2001).

Marker-Assisted Selection (MAS) in Sorghum

Molecular breeding is the application of molecular biology tools for the genetic manipulation of traits in crop or animal species. The term is generic and describes several modern breeding strategies like marker-assisted selection (MAS), marker-assisted backcrossing (MABC), marker-assisted recurrent selection (MARS) and genome-wide selection (GWS) or genomic selection (Ribaut *et al.*, 2010). However, in its general usage, molecular breeding refers more specifically to the application of DNA marker-assisted selection.

Markers assist in selecting a plant with required trait/s directly or indirectly. In plant breeding, different marker systems have been used for selecting desired plants. Morphological markers are the first genetic markers used for selecting plants with desired traits during the history of plant breeding. These are the visible plant traits like colour of flower, anther, stigma, pericarp, seed, leaf shape, awn, dwarf plant height, seed size, pubescence etc. The first association of a simply-inherited major effect gene with a quantitative trait in plants was reported several decades ago (Sax 1923), and the phenomenon has since been observed for a range of traits in many crops. Selection of semi-dwarf plants in rice and wheat are the most successful examples of use of major effect genes in modern plant breeding. However, the availability of such morphological markers is limited, many are not linked with economic traits, interact with environmental conditions, are less polymorphic etc. The next class of markers used with limited application in plant breeding is the biochemical or protein markers. Isozyme/proteins with their alternate forms and mobility have been utilized as molecular markers in seed purity testing. These markers also suffer from the limitations similar to those of morphological markers.

DNA markers are nothing but DNA sequence variations between individuals which can be seen using several tools like Southern blotting, PCR based techniques, microarray and by sequencing. Since 1980s, DNA markers have become important tools of genetic analysis and crop improvement. Unlike morphological and biochemical markers, DNA markers are abundant, available across the length of the genome, phenotypically neutral, stage and time independent, and therefore are considered to be ideal marker systems for application in molecular breeding of crop plants. During the past 2-3 decades, several marker systems have been developed, and some of the most important ones are RFLP (Restriction Fragment length polymorphism), RAPD (Random Amplified Polymorphic DNA), AFLP (Amplified Fragment length Polymorphism), SSR (Simple Sequence repeats), ESTs (Expressed Sequenced Tags), DArTs (Diversity Array Techniques) and SNPs (Single nucleotide Polymorphisms) etc. However, all these marker systems are not equally preferred for molecular breeding. SSR markers characterized by their hyper-variability, reproducibility, co-dominant nature, locus-specificity, and genome wide distribution make them excellent markers. SSRs are reported in an array of crop plants including sorghum. They are the markers of choice for high-throughput genotyping, high density linkage map construction and useful for gene mapping and marker-assisted selection. A number of linkage maps based on SSRs have been developed in many cereal species including sorghum. Thousands of sorghum SSRs have been developed and used for linkage map construction and QTL analysis in sorghum. However, with the developments in cheap genome sequencing technologies characterized by speed and efficiency, millions of SNPs are identified in several crop plants. SNPs are common in both animals and plants. They reveal a single nucleotide base difference between DNA sequences of two individuals. Typically, SNP frequencies are in a range of one SNP every 100-300 bp in plants (Edwards *et al.*, 2007). SNPs are co-dominant, often linked to genes, and have become very attractive and potential genetic markers in genetic analysis and moelcular breeding. Since they are available in millions per genome, easily detectable, amenable for automation, cover whole genome, it is expected that the SNPs will be increasingly used in most of the crop species for several genetic analyses including marker-assisted selection.

When to Adopt MAS?

There are several situations in which use of markers for trait improvement becomes advantageous over conventional phenotypic selection for higher genetic gains. Some of them are when the trait of interest is:

☆ Expressed in the later stage of plant development (Ex. Male sterility, seed traits)

☆ Recessive (Ex. Brown midrib in sorghum)

☆ Depending on its expression on specific environment (Ex. Cold, disease etc.)

☆ Difficult to measure (Ex. Moisture stress)

☆ Controlled by two or more unlinked genes (Ex. Multiple genes)

☆ Quantitative trait and show low heritability (Ex. Grain yield)

☆ With linkage drag

☆ Measured involving difficult assays (Ex. Biochemical traits)

☆ Also in Gene pyramiding (Ex. Genes for resistance)

☆ Locating a major effect gene

Pre-Requisites for MAS

The success of MAS depends on the strength of marker-trait associations established for a given trait. Therefore before the start of a MAS program, there is an essential need to identify, validate and establish a stable marker-trait association. This can be done either by using conventional QTL detection methods in a segregating biparental population or through an association mapping approach involving a diverse panel. For a successful MAS, critical information on component traits, accurate phenotyping, the identification of candidate genes and quantitative trait loci, the relationship between QTL and genes, the contribution of individual QTL to the phenotype, and their variability across different locations and different crop seasons are essentially required. Besides this, there are several essential requirements for MAS (Jiang 2013). Some of the important ones are:

☆ **Suitable marker system and its reliability**: Marker should be simple, high-throughput, low-cost, co-dominant, highly reproducible, show high levels of polymorphism and reliable.

☆ **DNA extraction method**: needs to be very quick and on high throughput basis.

☆ **Saturated Genetic maps**: Linkage maps provide the basis for the detection of marker-trait associations. Therefore, the maps should be highly saturated. A marker at every 3-5 cM is highly desirable in QTL analysis and for MAS.

☆ **Knowledge of marker-trait associations**: Tightly linked markers should be available for the successful MAS.

☆ **Quick and efficient data processing and management**: In MAS, since the decision on the selection of plants is time-bound, there should be a system for quick and efficient data analysis and its management.

Sorghum Genome

Sorghum is a C_4 monocot and predominantly self-pollinated species with out-crossing between 3-15 per cent. The nuclear DNA content of sorghum is 1.55 to 1.6 pg per 2C or 748 to 772 million base pairs (Mb) per 1C (Arumuganathan and Earle 1991), which is three times smaller than the maize and the pearl millet genome (2500 Mb per 1C and 2450 per 1C), twenty times smaller than the wheat genome (15,966 Mb per 1C), and nearly double the nuclear content of the rice genome (450 Mb per 1C). Therefore, sorghum genome is less complex than other C_4 crops like maize, pearl millet, sugarcane. Sorghum can act as an excellent model crop to study structural and functional genomics of C_4 cereals. Sorghum is the second cereal after rice for which the whole DNA sequence information was publicly available (Paterson *et al.*, 2009). Findings from this crop can therefore greatly help to investigate other cereals for synteny, plant architecture, genome evolution, understand stress resistance mechanisms at molecular, physiological and biochemical levels.

MAS in Sorghum

Sorghum genetic improvement through classical breeding approaches has been slow in addressing the causes of major loss and yield-destabilizing traits like susceptibility to insects and diseases, poor grain quality, drought and striga menace, as these traits are greatly influenced by environment and no reliable genetic clues have been available for recombination breeding (Bhat *et al.*, 2004). Therefore, the MAS approach is gaining importance in the improvement of sorghum crop. Several marker systems have been developed and used for tagging and mapping of major effect genes and also quantitative traits of economic importance like grain yield and its component traits, resistance to insect pests, diseases, striga, drought, salinity, cold and nutritional quality traits etc.

Grain Yield and its Component Traits

Genetic improvement of grain yield is a challenging task for plant breeders. Grain yield in sorghum is a quantitative trait (Beil and Atkins 1967) and is the outcome of several reproductive, morphological and phenological traits. Several DNA based markers such RFLPs, RAPDs, AFLPs, SSRs and DArTs have been developed in sorghum and used to construct linkage maps (Bhattramakki *et al.*, 2000; Mace *et al.*, 2008; Ramu *et al.*, 2009; Srinivas *et al.*, 2009) and marker-trait associations. QTL studies in sorghum identified several genomic regions associated with agronomically important traits *viz.*, plant height (Agrama *et al.*, 2002; Feltus *et al.*, 2006; Hart *et al.*, 2001; Klein *et al.*, 2001a; Lin *et al.*, 1995; Pereira and Lee 1995; Rami *et al.*, 1998; Srinivas *et al.*, 2009), maturity (Childs *et al.*, 1997; Crasta *et al.*, 1999; Feltus *et al.*, 2006; Lin *et al.*, 1995; Srinivas *et al.*, 2009), grain yield and related traits (Fakrudin *et al.*, 2013; Feltus *et al.*, 2006; Rami *et al.*, 1998; Reddy *et al.*, 2013).

A total of 771 individual QTL from 44 studies relating to 161 unique traits representing eight broad trait categories (grain, leaf, maturity, panicle, abiotic stress resistance, biotic stress resistance, stem composition and stem morphology) have been reported in sorghum and were projected onto the consensus map (Mace and Jordan 2011). Among them, 169 QTL related to the trait category stem morphology, 128 to biotic stress resistance, 121 QTL to grain, 93 to abiotic stress resistance, 62 to maturity, 96 to stem composition, 56 to panicle and 46 to the trait category leaf. It was found that the QTL distribution was uneven across the sorghum genome with SBI-01 containing almost 20 per cent of the total QTL and SBI-05 containing only 3.9 per cent of the QTL.

There were five main regions of high QTL density (20/0.5 cM): one on SBI-01 at approximately 70 cM, one on SBI-06 at approximately 84 cM, two on SBI-07, one at approximately 108 cM and the second at approximately 125 cM, and the final region of high QTL density was on SBI-10 at approximately 58 cM. The SBI-01 high QTL density region contained QTL for tiller number, endosperm colour and carotenoid content, cold tolerance, ergot resistance, kernel weight, panicle architecture, total number of leaves, panicle length, stay-green, maturity, protein digestibility and shoot fly resistance. The high QTL density region on SBI-06 contained QTL for kernel weight, grain yield, height, panicle weight, stay-green, ergot resistance, tillering, resistance to striga and shoot fly resistance. The first high QTL density region on SBI-07 contained QTL for height, leaf angle, kernel friability, stem yield, lodging, sugar-related traits, leaf hemi-cellulose, panicle architecture, tiller height and grain phosphorus. The second high-density QTL region on SBI-07 contained QTL for endosperm colour and carotenoid content, kernel weight, glume persistence, grain mold resistance, green bug resistance, height, leaf width, stay-green, stem cellulose and hemi-cellulose, sugar-related traits and tiller height. The high-density QTL region on SBI-10 contained QTL for ergot resistance, yield, head and kernel weight, grain mold resistance, green bug resistance, height, maturity, panicle architecture, rhizomatousness, shoot fly resistance, stay-green, sugar-related traits and tiller number (Mace and Jordan 2011).

Location of Major Effect Genes

Integration of previously mapped major effect genes onto a complete genome map, linked to the whole genome sequence was carried out by Mace and Jordan (2010), using common markers across populations, allowing sorghum breeders and researchers to link this information to QTL studies and to be aware of the consequences of selection for major genes. Readily scorable trait linked morphological traits and provides new opportunities for breeders to select the target traits indirectly, and develop more efficient breeding strategies. The list of major genes mapped in sorghum is listed in Table 12.1.

Biotic Stresses

Disease and insect management through host-plant resistance has been an effective means of reducing losses in sorghum. It is generally recognized that breeding for disease resistance is relatively simple than that for insect resistance. In sorghum, except for grain mold and stalk rots, resistance to most diseases has been reported to be controlled by major genes (Thakur *et al.*, 1997). However, on the other hand, for most of the sorghum insects, resistance is controlled by many genes. With the complexities involved in the inheritance of insect and disease resistance in sorghum, availability of DNA markers for these stress resistance would reduce the need for phenotypic screening. New resistance sources and alleles for insect and disease resistance can be explored and employed effectively through gene pyramiding into elite cultivars for their wider adaptation and effective cultivation. This target can be best achieved by deploying MAS in the conventional breeding programme.

Table 12.1: List of Major Genes Mapped in Sorghum

Sl.No.	Gene	Trait Involved	LG
1.	Tb1	Tillering	1
2.	Sh1	Grain shattering	1
3.	Y	Grain colour	1
4.	Ma3	Maturity	1
5.	Pericarp	Pericarp colour	1
6.	Rf2	Fertility restoration	2
7.	B2	Testa	2
8.	Z	Mesocarp	2
9.	Ma5	Maturity	2
10.	Pla	Downy mildew resistance	3
11.	R	Pericarp colour	3
12.	AltSB	Aluminium tolerance	3
13.	ms3	Male sterility	3
14.	A	Awn	3
15.	bmr6	brown midrib	4
16.	PlcorInt	Plant colour intensity	4
17.	Opr	Resistance to organophosphate	5
18.	dw2	Plant height	6
19.	Ma1	Maturity	6
20.	gc	Glume cover	6
21.	d	midrib	6
22.	Rs1	Coleoptile colour	6
23.	Lg	Ligule	6
24.	P	Plant colour	6
25.	Ymrco	Midrib colour	6
26.	bmr12	brown midrib	7
27.	I	Pericarp colour	7
28.	dw3	Plant colour	7
29.	Pu	Rust resistance	8
30.	Rf1	Fertility restoration	8
31.	Shs1	Head smut resistance	8
32.	Sb.Ht9.1	Plant height	9
33.	bm	Bloom	10
34.	rlf	Virus reaction	10
35.	wx	Endosperm	10
36.	Rs2	Coleoptile and leaf axil	10
37.	Ma4	Maturity	10
38.	Trit	Trichome morphology	10

Adapted from Mace and Jordan (2010)

Disease Resistance

Sorghum serves as host for over 100 pathogens, including fungi, bacteria and viruses (Thakur *et al.*, 1997). These pathogens either singly or in combination lead to considerable losses in yield of grain, fodder and quality. Among the diseases of global importance, grain mold, ergot, charcoal rot, and foliar diseases are important.

Grain Mold

Grain-mold incidence was observed to be influenced by five QTL each accounting for between 10 per cent and 23 per cent of the phenotypic variance (Klein *et al.*, 2001a). The effects and relative positions of QTL for grain-mold incidence were in accordance with the QTL distribution of several agronomic traits correlated with grain-mold incidence. Several genomic regions affected multiple traits including one region that affected grain-mold incidence, plant height, panicle peduncle length, and grain-milling hardness, and a second region that influenced grain mold and plant height. Collectively, QTLs detected in the population explained between 10 per cent and 55 per cent of the phenotypic variance observed. In a recent study involving an association mapping panel of 242 mini-core sorghum genotypes, two SNP loci linked to grain mold resistance have been identified (Upadhyaya *et al.*, 2013b). Among these, one contained a NB-ARCLRR class of R gene (Sb02g004900) that shares 37 per cent identity and 57 per cent similarity to the maize non-host resistance gene Rxo1. However, the map positions of the SNP markers did not overlap with the grain mold QTL from Klein *et al*. (2001a).

Ergot

Sorghum ergot is a disease of significant importance to sorghum seed industry. The pathogen manly infests unfertilized ovaries, leading to the total loss of developing grain in the spikelet. Resistance for ergot is controlled by many genes (Parh *et al.*, 2006) and is reported to act at two physiological levels, pollen mediated and non-pollen based. Nine, five and four QTLs were identified (Parh *et al.*, 2008) for percentage ergot infection (explaining 5-19 per cent PV), pollen quantity (explaining 6-19 per cent PV) and pollen viability (explaining 6-12 per cent PV) respectively. Two epistatic loci associated with ergot infection and pollen viability were also identified. Thus, the involvement of both additive and epistatic QTLs in ergot resistance has been reported.

Charcoal Rot

Charcoal rot is an economically important soil borne disease of post-rainy sorghum in India. The pathogen is most active under water stress conditions. Resistance is reported to be complex with involvement of quantitative inheritance. Two recent studies have reported QTL for charcoal rot resistance using the same RIL population evaluated over 3 locations and 4 years (Ayyanagouda *et al.*, 2012; Reddy *et al.*, 2008). The study using 93 RILs of a cross IS22380 × E36-1 was able to identify nine consistent QTL over locations and years for, three morphological traits (number of internodes crossed by the rot, length of infection and per cent lodging) and three for biochemical traits (lignin and total phenols). Candidate genes for each of the QTL influencing both morphological and biochemical traits have been reported.

Foliar Diseases

Foliar diseases of fungal origin are prevalent under warm humid conditions are highly destructive and drastically affect the green leaf area available for photosynthesis thereby reducing the grain yield and fodder yield and quality. Around 32-60 per cent of grain yield losses have been estimated.

A major gene conferring leaf blight resistance was linked with an RAPD primer OPD12 (Boora *et al.*, 1999) and by a SSR marker Xtxp309 on chromosome 10 in sorghum by Mittal and Boora (2005) which can be easily used in MAS. Search for QTL influencing foliar diseases resulted in the consistent detection of a major QTL on SBI-06 between SSR markers, Xtxp95-Xtxp57 (Klein *et al.*, 2001) influencing resistance against various unrelated pathogens causing foliar diseases. The phenotypic variation explained by the SBI-06 disease-response QTL ranged from 32 per cent (bacterial leaf blight, zonate leaf spot) to 55 per cent (anthracnose) indicating involvement of a key gene for disease resistance. Disease-response QTL for other foliar disease like oval leaf spot was also found to co-locate to this region on SBI-06. Consistent involvement of this QTL region in disease resistance against several foliar diseases was also reported (Murali Mohan *et al.*, 2010). In a recent study, Upadhyaya *et al.* (2013a) identified eight SNP marker loci (loci 1–8) to be linked with anthracnose resistance across environments. Genes known to be involved in plant defense mechanisms like NB-ARC class of R genes, HR-related genes, a transcription factor that functions in the R gene pathway, a gene that functions in the non-specific host resistance, and a gene for anti-microbial compound production were identified to be the putative genes for anthracnose disease resistance in sorghum. Of the eight SNPs identified for resistance to anthracnose, two SNPs were validated and were found to co-locate with the two major QTL (QAnt3 and QAnt2) reported (Murali Mohan *et al.*, 2010). Plant colour scored as a qualitative trait (tan vs purple) mapped to the same region of SBI-06 that contained the linked QTL for foliar diseases. These studies confirmed the strong correlation that was reported between plant colour and foliar disease resistance. Tan plant colour was associated with reduced foliar disease symptoms. Several breeders have noted the relationship between tan plant colour and apparent resistance to foliar and panicle diseases.

For anthracnose, two SCAR markers linked to recessive gene conferring resistance were reported (Singh *et al.*, 2006a; Singh *et al.*, 2006b), Ramasamy *et al.* (2009) have identified an AFLP marker Xtxa6227 on SBI-05 that co-segregates with *Cg1*, a dominant gene for resistance to anthracnose in sorghum. Similarly, Gowda *et al.* (1995) identified markers for resistance to downy mildew, and Oh *et al.* (1993) reported tagging of Acremonium wilt, downy mildew and head smut resistance genes in sorghum using RFLP and RAPD markers. Rust is another important foliar disease that affects the grain yield and the quality of fodder. QTL studies have identified four main regions of sorghum SBI-01, 2 and 3 with region on SBI-03 accounting 40 per cent of the phenotypic variation (Tao *et al.*, 1998).

Insect Resistance

More than 150 species of insect-pests damage sorghum from seed to seed stage. Of these insects, shoot fly, stem borer, midge, shoot bugs, head bugs and aphids are major yield constraints and cause economic damage. Plant resistance to insects is most often a quantitatively inherited trait with the involvement of different resistance mechanisms. Strong effects of both the environment and the genetic variability within insect pest populations on the assessment of bioassays have resulted in a high degree of genotype-by environment error (Smith *et al.*, 1994). Therefore MAS using QTL linked markers assume greater significance in breeding for insect resistance.

Shoot Fly Resistance

Shoot fly is one of the serious pests attacking the sorghum crop during seedling stage in Africa, Asia and Mediterranean Europe. In India, the losses due to shoot fly damage have been estimated to reach as high as 90 per cent of grain, and 45 per cent of fodder yield. In India, the annual economic losses in sorghum due to this pest have been estimated to be US$200 million.

Molecular markers linked to QTLs associated with component traits of shoot fly resistance have been detected using different genetic sources of resistance and susceptibility. Sajjanar (2002) reported 8 QTLs for shoot fly resistance components based on single environment analyses. One major QTL for glossiness located on linkage group J was identified which explained 34.3 per cent – 46.5 per cent of the phenotypic variance. This QTL also co-mapped with region associated with the frequency of 'dead hearts' under high shoot fly pressure indicating the usefulness of this QTL for MAS for shoot fly resistance in sorghum. Similarly, Satish *et al.* (2009) using a different RIL mapping population of 296B × IS18551 with multi-season experiments identified 29 QTLs for various component traits of shoot fly resistance. Two major genomic regions on SBI-10 between SSR markers, Xnhsbm1044-Xnhsbm1013 and Xgap1-Xnhsbm1011 were found to contribute the most for shoot fly resistance with their association with glossiness, seedling vigour, trichomes, oviposition and 'dead-hearts' traits. This study also mapped a gene controlling trichome morphological in sorghum, which was found to be very strongly associated with shoot fly resistance. A region on SBI-05 was found to be involved in leaf glossiness.

Major QTL regions identified in this study correspond to QTL/genes for insect resistance in maize. Leaf glossiness QTL on SBI-05 and 03 is syntenic to maize LG 4 and 3 respectively, and carry genes, glossy3 and glossy9 for leaf glossiness, and also harbor Long chain Acyl-CoA synthetase and wax synthase genes involved in wax biosynthesis. Seedling vigour QTL on SBI-03 is housing a gene for Indole 3 acetic acid-amino synthase GH3.5 which promotes plant growth, light and stress adaptation. Similarly, the QTL on SBI-10 where QTL for oviposition, dead-hearts, trichome density are co-located, putative candidate genes *viz.*, Cysteine protease Mir1, Homogentisate phytyl transferase vte2, Hydroxyproline-rich glycoprotein, NAC1, glossy15, mh11 responsible for biotic and abiotic stress resistance, trichome density have been identified. The study was successful in identifying important QTL, putative candidate genes. The involvement of QTL in shoot fly resistance on SBI-10 were further validated by Aruna *et al.*, 2011 using a different genetic background - RIL population of

27B × IS2122. Few more new QTL were also detected in this study. In the recent study by Apotikar *et al.*, 2011, using a reciprocal cross IS18551 × 296B, QTL for glossiness, oviposition and dead-hearts have been reported on SBI-01 between Xtxp248-Xtxp316 SSR markers on SBI-01.

Midge Resistance

Sorghum midge is one of the most damaging pests of grain sorghum worldwide. Quantitative trait loci associated with two of the mechanisms of midge resistance, antixenosis and antibiosis, were identified in a RIL population from the cross of sorghum lines ICSV745x 90562 (Tao *et al.*, 2003). Two QTL on separate linkage groups (SBI-03 and SBI-09) were found to be associated with antixenosis and explained 12 per cent and 15 per cent, respectively, of the total variation in egg numbers/spikelet. One region was significantly associated with antibiosis on SBI-07 and explained 34.5 per cent of the variation of the difference of egg and pupal counts. The identification of DNA makers for both antixenosis and antibiosis mechanisms of midge resistance will be particularly useful for exploring new sources of midge resistance and for gene pyramiding of these mechanisms for achieving durable resistance through MAS.

Green Bug Resistance

Four QTL studies have been reported for green bug resistance in sorghum (Agrama *et al.*, 2002; Katsar *et al.*, 2002; Nagaraj *et al.*, 2005; Wu and Huang 2008). The association experiments of sorghum phenotypic resistance to biotypes C, E, I and K with restriction fragment length polymorphisms (RFLP) indicated that nine resistance loci in eight linkage groups in the sorghum genome independently explained 3–49 per cent phenotypic resistance variation, and that epistasis accounted for 3–56 per cent of the variation (Katsar *et al.*, 2002). Agrama *et al.* (2002) observed nine QTLs in seven linkage groups responsible for resistance to biotypes I and K using simple sequence repeat (SSR) markers. Another similar experiment using a different resistant sorghum source identified eight QTLs on two linkage groups expressing resistance to both biotypes I and K Nagaraj *et al.* (2005). Wu and Huang (2008) reported two QTLs which consistently conditioned the resistance of host plant to the green bug explaining 55-80 per cent and 1-6 per cent of the phenotypic variation for the green bug resistance.

Weed Management

Striga spp.

Striga spp. is a devastating parasitic weed in Africa and parts of Asia. Low *Striga* germination stimulant activity, a well-known resistance mechanism in sorghum, is controlled by a single recessive gene (lgs). Molecular markers linked to the lgs gene can accelerate development of Striga-resistant cultivars. Using a high density linkage map constructed with 367 markers (DArT and SSRs) and an *in vitro* assay for germination stimulant activity towards *Striga asiatica* in 354 recombinant inbred lines derived from SRN39 (low stimulant) 9 Shanqui Red (high stimulant), Satish *et al.* (2012) precisely tagged and mapped the lgs gene on SBI-05 between two tightly linked microsatellite markers SB3344 and SB3352 at a distance of 0.5 and 1.5 cM, respectively.

Abiotic stresses

Post-Flowering Drought

The term stay-green has been used to describe the post–flowering drought tolerance response in sorghum (Rosenow *et al.*, 1981). The staygreen trait in sorghum, which is an important component of the post-flowering drought resistance mechanism is characterized by the plant's ability to maintain functional photosynthetic leaf area during the grain filling stage even under severe post-flowering drought stress. Sorghum genotypes with this trait continue to fill their grain normally under drought and exhibit increased resistance to charcoal rot and lodging. Several sorghum genotypes (BTx642, SC56, and E36-1) have been identified that exhibit the stay-green trait (Haussmann *et al.*, 2002; Kebede *et al.*, 2001; Rosenow and Clark 1983).

QTL studies have resulted in the identification of several genomic regions associated with stay-green trait. Comparison of the stay-green QTL from Xu *et al.* (2000) and Subudhi *et al.* (2000) along with results obtained by other workers (Tao *et al.*, 2000; Tuinstra *et al.*, 1997) using B35 as a stay-green source resulted in the consistent identification of four major QTL, namely *Stg1* and *Stg2* (on LG SBI-03), *Stg3* (on LG SBI-02) and *Stg4* (on LG SBI-05) in different genetic and environment backgrounds which together accounted for up to 53.5 per cent phenotype variance (Subudhi *et al.*, 2000). The *Stg1*, *Stg2* and *Stg3* QTL overlap with the QTL for chlorophyll content and molecular markers linked to these QTL are available. Stay-green QTL individually reduced leaf senescence in introgression lines, and may contribute significantly towards breeding drought tolerance (Harris *et al.*, 2007; Hash *et al.*, 2003; Kassahun *et al.*, 2010). More recently, potential use of stay-green QTL in improving transpiration efficiency and water extraction capacity has been demonstrated in sorghum for terminal drought tolerance (Vadez *et al.*, 2011) and contribution of stay-green to grain yield, particularly under low yield environments is demonstrated (Jordan *et al.*, 2012).

Cold Tolerance

Sorghum is a tropical crop adapted to warmer environments. Germination and early crop establishment is an important growth stage requiring optimum soil moisture and temperature. Cool temperature (15C or less) especially during the early growth stages is one of the major abiotic stress limitations to sorghum cultivation in temperate and higher elevation regions. Knoll *et al.* (2008) carried out genetic mapping and identification of genome regions associated with cold tolerance using a population of 153 RI lines, developed from a cross between Chinese landrace 'Shan Qui Red,' (cold-tolerant) and SRN39 (cold-sensitive). Two QTL for germination were identified, with one (on SBI-03) contributing 12 per cent – 15 per cent of variation to germination under both cold and optimal temperatures, while the QTL on SBI-07 showed greater significance only under cold temperature accounting 10 per cent trait variation. A major QTL with 8 per cent – 27 per cent trait contribution was identified on SBI-01 showed strong associations with seedling emergence and seedling vigour under both early and late field plantings. Similarly, one QTL for both early and late seedling emergence was identified on SBI-02 explaining 8 per cent – 10 per cent of trait variation. New source of cold tolerance PI610727 was used to tag genome regions that showed significant contributions to traits for early-season cold tolerance (Burow *et al.*, 2011). A total of 14 QTL for four component traits of cold tolerance (germination at low and optimum temperature, field emergence and seedling vigour) were detected on five linkage groups (1, 2, 4, 7 and 9). Vigorous germination was found to be an important component of cold germinability in sorghum (Knoll and Ejeta 2008). This strong relation was also reinforced by the co-location of QTL for cold and optimal temperature germinability detected in chromosome 2. PI617027 was found to share common loci with other known early-season cold-tolerant sorghum germplasm (Knoll *et al.*, 2008) and also harbouring novel QTL for enhanced germination and field emergence. Further investigations would be required to validate these results and use of other types of markers for use in MAS.

MAS: Challenges

MAS is a great tool in the scheme of plant breeding. Compared to conventional phenotypic selection strategies, MAS has several significant advantages. However, so far the successful applications of MAS in plant breeding are limited mostly to simple traits with monogenic or olegogenic inheritance. The application of MAS in plant breeding has not achieved the expected results. Improvement of traits of complex inheritance through MAS is still a challenge. Non-availability of robust markers, non-validation of marker-trait associations, imprecise estimates of QTL locations and effects, epistasis, genetic background, g x e, lack of cost-effective marker genotyping systems, lack of wet-lab facilities, knowledge gap in plant breeders etc. are some of the reasons that can account for the low visible impact of MAS in plant breeding.

Over the past two decades, considerable progress has been made in the development of genomic resources in sorghum. Several DNA marker systems have been developed and are effectively used in developing linkage maps. Significant efforts have also gone into integrating various linkage maps and constructing a highly saturated consensus map. Several studies have been undertaken to identify QTL for many traits. Fine mapping of the few traits resulted in identifying candidate genes involved in trait expression. Several of the QTL have been validated in different genetic backgrounds and are therefore ready for MAS applications in sorghum. The time has come for plant breeders to use these molecular tools for improving sorghum and making MAS an integral part of conventional breeding programmes.

Chapter 13
Sorghum Food and Industrial Utilization

Sorghum is a staple food in African and Asian subcontinents. Most of the grain produced in these countries is utilized for human consumption. The grain sorghum is utilized in preparation of many traditional foods and in bakery preparations like bread, cakes and biscuits. Though sorghum is known for its nutritional quality, the consumption of this cereal is decreasing due to easy availability of rice and wheat through public distribution system and easy methods of processing and cooking of fine cereals (such as rice). The requirement of special skill in preparing sorghum *roti*s and non-availability of ready-made sorghum flour and *suji* in the market are deterrents for wider use of sorghum as food.

Semi-Processed Products of Sorghum

The traditionally consumed foods of sorghum in India were discussed earlier. Absence of appropriate primary processing technologies to yield shelf-stable flour/products has been the major limiting factor in their utilization for diversified food uses and development of value-added products. Some recent works have shown this possibility. Technologies for production of shelf-stable refined flour, grits and semolina from sorghum and millet have been developed and laboratory studies have demonstrated their successful utilization and incorporation into various traditional foods (like idli, dosa, chakli, papad, etc.) and newer convenience health products (vermicelli, noodles, plain and ready-to-eat flakes, extruded products, weaning and supplementary foods, and bakery products). Efforts are needed for popularization and wider adoption of the successful technologies to promote these grains for diversification of their utilization among the non-traditional urban population (Ali *et al.*, 2003)

However, sorghum can be replaced with rice or wheat in many household food dishes that are commonly made. Sorghum grains are polished with a pearling machine and processed in to flour as well as semolina (*suji*) of different particle size (coarse *rawa*, medium *rawa* and fine *rawa*). Pearling/polishing reduces the coarseness of the product and also removes the bitterness that is associated with the pericarp of the grain. Sorghum does not have gluten and therefore becomes an ideal gluten free energy source for the people suffering from wheat or gluten allergies.

The milled products that are commonly made from wheat can be made from sorghum also. *Rawa* types of different particle sizes (coarse *rawa*, medium *rawa* and fine *rawa*) can be prepared to suit the special food product that is made. For preparation of bakery products, sorghum grain has to be polished and made into very fine flour. Recovery of the different grades of *rawa* was compared among elite genotypes of sorghum and cultivars with corneous endosperm are more suitable for semolina/ *rawa* processing. The recovery of *rawa* (coarse one) would be 60-70 per cent where as medium one would be approximately 40-45 per cent. However the quality of *rawa* made from corneous grain of sorghum would be hard in texture unlike wheat *rawa*. The cooking quality of sorghum *rawa* is quite different from that of wheat *rawa*. Unlike wheat *rawa* sorghum *rawa* becomes harder after roasting before it is processed into a food product (Anonymous, 2007).

With regard to shelf-life of these products, coarse *rawa* has a good shelf-life which is up to 45 days (6 weeks). The medium and fine *rawa* have a shelf life of 30 days when tightly packed in polythene bags. These *rawas* have a shelf life for a week when kept open in polythene bags without sealing. A study on the percent recovery of these products was compared in 20 elite genotypes. Among released genotypes, C-43, CSV 14R, CSV 216 R, M 35-1 were having percent recovery as 48 per cent. Among advanced *rabi* hybrids, SPH 1581, SPH 1582, SPV 1709, SPV 1758, SPV 1760, SPV 1762 and SPV 1768 were having recovery of 49 per cent. These products were also tested for their suitability to make different sweet recipes like *kesari, laddu* and *appam* etc.

Some of the processed products like parboiled *rawa*, flakes, extruded products, and pops were also prepared from sorghum at laboratory scale at NRCS. Further, the commercial production and suitability of wheat or rice machinery for producing these products from sorghum are being studied.

Traditional Foods in India

The various traditional food preparations in India encompass the following:

1. Roti
2. Annam
3. Sankati
4. *Kanji*

Roti

The most preferred form of sorghum used traditionally is *roti* or *bhakri* (unleavened pan cake). *Roti* is consumed along with different kinds of dishes depending on the socio economic status of the consumer (Subramanian and Jambunathan 1980). The consumption of sorghum *roti* is a traditional practice in Maharashtra, Karnataka and Andhra Pradesh. There is a decline in the consumption pattern of sorghum mainly due to the urbanization and easy availability of fine cereals like rice through public distribution system. Further, special skill is required to make sorghum *roti*.

However, recently (for the past 1-2 years), there is a growing awareness among the urban population that sorghum is a health food for diabetics. This is due to the higher dietary fibre and prolonged release of energy leading to a low pressure on insulin. Thus there is an increase in the consumption of sorghum and now sorghum *roti* has become popular health food in Andhra Pradesh. The consumption of sorghum as a staple diet in Africa proved that, the risk of cancer and arthritis are fairly low among the African population (Tariq M. Sawandi) and the presence of nitrilosides in sorghum is the reason for this. The flour from sorghum is gluten free and therefore is a safe energy source for people allergic to gluten.

Sorghum flour can be made using a grinding mill and sieving the flour to make it fine and used in *roti* making. Since sorghum does not contain gluten and the dough does not have stickiness, it is difficult to roll with the chapatti roller. Rolling *roti* with sorghum dough needs special skill. Traditionally it was done by hand tapping on a flat stone. The *roti* rolling is not only time consuming, but the *rotis* will also be thick and unpalatable for some.

To overcome this, a machine is developed to facilitate rolling wet *rotis* on a commercial scale. The electric machine consists of a revolving rotary circular flat plate with an upper rolling pin. A foot operated lever applies pressure gradually on the rotating dough, flattening it uniformly. A thin *roti* is formed between two plastic sheets which is removed carefully and baked on a hot pan. Using this machine, 40-45 *rotis* can be made in one hour. Thirty thin *rotis* each weighing 25-30 gm can be made per Kg. flour using the machine. Polishing of the grains in a pearling machine prior to milling removes the bitterness associated with pericarp and reduces insoluble fibre thereby increasing digestibility. However the shelf life of the polished grains is lower than that of whole grain (Ratnavathi *et al.*, 2008).

A comparison of four independent studies made on the dough and *roti* quality analysis of sorghum genotypes was done using M 35-1 as control. For the preparation of *roti*, the quality of the dough is very important. The dough quality is assessed by following parameters: a) water requirement, b) kneading quality c) time required for baking, d) rolling quality (diameter of the *roti* that is expanded with an equal amount of flour), and diameter of the *roti* after baking and f) per cent moisture retained in the *roti*. The kneading quality was scored in a scale of 1-3 (1= poor, 2= medium to good and 3= very good). *Roti* quality was assessed for the taste and sensory properties which were measured on a hedonic scale. The properties used for sensory evaluation were a) *roti* colour and appearance, b) *roti* texture, c) *roti* flavour, d) grade and e) acceptability of the *roti*. This comparative study based on four independent analyses showed that more than 20 improved breeding lines out of 77 genotypes (genotypes pooled from elite breeding lines and also released genotypes) tested were superior to M 35-1 for *roti* quality (Ratnavathi *et al.*, 2008).

Annam

In India, particularly in southern regions, boiled sorghum (rice-like) called *annam* or *soru* is one of the common items cooked, and it accounts for about 10 per cent of the total sorghum grain produced. The freshly made product is consumed with *dhal*, *sambar*, buttermilk with pickles, or onion and green chillies for lunch or supper. Sometimes, it is stored overnight by adding water and consumed the next morning with buttermilk.

Sorghum is traditionally used as boiled sorghum after dehulling the grains. The dehulled grain is cooked in water in the proportion of 1:3. Sometimes the grains are also soaked overnight in water and cooked next day morning. The cooking is preferably done in an earthen pot, which is heated using firewood. The grains are cooked to softness and the excess water is drained off. The cooked product has to be fluffy, uniform yellow or creamy white in colour with a sweet taste.

Sankati

Sorghum *sankati* is a type of thick porridge consumed in South India. It is called by different names in various regional languages, *e.g.*, *mudda* (Telugu), *mudde* (Kannada), and *kali* (Tamil). Sorghum *sankati* is consumed in the Rayalaseema tracts of Andhra Pradesh, the southern tracts of Karnataka, and all over Tamil Nadu. About 60 per cent – 70 per cent of sorghum consumed is eaten in the form of *sankati* in Tamil Nadu, 50 per cent in Andhra Pradesh and 30 per cent in Karnataka. It is usually consumed with a range of side dishes such as *sauce*, *dhal* from *pulses*, *pickles*, *chutneys*, *buttermilk*, curd *curries*, etc.

Sorghum grits/flour and water in a ratio of 1:3 are used for preparing *sankati*. Water is allowed to boil in a vessel and grits are added to boiling water coupled with stirring. After 10 min, fines are added followed by stirring and this is continued for 3 min. The vessel is removed from fire and poured on to a moist plate and made into balls of 10 cm diameter by hand. *Sankati* is eaten fresh or stored overnight in water or buttermilk.

Kanji

Kanji is a thin porridge, mostly consumed in the southern parts of India, Africa and Central America. However, the local names are different. This is also called as *ambali* and is prepared from flour. Ambali is consumed after fermentation (Ali *et al.*, 2003).

Upma

Upma is a very important South Indian breakfast food or snack food item that can be prepared in a very short time. This is usually prepared with wheat or rice semolina. Semolina should not contain flour and it can be either coarse or be fine like wheat semolina. This is usually eaten hot with either sauce or chutney made with coconut and chana dal (chick pea) or groundnut. *Upma* is made with semolina that is prepared with polished sorghum grain. A little oil is taken on a sauce pan and seasoning is done with grains like chick pea and black gram along with mustard and cumin seeds. Curry leaves and green chilies are also added for taste. Then water is added (one and half times to the quantity of semolina) and allowed to boil before the addition of semolina. Then it is cooked under reduced heat till it becomes solid.

Dosa and *Idli* are fermented breakfast foods mainly consumed in South India. *Idli* is made in moulds and is a steam cooked food while *dosa* is a thin oily pan cake made with black gram dal and rice. However, in place of rice, sorghum grain can be used.

Sweets that are prepared commonly from wheat semolina can also be prepared from sorghum semolina. *Rawa* laddu, *rawa* kesari and *appam* are the sweet dishes that can be prepared from sorghum. *Rawa laddu* is prepared with roasted semolina, sugar and ghee. Nuts and grated and de-oiled coconut are added for taste. This mixture is made into *laddus* with ghee and milk. *Rawa kesari* is prepared by cooking roasted semolina and sugar with little ghee and nuts. *Appam* is made by making small portions of kesari into round and thin shaped biscuit like products and are fried in oil.

Snack foods like *muruku*, *chakkalu* and *namak para* can be made from sorghum flour by blending with chick pea flour. These are fried items containing high amount of fat. However, they have commercial value and potential to compete with other snack foods made from rice and wheat.

Bakery Products

Substitution of wheat with local cereals like maize and sorghum in biscuit production was studied to have improved the nutritional quality of biscuits. At NRCS, efforts were made to prepare common bakery products like bread, cakes and biscuits. Fine sorghum flour made out of kharif grain (pearled) equal to the consistency of *maida* (refined wheat flour) is used in combination with *Maida* for the preparation of various bakery products like bread (whole sorghum), mixed bread (bread made from sorghum, ragi and bajra in 2:1:1 ratio), plum cake and biscuits. The method of preparation of these products is similar to that of the one used for wheat flour (Ratnavathi *et al*, 2003).

Bread

Bread can be made with sorghum flour by blending it with maida up to 40-60 per cent. Very fine flour of sorghum is mixed with salt, sugar, fat and bread improvers and is made into a dough. Baker's yeast is added to the dough and allowed for fermentation for longer period compared to the normal wheat bread. After the fermentation the dough is ready for baking. The dough is then kept in the mould and baked for one hour. To improve the leavening and softness comparable to wheat bread, more yeast and external gluten are added. 30 per cent - 40 per cent of maida blended with sorghum might result in producing a tasty product. Studies on the shelf life are very important, as it is a key factor that is directly related to economy of bakery industry. Bread can be made using the modified starches like carboxy methyl starch. The shelf life varies from 24 to 72 hrs.

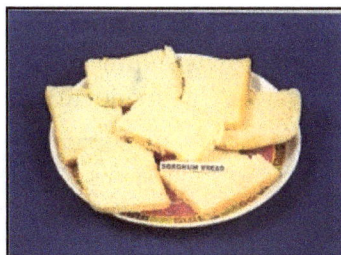

Bread made with a composite flour containing sorghum is nutritionally valuable. However, sorghum alone lacks the functional proteins for bread making. Carson and Sun (2000) investigated the rheological properties and bread baking potential of a sorghum-based composite flour system containing various amounts of vital wheat gluten (exogenous gluten protein). Mixograph and Kieffer test results showed that exogenous gluten protein significantly enhanced the composite dough's strength. At fixed gluten protein levels, as sorghum flour increased, water absorption decreased slightly, dough strength and extensibility decreased, and mixing time increased significantly. Exogenous gluten proteins when added in the form of vital wheat gluten into the composite flour, which was without wheat flour, could not form an appropriate gluten network for bread making. The interaction between exogenous and endogenous proteins in wheat flour and in the composite flour contributed greatly to the rheological properties of the sorghum composite dough and bread volume.

Organoleptic tests of the composite bread showed that 70 per cent of the taste panelists rated the overall quality of 70 (wheat) : 30 (sorghum), composite bread as good. Proximate composition of the composite bread showed that it contained much lower protein, and higher crude fibre contents than 100 per cent wheat bread. The shelf life of composite bread at room temperature was lower than that of 100 per cent wheat bread. It was found that an addition of 2-4 per cent pentosans to composite flour (up to 50 per cent substitution level) improved the quality of the bread. Pre fermentation of the sorghum flour up to 20 hours was found to have positive effects on the baking quality of the wheat and sorghum composite flour. Experience showed that composite flour required additional quantities of sugar, yeast, and water as compared to 100 per cent wheat, to make the bread tasty. Baking of composite dough required higher temperatures and the texture of composite bread was less acceptable. One of the major problems faced by bakers is the smaller volume of composite bread as compared to 100 per cent wheat bread from similar quantities of composite flours and wheat flours (Idowu, 1989).

Cake

Preparation of cakes is similar to that of cakes prepared from wheat *maida*. Fine sorghum grain flour is used for the preparation of cakes. Sorghum flour is comparatively superior to the wheat flour for cake preparation. Fine sorghum grain

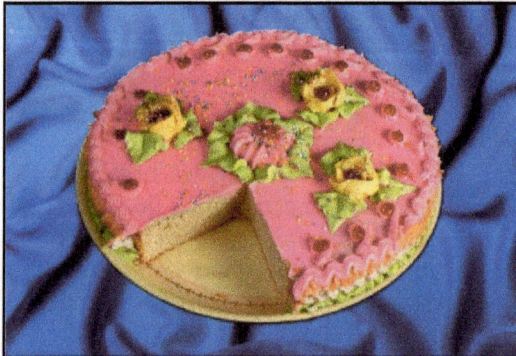

flour is mixed with required quantities of sugar, egg, emulsifiers and fat. The batter is made a little soft and nuts are added to decorate on the top. This batter is then poured in a mould kept in the oven for baking.

Biscuits

Biscuits are prepared from fine sorghum flour in combination with maida to an extent of 15 per cent. Biscuits are prepared by mixing sorghum flour with *maida*, vegetable fat, sugar, baking powder (15 per cent) and essences required. The mixed dough is then compressed in a mould and baked at the required temperature. Studies on the parameters like compressibility, breaking strength etc. showed that sorghum biscuits had lesser breaking strength. Biscuits are good in taste and taste panel acceptability score is high for cakes and biscuits at NRCS, pilot studies are in progress in collaboration with a food Industry in Hyderabad. It is possible to produce biscuits of acceptable quality using 50:50 wheat and sorghum composite flour.

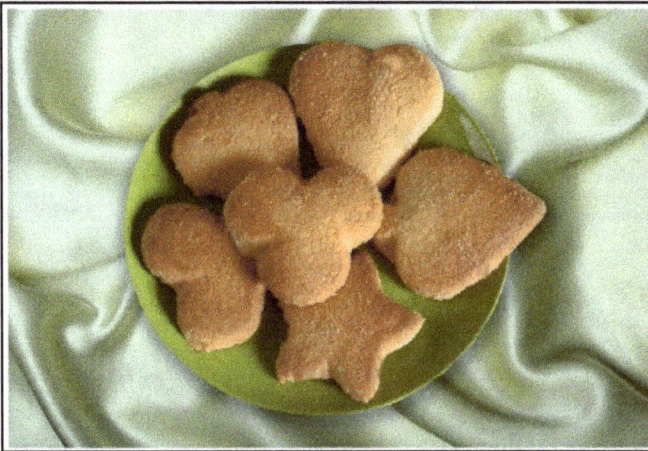

Substitution of 25 per cent of wheat flour with sorghum flour in production of short and hard dough biscuits and wafers was cost effective without affecting quality, breakages, and plant efficiency. It was suggested that improved milling techniques to produce sorghum flour with particle size comparable to that of wheat flour can increase the possibility of higher substitution (Priyolkar, 1989). The special taste property of sorghum bakery products is its non-stickiness to the mouth. Sorghum-soy flour blends, recorded the highest peak viscosities compared to other blends. Each flour blend showed a decline in its cooking properties, as the level of soy was increased from 20 to 30 per cent while the biscuits from sorghum-soy blends were brown in colour with a slight spread (Ogundipe *et al.*, 1989).

Noodles and Pasta

Noodles of acceptable quality could be made from hard endosperm sorghums while pasta could be made from sorghum and wheat composite flours. Sorghums with soft texture, yellow endosperm, and white pericarp and without pigmented testa produce best pasta products (Rooney and Waniska, 2000). The technology for making noodles and pasta from sorghum makes the product cheaper and healthier as sorghum products are known for high B vitamin and dietary fibre.

Extruded Products

Extruded products are very important nutritional snack food items which have a very high commercial value. The extrusion properties of sorghum are excellent and is equal to maize and rice. Though the machinery and other infra structure costs are very high, the major advantage of extruded products is the larger output of the final product from the raw flour. Low amylose content yielded brittle extruded products and digestibility of extruded products for high amylopectin starch increased (Gomez *et al.*, 1988). High amylopectin (Waxy) lines are suitable for production snacks, dry breakfast cereals and beverages (Gomez *et al.*, 1986).

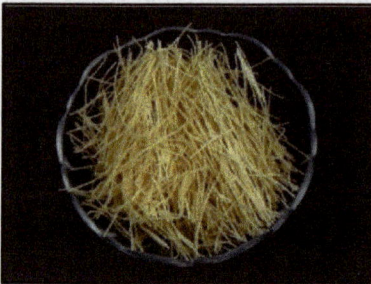 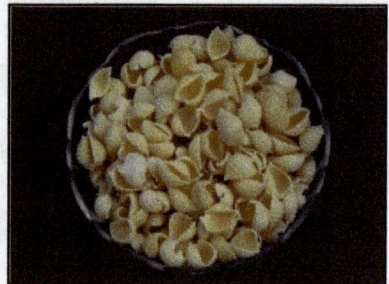

| Pasta | Vermicelli |

Industrial Utilization

Production of Natural Syrup from Sweet Sorghum Stalk Juice (NARI, Phaltan, India) (Small Scale)

Generally, good quality syrup can be produced from sorghum genotypes with high percentage of reducing sugars and low percentage of sucrose in their juice, while high quality jaggery production requires just the opposite composition. For ethanol production the total sugar content of juice is important and not its composition.

Sweet sorghum syrup production offers farmers an excellent opportunity to improve their income from sorghum crop. The marketing outlook for sorghum syrup is also very favourable, but the processing of sweet sorghum juice is the most critical aspect of making high quality syrup. The yield and quality of sorghum syrup is influenced by the equipment and process used in manufacturing and by the syrup maker's knowledge and skill.

A protocol was developed for the production of natural, chemical-free, quality syrup from the juice of sweet sorghum hybrid "Madhura". Nearly 500 kg syrup prepared from juice of hybrid "Madhura" has been test marketed mainly in Phaltan and Pune during last three years. A bottling machine has been used successfully to package the syrup so that its shelf-life is increased. The response of consumers to the coloured syrup has been very encouraging. Also the syrup is entirely chemical-free as only natural ingredients such as the aqueous extracts of okra fruits or plants are used for facilitating scum removal. The nutritional quality of syrup was also found to be excellent. When extensive screening of a large number of sweet sorghum genotypes was done, it was found that the entries RSSV-9, RSSV-24, RSSV-45, NSS-221, NSS-104 and SSV-84 gave good quality syrup. Also the hybrids developed at NARI such as Madhura, NARI-SSH-3, NARI-SSH-15, NARI-SSH-40 and NARI-SSH-21 produced good quality syrup.

Economic analysis of table syrup production from sweet sorghum hybrid "Madhura" was carried out for one hectare during one season for a processor as well as a farmer by considering all the costs of a syrup processing unit as well as raw material and transport. The study revealed that the total cost of production of table syrup from 22.5 t/ha of stripped stalks of Madhura for a farmer is about Rs. 55,000 and about Rs. 64,000 for a processor producing 2000 kg of syrup (9 per cent recovery) in one season. If calculated on per kg basis, the cost of table syrup for a farmer and a processor would be about Rs. 27 and Rs. 31 respectively. The sensitivity analysis of costs based on variable stalk production shows that the costs of syrup production for a farmer as well as a processor could be reduced linearly with a linear increase in stalk yields of sweet sorghum. For example, for 35 t/ha of stripped stalks of sweet sorghum with 9 per cent syrup recovery, the costs would be Rs. 18 and Rs. 6 per kg for a farmer preparing table and crude syrup respectively.

Table 13.1: Chemical Composition of Sweet Sorghum Syrup Compared with Honey

Parameters	Sweet Sorghum Syrup	Honey
Calorific value, Cal/g	2.60	3.26
Total soluble solids, per cent wt	77.00	81.00
Proteins (N X 6.25), per cent wt	1.65	–
Ash, per cent wt	3.69	0.59
(values are in mg/100 g)		
Calcium	160.00	5.00
Phosphorous	11.00	4.10
Riboflavin (Vitamin B2)	10.00	0.06
Vitamin C	11.50	5.00
Nicotinic acid	153.00	32.00
Iron	0.86	0.59
Sodium	86.00	4.70
Potassium	1810.00	90.00
Sulphur	Not detected	8.00
Benzoic acid	Not detected	
Added colouring matter	None	
Pesticide residues	Not detected	

Data for Honey is from literature.

Analysis of sample of Madhura by CFTRI, Mysore and ITALAB Pvt. Ltd., Mumbai

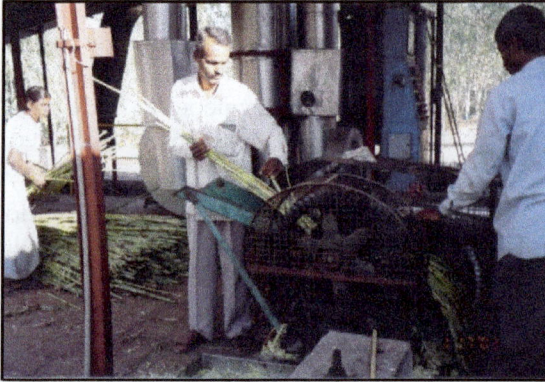

Figure 13.1: Extracted 'Madhura' Juice being Strained into a Settling Tank.

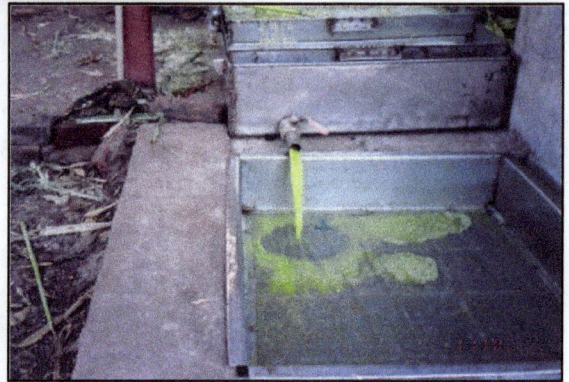

Figure 13.2: Crushing of 'Madhura' Stripped Stalks.

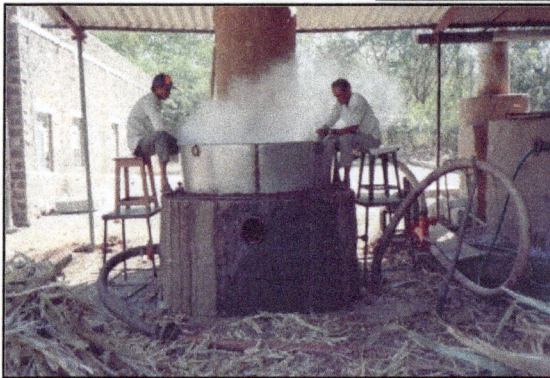

Figure 13.3: Syrup Preparation from 'Madhura' Juice.

Glucose and High Fructose Syrup

Production of Glucose Syrup by Saccharification Using Native Gluco-amylase at Optimum Condition

Attempts were made under NATP project to undertake the optimum production of glucose-syrup by saccharification, employing purified gluco-amylase at optimum experimental condition in the present study. It is evident from the results that the sorghum starch dextrin syrup to the extent of 25 per cent dry solids was used employing

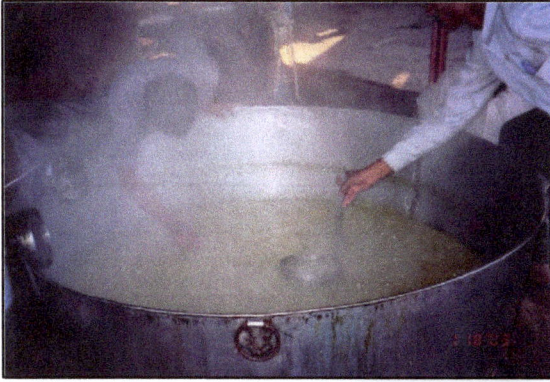

Figure 13.4: Temperature Recoding and Scum Removal from Juice.

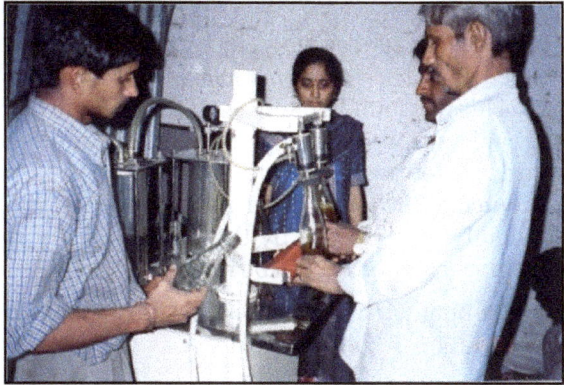

Figure 13.5: Bottling of 'Madhura' Syrup with Filling Machine.

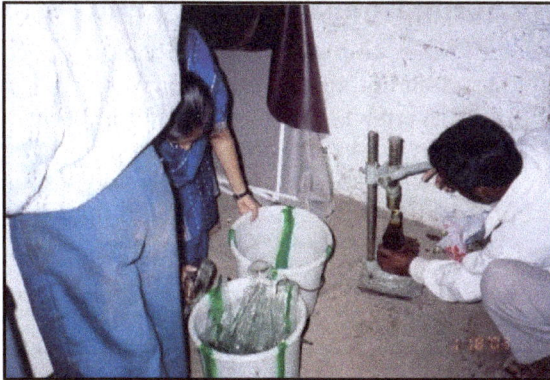

Figure 13.6: Crown Capping of Filled Bottles of 'Madhura' Syrup.

gluco-amylase at optimum enzyme activity (115 units) to produce glucose syrup. The yield of saccharification (*i.e.* dextrose yield) was found to be 94.5 per cent on laboratory scale in batch type operation.

Production of glucose syrup employing immobilized gluco-amylase (*Aspergillus niger*) at optimum conditions is experimented. The production of glucose syrup (*i.e.* saccharification) was under taken using immobilized gluco-amylase (*Aspergillus niger*) at isomaltose.

Production of Glucose Syrup by Saccharification Using Native Gluco-Amylase at Optimum Condition

Sl.No.	Sorghum Starch Dextrin Syrup (Dry Solids Percentage)**	Enzyme Concentration (Units)	Saccharification (per cent)	Glucose (g)
1	25	115	94.5	23.62

*   Unless otherwise mentioned Per cent dry solids of dextrin syrup of sorghum starch, time, temperature, enzyme concentration are 25 per cent, 10 hrs.

60°C and 115 units respectively kept constant throughout the study.

** The Dextrose equivalent (DE) - 11.5.

The effect of recycling gluco-amylase on the production of glucose-syrup was studied. It is observed from the data, the optimum production of glucose-syrup at 0 and 24 hrs was found to be 94.5 and 93.0 per cent respectively in first cycling. However, it is evident from the result that the saccharifying activity of sorghum dextrinized syrup was found to be comparatively lower during second recycling. This may be attributed to the lowering of gluco-amylase activity during cycling operation. The possibility of inhibition by the desired other products (Sugar derivative) due to transglucosidation cannot be ruled out.

The optimal conditions for the isomerization were found to be 125 units of enzyme concentration at 65°C with pH 7.0.

Production of High Fructose Syrup from Sweet Sorghum Juice

Attempts have been made to identify the promising and high yielding juice genotypes of sweet sorghum. The highest and significant juice extraction was recorded in RSSV-9 and the brix up to tune of 16.70 per cent was recorded in genotype Keller. Similarly it has been reported that the maximum value (3.56), higher total sugar content and non-reducing sugar content was reported in RSSV-9 and Keller respectively. Thus the production of high fructose syrup using *invertase* was performed.

Selection of Promising Genotypes of Sweet Sorghum for the Production of High Fructose Syrup

Sl.No.	Genotype	Per cent Total Sugar	Per cent Non-Reducing Sugar
1.	RSSV-9	18.8	15.76
2.	Keller	18.5	16.30

Production of High Fructose Syrup from Juice of Sweet Sorghum Genotype

It is well known that the sweet sorghum juice was found to contain glucose, fructose and sucrose. The hydrolysis of sucrose can be achieved by acid hydrolysis. However, it has been observed that it has got several demerits such as caramelized colour formation, inhibiting by product formation, corrosion of the reactor etc. Moreover, the involvement of costly refining process, relatively low degree of hydrolysis and usages of highly purified chemical as a starting material for hydrolysis will lead to uneconomical and costly process. Therefore the attempts were made on laboratory scale as a trial using *invertase* enzyme.

Production of HFS Using Native Invertase, a Batch Type on Laboratory Scale at 65 °C for 48 hrs and pH 4.5

Sl.No.	Genotype	Initial Fructose	Final Fructose
1.	RSSV-9	3.15	9.32
2.	Keller	3.26	9.78

In the typical experiment, 250 ml of juice of above varieties were subjected to *invertase* hydrolysis in the Pharmacia double jacketted glass (quartz) columns (2.5 × 55 cm) at sugar concentration of 40 per cent at 65°C for 48 hrs. The results revealed that the fructose concentration was found to increase considerably in the resultant reaction mixture.

Studies on the Production of Sorbitol from Purified Sorghum Starch Glucose

The results on sorbitol production indicated that the glucose was converted to sorbitol using Raney Nickel catalyst under experimental conditions. It is evident from data that the conversion of glucose to sorbitol was found to the extent of 90 per cent. The hydrogenation kinetics was investigated using various parameters. Hydrogenation of purified sorghum starch glucose (50 per cent in 200 ml) was carried out in presence of Nickel catalyst (4 per cent) and hydrogen gas pressure (400 psi) at temperature of 140°C.

The sorbitol salt obtained from hydrogenation of glucose was analyzed and found that it has various impurities such as Nickel catalyst, colour, organic acid, and break down product of glucose. Removal of all these impurities is necessary for recovering pure sorbitol with good yield. Raney Nickel catalyst is removed from the solution by filtration and the other organic impurities are removed by passing hydrogenated syrup. Successively through column of a strong acid cation exchange resin and a weak base anion exchange resin. The pure sorbitol crystals in stable form were obtained by cooling sorbitol syrup of 68 Brix from 25°C to 15°C within 30 min with stirring.

Properties of Sorbitol

Solubility

The concentration of saturated solution of sorbitol at 40°C is 75 per cent (w/w).

Relative Sweetness

10 per cent aqueous solution of sorbitol at 25 per cent is 60 per cent relative to sucrose.

Hygroscopicity

Sorbitol powder is not very hygroscopic. It absorbs less than 10 per cent water at relative humidity 40 to 75 per cent.

Cooling Effect

When Sorbitol (70 per cent) dissolved in mouth saliva it gives cooling effect in 6 seconds.

Sorghum Starch

1. Standardization of Suitable Process for the Extraction and Recovery of Starch from Moulded and Blackened Sorghum Grains

a. Extraction and Recovery of Starch

The black sorghum grains were soaked in distilled water for 24 hrs to 168 hrs separately at ambient temperature ($27 \pm 2^{\circ}$C) and 60°C. The soaking water was changed after every 24 hrs. The soaking grains were blended with water (1:2, w/v) in a laboratory for 2 min. The blending was repeated for two more minutes after a pause of one minute. The slurry was screened through a double-layered muslin cloth. The residue on the muslin cloth was washed with additional water to solubilize and filterate out the remaining starch. The filterate was centrifuged at 8000 x g for 30 min. The supernatants were discarded and the residue was suspended in 0.2 percent sodium hydroxide solution to solubilize the proteins. The contents were allowed to stand for 3 to 4 hrs to settle the starch. The yellowish upper sodium hydroxide layer was decanted and the settled starch was re-suspended in sodium hydroxide until the sodium hydroxide layer became colourless. The settled starch was then washed with water and the contents were screened through the 0.045 mm sieve. The filtrate was centrifuged and the starch obtained was recorded as 'residue' in centrifuge tubes and dried at ambient temperature (Figure 13.1).

A maximum absorption of water was observed in the grins soaked at 60°C for 96 hrs. However, the highest starch yield was obtained when the grains were soaked at 60°C for 144 hrs. The dilute alkali (0.2 per cent) was found to be superior grain soaking and residue washing medium than the dilute acids or water. A significant higher starch yield was obtained with the use of 0.045 mm sieve (59.3 per cent) as a slurry filtration device as compared to that of muslin cloth (33.8 per cent).

The starch obtained with muslin cloth exhibited slightly higher purity but significantly lower recovery. A soaking of grains for 144 hrs at 60°C in 0.2 percent NaOH followed by grinding in water and filtration of the slurry through 0.045 mm sieve, centrifugation of the filtrate at 8000 x g for 30 min, washing of the residue in 0.2 percent NaOH followed by water washing, centrifugation and drying of the residue, has been standardized to obtain a maximum of 62.2 per cent bright starch from molded and blackened sorghum. The product contained 91.6 per cent starch (Plate 13.1).

A process to get white starch from the mould-infected sorghum with black or red/brown discolouration is described here. It involves soaking of grains in 0.2 per

Black Sorghum
↓
Soaking in water
↓
Blending of grains

Screening through	Screening through
↓	↓
Muslin cloth	0.045 mm sieve
↓ Centrifugation	↓ Centrifugation
Filtrate	Filtrate
↓	↓
Residue	Residue
↓	↓
Alkali washing and decanting	Alkali washing and decanting
↓	↓
Settled material	Settled material
↓	↓
Water washing and Screening through 0.045 mm sieve	Water washing and centrifugation
↓	↓
Filterate	Residue
↓	↓ Dry at ambient temperature
Residue	Starch
↓ Dry at ambient temperature	
Starch	

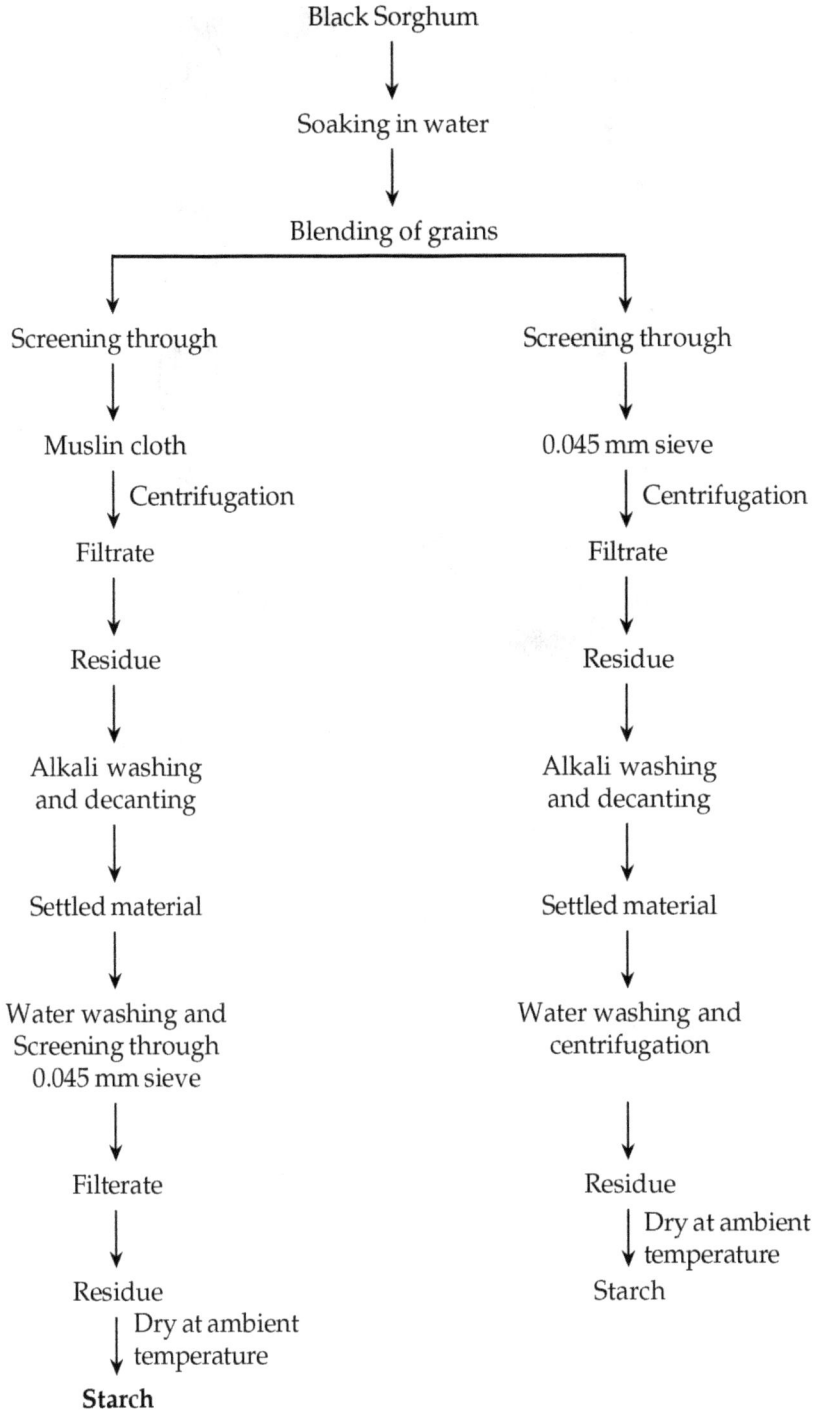

Figure 13.1: Standardization of starch extraction processes from sorghum.

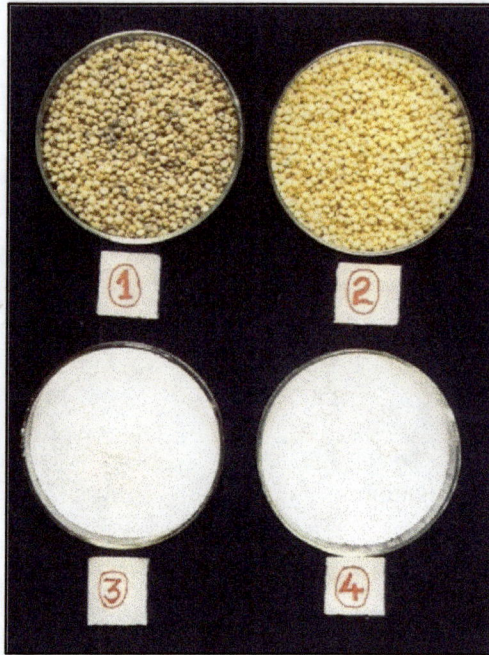

Plate 13.1

1: Moulded grains; 2; Sound grains; 3; Starch from 1 and 4; Starch from 2.

cent solution of H_2SO_4 or NaOH (1:2 w/v) for 12 hrs at 60°C followed by blending in the same extract for 2-3 min and filtration of slurry through 0.045 mm sieve (**Figure 13.2**). The extracted starch is recovered by centrifugation of the filtrate at 8000 x g for 20 min, washing the starch-pellet with water to remove residual acid/alkali and drying the product at 40°C. Sodium hydroxide was suitable for extraction of starch from grains with both black and red/brown discolouration while H_2SO_4 was suitable for only blackened grains. The physico-chemical properties of sorghum starch are given in **Tables 13.2 to 13.8 and Plates 13.2 and 13.3**.

Table 13.2: Water Absorption by Mould Infected Blackened Sorghum

Grain Soaking Temperature °C	Weight Gain after Soaking of Grains (hrs)			
	6	12	24	Mean
30	24.8 + 0.6	31.9 + 0.7	38.7 + 0.8	31.8
40	27.2 + 0.7	33.6 + 0.6	40.1 + 0.4	33.7
50	37.7 + 0.6	36.4 + 0.8	42.6 + 0.7	38.9
60	39.9 + 0.7	42.9 + 0.6	43.0 + 0.4	41.9
70	41.1 + 0.4	43.0 + 0.5	43.1 + 0.6	42.4
Mean	33.1	37.6	41.5	37.7

Table 13.3: Effect of 'Soaking Medium' on Extraction and Recovery of Starch from Black Sorghum

Grain Soaking Medium (per cent)	Extracted Starch (per cent)
NaOH, 0.1	52.00 ± 2.4
H_2SO_4, 0.1	23.38 ± 1.8
Lactic acid, 0.1	34.4 ± 1.9
Water	33.8 ± 2.1

Table 13.4: Effect of different Soaking Periods and Extraction Media on Yield of Starch from Black Sorghum

Soaking and Extraction Medium	Starch Yield (Per cent) after Soaking Grains (hrs)		
	6	12	24
Water	45.7 ± 1.6	52.2 ± 1.8	53.0 ± 1.7
Lactic acid, 0.2 per cent	49.4 ± 1.9	56.7 ± 1.5	57.2 ± 1.5
Potassium metabisulphite, 0.2 per cent	50.0 ± 1.8	59.2 ± 1.6	60.0 ± 1.7
Sodium hydroxide, 0.2 per cent	52.8 ± 1.7	64.0 ± 1.4	64.3 ± 1.6
Sulphuric acid, 0.2 per cent	53.7 ± 1.9	63.8 ± 1.8	64.1 ± 1.5

Table 13.5: Effect of Increasing Concentration of Alkali as Soaking Medium on Starch Extraction and Recovery

NaOH Concentration (per cent)	Starch Recovery (per cent)
0.1	52.0 ± 2.4
0.2	54.4 ± 2.6
0.5	54.8 ± 2.8

Table 13.6: Effect of Screening Method on Recovery of Starch

Screening Method	Starch Recovery (per cent)
Muslin cloth	33.8 ± 1.6
Sieve (0.045 mm)	59.3 ± 2.7

Table 13.7: Effect of Period and Temperature of Soaking of Grains on the Extraction and Recovery of Starch from Black Sorghum Grains

Soaking Period (hrs)	Starch Recovery (per cent) at	
	27 ± 2 °C	60 °C
24	17.9 ± 0.50	18.4 ± 0.90
48	20.2 ± 1.30	20.8 ± 1.10
72	23.7 ± 0.80	24.7 ± 0.80

Contd...

Table 13.7–*Contd...*

Soaking Period (hrs)	Starch Recovery (per cent) at	
	27 ± 2 °C	*60 °C*
96	27.2 ± 1.60	27.6 ± 1.20
120	28.5 ± 0.80	32.1 ± 1.60
144	32.0 ± 0.95	33.8 ± 0.85
168	32.4 ± 0.80	34.0 ± 0.60

Table 13.8: The yield, content and recovery of starch by different methods of extraction

Sl.No	Type of Method Used			Per cent Starch in Black Grain	Starch Product from Grain, Per cent	Actual Starch Content in Extracted Product, per cent	Starch Recovery on Initial Grain Basis, Per cent
	SM	*BM*	*RW*				
1.	W	W	N	64.7	33.8 ± 1.20	96.0 ± 1.59	50.2 ± 1.60
2.	N	W	N	64.7	52.0 ± 1.80	93.8 ± 1.65	75.4 ± 1.75
3.	N	N	W	64.7	48.3 ± 1.90	94.7 ± 1.57	70.7 ± 1.70
4.	W	W	N	64.7	59.3 ± 1.80	92.0 ± 1.83	84.3 ± 1.81
5.	N	W	N	64.7	62.2 ± 1.95	91.6 ± 1.92	88.0 ± 1.79
6.	N	N	W	64.7	61.8 ± 1.10	92.2 ± 1.50	88.1 ± 1.67

Method 1 to 3 with muslin cloth, Method 4 to 6 with 0.045 mm sieve.

SM = Soaking medium, BM = Blending medium, RW = Residue washing medium, W = Water, N = NaOH (0.2 per cent).

Black/Mould infected discoloured sorghum grains

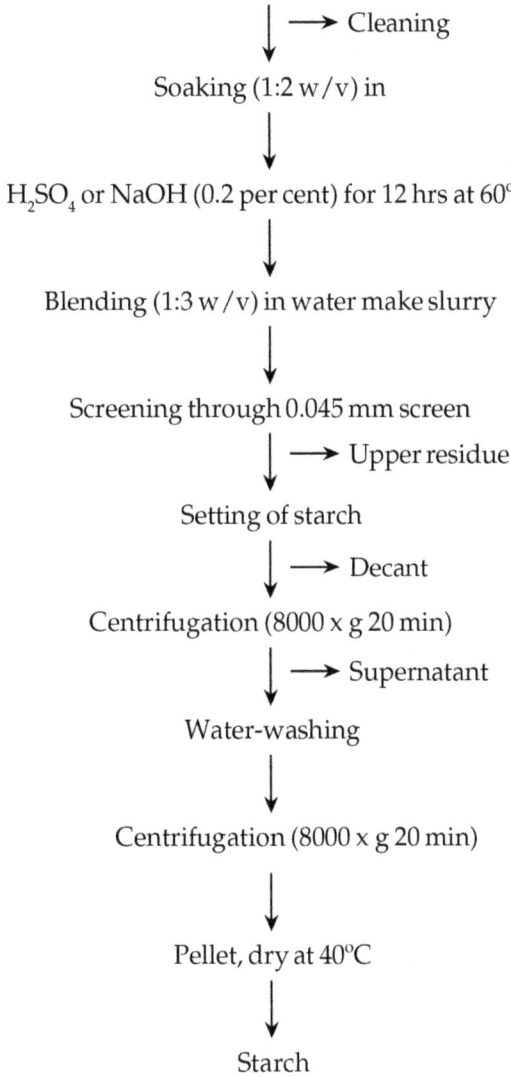

↓ ⟶ Cleaning

Soaking (1:2 w/v) in

↓

H_2SO_4 or NaOH (0.2 per cent) for 12 hrs at 60°C

↓

Blending (1:3 w/v) in water make slurry

↓

Screening through 0.045 mm screen

↓ ⟶ Upper residue

Setting of starch

↓ ⟶ Decant

Centrifugation (8000 x g 20 min)

↓ ⟶ Supernatant

Water-washing

↓

Centrifugation (8000 x g 20 min)

↓

Pellet, dry at 40°C

↓

Starch

Chapter 14

Value of Sorghum and Sorghum Co-products in Diets for Livestock

Sorghum was domesticated as a human foodstuff and animal feed nearly 3000 to 5000 years ago in Africa and from there it spread subsequently into India and China. This hardy crop, with its relatively low requirement for rainfall, became a staple human foodstuff in drought-prone regions of third world countries. Despite the lack of direct selection for nutritional value, good quality sorghum grain is available as a feedstuff for livestock, with an average feeding value that is 96 per cent to 98 per cent that of corn.

Nutrient Content of Sorghum Grain

The objectives in use of sorghum grain for livestock feeding of ruminants (*e.g.*, cattle, sheep and goats) than non-ruminants (*e.g.*, swine, poultry and fish). In ruminants, microflora of the rumen can upgrade poor-quality proteins and nonprotein nitrogen to the protein quality of the microflora itself. Therefore, ruminant nutritionists view sorghum and other cereal grains primarily as sources of starch. In non-ruminats, sorghum also is viewed as an energy source, but its quality and quantity of protein is important because in sorghum-based diets, it can contribute more than one-third of the dietary crude protein for chicks and more than one half of the dietary crude protein for growing and maturing pigs.

Digestible energy (DE), metabolizable energy (ME), and net energy (NE) are used to express the energy value of feedstuffs, but the ultimate measure of suitability for livestock feeding is growth performance. A compilation of university experiments comparing sorghum and corn for pig feeding was made. The feeding value (*i.e.*, efficiency of gain) of sorghum, as compared to corn ranged from 91 to 99 per cent with an average of 95 per cent. Riley (1985) proposed the same feeding value (*i.e.*, 95 per cent) for sorghum grain in relation to corn in a review of literature from feedlot cattle experiments.

Seed Coat and Endosperm Characteristics and Nutritional Value of Sorghum Grain

Noland *et al.* (1977) reported that sorghums with yellow pericarp were better utilized by nursery pigs (fed from 10 to 20 kg of body weight) than sorghums with brown pericarp, but the latter had high tannin content. Richert *et al.* (1991) reported that, data from 'chick growth' assays by comparing the nutritional value of sorghums with low tannin content but with bronze and yellow pericarp colour. The bronze sorghum had 5 per cent more ME, but chicks fed with the yellow sorghum, had 4 per cent greater protein utilization. Grabouski *et al.* (1987) evaluated the feeding value of corn and sorghums with bronze, cream, and yellow pericarp colours (all with low tannin concentrations) in nursery and finishing pigs. Nursery pigs eat less feed and gained 5 to 8 per cent slower when fed the sorghums compared to corn. In the finishing pigs, those fed with sorghums gained 4 per cent slower and also were 4 per cent to 9 per cent less efficient than pigs fed corn. Combining the nursery, growing and finishing results, corn generally supported improved gains. Efficiency of gain was similar in nursery pigs fed corn and the sorghums, but finishing pigs consumed more of the diets with sorghum and converted feed to weight gain with less efficiency. However, the authors could find no consistent differences due to pericarp colour.

Nutritional Value of Sorghum Based Co-products

Distillers dried grains with soluble (DDGS) is a co product of the brewing industry that has been sued in diets for swine and poultry for many years. After fermentation of grain to make ethanol, the alcohol is removed and the residue is dried to yield DDGS that can be used as a source of energy and protein for animal diets. Currently, use of DDGS for swine feeding is limited to diets of gestating sows and finishing pigs, with maximum inclusion rates of only 5 to 10 per cent of the formulation. However, with increasing emphasis on the use of oxygenated fuels, large quantities of DDGS likely will become available for use in animal diets. This has prompted concern from feed manufacturers, nutritionists, and livestock producers about accurate and complete data needed to make decisions on feed formulation and feeding practices that will optimize the use of these ethanol industry co-products.

Cabera (1994) reported that crude protein of sorghums and DDGS made from sorghums was greater than that of corn and DDGS made from corn (Table 14.1) with bronze sorghum have the greatest values (*i.e.*, 9.8 per cent for the grain and 26.6 per cent for the DDGS). Ether extract was greater for corn than for the sorghums, but DDGS made from the three cereal grains had similar ether extract values. In broiler chicks, neither grain source nor distillation treatment affected the food intake. However, birds who fed ground grains tended to gain more weight than birds who fed distillers grains. Interestingly, they were 10 per cent more efficient too. The Men values were 38 per cent greater for all of the grains compared to all of the DDGS and were 24 per cent greater for DDGS from the two sorghums versus that of the DDGS from corn. Finally,

Table 14.1: Chemical Composition of Grain and Distillers Dried Grains with Solubles (DDGS) from Corn, Bronze Sorghum, and Yellow Sorghum

Item	Corn		Bronze Sorghum		Yellow Sorghum	
	Grain	DDGS	Grain	DDGS	Grain	DDGS
CP, per cent	8.0	23.9	9.8	26.6	9.3	25.6
Ether extract per cent	3.9	8.1	3.0	8.1	3.0	8.0
Crude fiber per cent	3.2	11.0	2.6	8.5	2.4	9.5
Ash per cent	1.3	4.4	1.2	4.9	1.4	4.2
GE, Mcal/kg	4.0	4.6	4.2	4.5	4.0	4.3
Amino acids, per cent						
Arginine	0.42	0.94	0.31	0.97	0.35	0.91
Histidine	0.26	0.55	0.19	0.57	0.22	0.55
Isoleucine	0.30	0.88	0.30	0.99	0.37	0.95
Leucine	0.97	2.30	0.94	2.55	1.12	2.39
Lysine	0.29	0.59	0.21	0.60	0.25	0.55
Methionine and Cystine	0.42	0.95	0.32	1.00	0.35	0.93
Phenylalanine+tyrosine	0.66	1.77	0.61	2.02	0.74	1.83
Threonine	0.28	0.77	0.24	0.87	0.29	0.79
Tryptophan	0.06	0.19	0.07	0.22	0.09	0.21
Valine	0.41	1.15	0.39	1.25	0.47	1.24

Men were 12 per cent greater for grain and DDGS from yellow sorghum than for grain and DDGS from bronze sorghum. Lysine availabilities were 77 per cent, 74 per cent and 65 per cent for corn and bronze sorghum grain, respectively. Lysine availabilities for the DDGS made from those grains were 76 per cent, 73 per cent and 71 per cent for the corn, bronze sorghum, and yellow sorghum. Thus, lysine availability of corn was greater than that of the sorghums and distillation process had minimal effect on the availability of Lysine in the cereals. In further experiments from our laboratory, Senne *et al.* (1996) reported that ADG, ADFI and gain/feed were not affected by increasing the concentration of sorghum based DDGS to 30 per cent in isocaloric diets for nursery pigs. These results are in sharp contrast to the rule of thumb that limits use of DDGS to 5 per cent of nursery diets. Similarly surprising results were observed in finishing pits, with no adverse effects on ADG, adfi, and gain/feed with concentration of sorghum-based DDGS up to 60 per cent in isocaloric diets. Thus, when priced acceptably and as long as diets are adjusted to the same ME concentration, sorghum-based DDGS are well utilized by pigs of all ages and sizes.

Nutritional Consequences of Tannins

Sorghum grain is relatively free of potential anti nutritional factors. Indeed, because of the dry climate in which sorghum is produced, it is less prone to infestation with mycotoxins than corn. However, there is one group of problematic compounds

– tannins - that are sometimes associated with sorghum grain. Tannins actually have beneficial effects, such as prevention of molds and bird predatation. However, they are best known for their negative influence on the nutritional value of sorghum grain (Table 14.1). Tannins are water-soluble phenolic compounds that have the ability to bind and/or precipitate proteins from queous solutions. Tannins can be generalized into two categories; hydrolysable and condensed. Hydrolysable tannins also are referred to as tannic acid, and these compounds are not present in sorghum. Thus references to high tannin grain sorghums refer to the presence of condensed tannins that are concentrated in the seed testa.

Generally, sorghums with more than 1 per cent condensed tannins are considered high tannin varieties. These tannins bind with the proline-rich storage proteins of sorghum and inhibit their digestion. In nearly all experiments where high tannin sorghums are fed to the animals, an increased excretion of N and DM in the feces was observed. Thus, researchers speculate that digestibility is decreased by tannins binding to either digestive enzymes or to the proteins themselves.

Table 14.2: Effects of High Tannin Sorghum on Poultry and Swine Performance

Item	Percentage difference Relative to Control			
	ADG	ADFI	Grain/feed	N Digestibility
BROILERS				
0.4 per cent tannin*	99	98	101	100
1.3 per cent tannin*	98	101	96	100
2.0 per cent tannin*	93	100	92	97
2.26 per cent tannin acid equivalents**	63	70		
3.1 per cent tannin***	95	100	95	
SWINE***	Apparent			
3.1 per cent tannin	95	109	85	84
0.9 per cent tannin	98	101	96	101
0.6 per cent tannin	88			
1.0 per cent tannin	85			
1.5 per cent tannin	87			
3.1 per cent tannin				82

*: Control sorghum vs sorghum with tannin; **: Control sorghum vs bird resistant sorghum; ***: Compared to corn control; ***: Expressed as mg catechin/100 mg grain DM.

The first step in dealing with high-tannin sorghum is to identify if, in fact, the grain actually contains tannin. The Federal Grain Inspection Service (FGIS) uses a bleach test to identify sorghums with tannins. Briefly, 15 g of sorghum grain is soaked for 3 minutes in a flask with 5 g of potassium hydroxide and 40 ml of 5 per cent bleach. The grain is then rinsed with water and blotted dry. Warm air is used to dry the sample until the kernels are not tacky (sticky). Kernels that turn black have a pigmented testa, contain condensed tannins. If a sorghum is found to have condensed tannins, a more sophisticated test must be used to determine the actual concentration. The vanillin assay is used extensively to obtain quantitative values for tannin content in sorghum samples. This test measures catechin equivalents (monomeric units of condensed tannins) that are expressed as mg of catechin/100 mg of sorghum grain DM. Catechin equivalents are multiplied by a constant to estimate actual percentage tannins.

Research suggests that high tannin sorghum can be detoxified by using ammonia. The ammonia converts tannins to an inert form that can be fed to animals within 12 to 24 hours of treatment. However, this procedure is viewed as impractical for the large amounts of grain that would be used on a commercial livestock operation. Thus, the most prudent way to avoid loss of animal performance which is at the mercy of tannins, is to reject any sorghum that tests positive with the bleach test.

Chapter 15

Fermented Products

Sweet sorghum can be used as an alternative feedstock for ethanol production because, it has higher tolerance to salt and drought as compared to sugarcane and corn that are currently used for biofuel production. In addition, high content of carbohydrates and fermentable sugars in sweet sorghum stalk makes it, more suitable for fermentation to ethanol. Therefore, it is suggested to plant sweet sorghum for bio-fuel production in hot and dry countries to solve problems such as, increasing octane of gasoline and reducing greenhouse gases and gasoline imports (Almodares and Hadi, 2009). Sweet sorghum is currently being looked for the production of bioethanol due to its several advantages over other crops like:

1. It contains large amounts of sugars in its stalk that are directly fermentable.
2. It has a short growing period of 4–5 months.
3. It not only tolerates drought but also grows in colder regions of the temperate zones and hence has wider growing areas.
4. The whole plant (grain, stalk juice and lignocellulosic biomass) can be used for fuel ethanol production.

Previous barriers to commercialization of sweet sorghum to ethanol have primarily been the high capital cost involved in building a central processing plant that may be operated only seasonally. Technical challenges of using sweet sorghum for biofuel are a short harvest period for highest sugar content and fast sugar degradation during storage.

Alcohol from Sweet Sorghum (DSR, Hyderabad)

Initially five sweet sorghum genotypes, Keller, SSV 84, BJ 248, NSSH 104 and Wray were evaluated for total sugar, alcohol production and fermentation efficiency using batch fermentation with *Saccharomyces cerevisiae*. Higher amounts of total sugar per 100 ml of extractable juice were obtained from Keller. High juice extractability was observed with SSV-84 (34368 L/ha). Total sugar yield was found to be high in SSV-84 (7.35 Mg/ha) and Keller (4.66 Mg/ha). Highest alcohol yields of 4502.2 L/ha was observed in SSV 84, whereas high fermentation efficiency (FE) of 91.0 per cent was observed with Keller.

Ten strains of yeast (*Saccharomyces* sp.) were isolated from sorghum and evaluated for their alcohol production and tolerance to alcohol. Four strains were found to be superior for the alcohol production and out of which one strain (Strain 2) was having highest alcohol tolerance (20 per cent). These strains were evaluated for their performance in the production of alcohol and fermentation efficiency in comparison to the strain (*Schizosaccharomyces pombe*) obtained from distilleries. Strains 2 and 3 have recorded highest percentage of alcohol production. Strains 1 and 2 have the superior mean fermentation efficiency (81.42 and 79.82 per cent respectively) as compared to the fermentation efficiency of strain 5 (75.7 per cent) (Distiller's strain) (Figure 15.1).

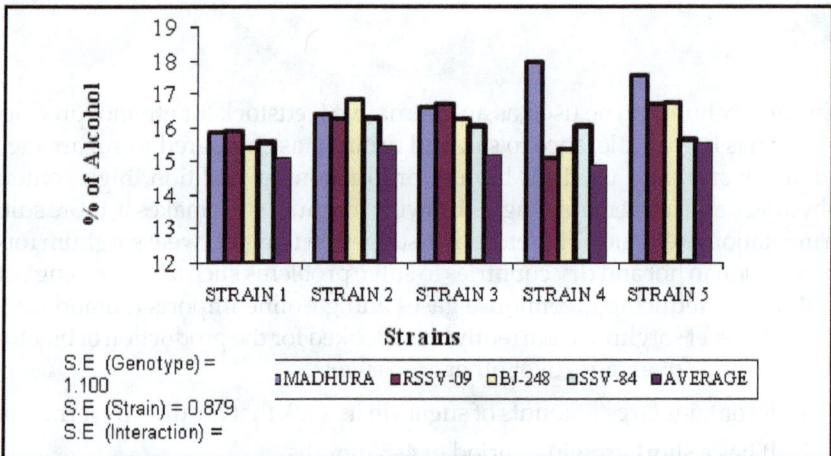

Figure 15.1: Fermentation Efficiency of different Strains of Yeasts.

Recovery of Ethanol at different Crop Growth Stages with different Yeast Strains (at DSR, Hyderabad)

Ethanol was produced in laboratory with four different yeast strains *viz.* 1) *Saccharomyces cerevisiae* 2) *Candida tropicalis*, 3) *Saccharomyces pombe* and 4) *Cryptococcus albidus* by fermenting the juice obtained at different crops growth stages like milky stage, physiological maturity and harvesting stage or normal maturity stage. The study was conducted with 18 promising sweet sorghum genotypes. The total soluble sugars left out in the medium were also estimated after 72 hours of fermentation, (Figure 15.2).

At harvesting, high recovery of ethanol was obtained with all the four yeast strains followed by physiological maturity and milky stages respectively. The yeast strain *Candida tropicalis* and *Cryptococcus albidus* have produced higher ethanol (25 per cent and 21.9) compared to the distillery strain *Saccharomyces pombe* (20 per cent)

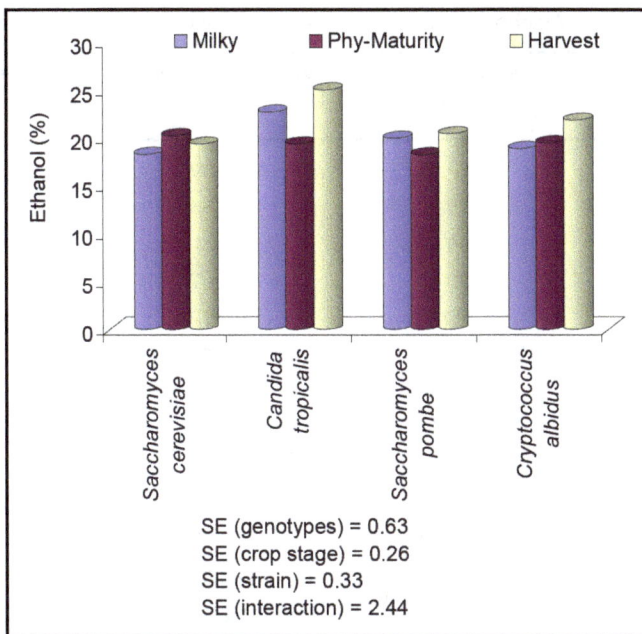

Figure 15.2: Recovery of Ethanol in different Crop Stages.

and *Saccharomyces cerevisiae* (20 per cent). Among the genotypes NSSV-21, NSSV-254, NSSV-216 and NSSV-219 from NRCS, RSSV-59, RSSV-46 and RSSV-91 from MPKV Rahuri are promising for ethanol recovery.

Aldehyde is by-product produced during fermentation. The production of aldehydes and fused oil should be minimal. In the fermentor experiment using two genotypes NSSH 104 and BM 09, percent aldehyde content was in the range of 0.0005 to 0.0008 per cent. Lowest amount of aldehyde content was reported in strain Svt after 48 hours of fermentation. The content of aldehyde in alcohol from sweet sorghum is minimal.

Total Alcohol Recovery (Stalk and Grain) in Sweet Sorghum

Advance sweet sorghum genotypes from breeding performance trials were evaluated for the total alcohol recovery from sweet sorghum stalk juice and grain. The data presented in table 4 shows that, the genotype RSSV-91 (1709.28 l ha^{-1}) and NSSV-218 (1572.73 l ha^{-1}) were found to be highest in recovery of alcohol from stalk juice, however, maximum grain alcohol was obtained from NARISSH-43 (2014.65 lit.ha^{-1}) followed by AKSSV-21 (2006.54 l ha^{-1}) and NSSV-219 (1969.51 l ha^{-1}). With regards to total alcohol yield from stalk juice and grain, AKSSV-22 recorded highest recovery (3354.67 l ha^{-1}) followed by RSSV-91 (3161.35 l ha^{-1}) and NARISSH-43 (3136.82 l ha^{-1}).

Table 15.1: Average Alcohol Yield (lit. ha⁻¹) from Advanced Sweet Sorghum Genotypes

Cultivars	Alcohol Yield from Stalk Juice (lit ha⁻¹)	Alcohol Yield from Grain (lit ha⁻¹)	Total Alcohol Yield (lit ha⁻¹)
RSSV-24	684.61	1021.63	1706.24
RSSV-44	670.77	1729.69	2400.46
RSSV-45	490.72	783.60	1274.32
RSSV-46	890.69	1720.87	2611.56
RSSV-57	1018.91	1009.72	2028.63
RSSV-58	987.37	1635.23	2622.60
RSSV-59	1439.82	877.59	2317.41
NSSV-216	568.54	1547.13	2115.67
NSSV-218	1572.73	1532.43	3105.16
NSSV-219	857.51	1969.51	2827.02
RSSV-91	1709.28	1452.07	3161.35
RSSV-106	1275.38	1286.08	2561.46
RSSV-120	877.60	1359.89	2237.49
NSSV-13	994.12	767.33	1761.45
NSSV-253	1091.47	950.81	2042.28
NSSV-254	1502.55	967.99	2470.54
NARISSH-43	1122.17	2014.65	3136.82
AKSSV-22	1492.66	1862.01	3354.67
AKSSV-21	868.61	2006.54	2875.15
SSV-84	1020.07	854.16	1874.86

Pilot Scale Evaluation of Ethanol Production from Sweet Sorghum Stalk Juice

A pilot study was conducted during the year 2002 with Sri Renuka sugar factory located at Munoli, Belgaum Dist, Karnataka to determine the feasibility of ethanol production from sweet sorghum juice. Two varieties of sweet sorghum (SSV 74 and SSV 84) and one hybrid (Madhura) were grown during *kharif* 2002 in more than 600 acres of dryland in and around the factory. Year, 2002, being a drought year, green cane yield and grain yield were 25 tons/ha and 2 tons/ha respectively. The juice brix was 18 per cent and was brought down to 12 per cent for fermentation. About 112 tons of cane was used for one fermentor with a capacity of 60 KL. Fermentation was carried out for 48 hrs. The recovery of ethanol was approximately 9 per cent of the juice. The bagasse (46.44 per cent of stalks with 2.58 per cent sugars) obtained, was used for the cogeneration of electricity.

In another pilot study, carried out with Sagar Sugars and Allied Products at Nelavoy in Chittoor district of Andhra Pradesh, SSV 84 was grown in *kharif* 2004 on about 378 hectares. In Nallatur village in Tamil Nadu SSV 84 was sown during the last week of May and harvested during first week of October. The green cane yield and grain yield were 40 tonnes per hectare and 2 tonnes per hectare respectively however, the diffuser machinery was listed for sweet sorghum in *rabi* season and it was tested suitable

Use of Sorghum as Malt

In India sorghum is used largely as a food grain, while in many African states it is also important for commercial brewing. Recent studies have indicated the feasibility of using sorghum malt for brewing lager beer. While production of lager beer from barley malt along with sorghum as a cereal adjunct poses no problem, lager beer brewing from 100 per cent sorghum is confronted with problems relating to equipment, sorghum malting, mash gelatinization, saccharification, lautering, wort fermentability, body fullness and acceptability. Development of non-biological haze caused by polyphones and insoluble proteins present in sorghum malt and the presence of high lipid content are other unfavourable aspects encountered during sorghum brewing. There is scope, however, to identify sorghum cultivars with desirable malting qualities through searching for natural variability or identify sorghum cultivars with desirable malting qualities barley malt with sorghum malt may provide a cheaper indigenous cereal alternative for lager beer brewing in countries having substantial sorghum production.

Lager Beer from 100 per cent Sorghum

Lager beer is now possible to be produced from 100 per cent sorghum using exogenous enzymes (Arri, 1989). Properties of sorghum malt were in general poor compared to barley malt, but total soluble sugars and cold water (per cent) extract of the sorghum malt were relatively higher than those of barley malt (Ogundiwin *et al.*, 1989). Production of lager beer from 100 per cent sorghum grain is an entirely new concept. The cultivars that have low gelatinization temperature, low polypeptides, low lipid, high diastatic power and readily soluble protein are good for lager beer preparation. Beer was prepared using 100 per cent sorghum malt, sorghum adjuncts and hops in the ratio 96:3:1 (Ratnavathi *et al.*, 2000). Current sorghum brewing techniques have been based on barley brewing technologies with suitable modifications. Sorghum beer had 4 per cent alcohol and higher free amino nitrogen content than in sole sorghum malt beer. The pentosanase complex of the sorghums, unlike that of barley does not embody a xylosidase, but as in barley, displays arabinosidase activity. Polymeric pentosans of barley worts were found to range from 162 mg/100 ml in the un-malted grains to 239 mg/100 ml in the 6 day malts while that of the sorghum over the same period was from 41 to 79 mg/ml (Etokakpan, 2004a). The diastatic power of the freshly kilned sorghum malt at 68.1°WK had a 29 per cent drop after six months of storage. Freshly kilned sorghum malt displayed high wort turbidity (4.9 EBC) which dropped to 0.95 EBC and 1 EBC after 2 and 6 months of storage respectively (Etokakpan, 2004b).

The composition of lager beer made from sorghum malt and sorghum adjunct are shown in Table 15.2. The lager beer from sorghum malt and adjunct showed superiority in composition in terms of increased free alpha amino nitrogen and colour units in sorghum malt and adjunct beer.

Table 15.2: Analysis of Lager Beer from Sorghum

Component	Malt Beer	Adjunct Beer
Reducing Sugars (per cent)	0.05±0	0.02±0.02
Total Sugars (per cent)	1.54±0.13	0.95±0.07
Alcohol (per cent)	4.66±0.12	4.5±0.17
Colour (EBC)	5.89±0.03	8.58±0.14
Specific Gravity	1.03±0.002	0.98±0.03
Bitterness (BU)	6.56±0.08	7.58±0.15
Proteins (per cent)	2.68±0.07	1.98±0.07
Free α amino nitrogen (mg/L)	74.61±5.18	119.01±2.63

Germinated sorghum flour had lower fat, protein and carbohydrate contents but higher ash and fibre than non-germinated sorghum flour. Germinated millet flour had higher moisture, protein and fibre compared to the non-germinated flour while the latter had higher ash and carbohydrate contents. Germination resulted in an increase in the concentration of sugars in both sorghum and millet grains (Muyanja *et al.*, 2003).

In Nigeria, use of malted sorghum rather than raw grains, as a source of fermentable sugars was found to be advantageous. Grains of sorghum varieties SK 5912, Farafara, and HQSV are currently being used for malting. HQSV variety was found to be superior to other varieties for malting purposes. The byproduct of malting - namely sprout (dried shoot and root), is currently being used as organic fertilizer and can be a rich source of dhurrin. The increased use of white grain sorghum by breweries might result in competition in the market between, grain for food and grain for brewing purpose (Ikediobi, 1989).

Malting and Brewing

In Nigeria following the ban on the import of barley malt in 1988, the brewing industry there has been utilizing sorghum and maize as raw material for lager beer production. Sorghum can be used as raw grains, grits or malted material. The bulk of the sorghum grain currently used by the brewers in Nigeria is from the varieties, SK 5912 and farafara. The malting processes in use are still empirical. In contrast to barley, sorghum malt has low levels of β-amylase, β -1, 3, 1, 4-glucanase, and β -D glucans. During the mashing operations, external 'heat stable' enzymes, namely, α-amylase, neutral protease, β -glucanase, cellulose and amyloglucosidase are required.

Lager beer can be produced from barley malt and any cereal adjunct including sorghum. It is now possible to brew some sort of beer from 100 per cent sorghum using exogenous enzymes. Good quality lager beer, similar to one prepared from barley, can be prepared from sorghum malt and sorghum adjunct. Rain damaged lower grain and mold infected grain can be conveniently used as raw material for the purpose. At DSR Lager beer was prepared using sorghum malt and sorghum as an adjunct, in the ratio of 96:3:1. Hops were used up to 1 per cent. Malt was used as ground and gritted sorghum (CSH 9) and was gelatinized to get 'wort'. Then wort was cooled and fermented with yeast for 7-8 days. Later it was filtered and carbonized with CO_2 and bottled. The chemical composition of beer was analyzed as per the EBC methodology (table). Sorghum beer had 4 per cent alcohol and a higher free alpha amino nitrogen (FAN) content than, sole sorghum malt beer. Higher ratio of adjunct use (up to 8-10 per cent) would achieve the required FAN content (140 mg/L).

Table 15.3: Sorghum Beer Analysis

Component	Malt Beer*	Adjunct Beer*
Reducing Sugars (per cent)	0.05± 0	0.02±0.02
Total Sugars (per cent)	1.54±0.13	0.95±0.07
Alcohol (per cent)	4.66±0.12	4.5±0.17
Colour (EBC)	5.89±0.03	8.58±0.14
Specific gravity	1.03±0.002	0.98±0.03
Bitterness (BU)	6.56±0.08	7.58±0.15
Proteins (per cent)	2.68±0.07	1.98±0.07
Free alpha amino Nitrogen (mg/L)	74.61±5.18	119.01±2.63

Properties of sorghum malt were in general poor, in comparison to barley malt, but total soluble sugars and cold water (per cent) extract of the sorghum malt were relatively higher than those of barley malt (Ogundiwin *et al.* 1989)

Use of malted sorghum, rather than raw grains, as a source of fermentable sugars was found to be advantageous. Grains of sorghum varieties SK 5912, Farafara, and HQSV are currently being used for malting. HQSV was found to be superior to other varieties for malting purposes. The byproduct of malting, namely sprouts (dried shoots and roots), currently being used as organic fertilizer can be a rich source of dhurrin. The increased use of white grain sorghum by breweries might result in competition in the market between grain for food and grain for brewing purpose (Ikediobi, 1989).

Chapter 16
Forage Sorghum

Sorghum is an important forage crop of semiarid regions due to its high adaptability and suitability to rain-fed low input agriculture. It has a substantial popularity amongst farmers due to its greater adaptability and various forms of utilization like green fodder, stover, silage and hay to suit the diverse needs of farming system. Forage sorghum is characterized by quick growth, high green biomass yield and drymatter content, leafiness as well as better palatability and intake. Sorghum for green forage is grown over 2.6 m ha area in Western Uttar Pradesh, Punjab, Haryana, Delhi, Gujarat, Rajasthan and is fast becoming popular with farmers from other states. Almost 60-70 per cent of total forage demand in *kharif* is met from sorghum. Multi-cut sorghum under irrigation in summer and single-cut as rainfed crop in *kharif* are popular. Its quick growth, high yielding ability, high dry matter content, leafiness, wider adaptability and drought resistance make sorghum an ideal forage crop. Sorghum is suitable for silage and hay making and thus supplements the nutritious supply in lean season.

Types of Forage Sorghum

The main types of forage sorghums are; Sudan grass varieties, grain sorghum × sudan grass hybrids, and dual purpose varieties. In general, sudan grass varieties, grain sorghum × sudan grass hybrids are more popular in northern belt of India.

Sorghum (*Sorghum bicolor*)

Tall forage types have high dry matter yields, large stalks and sparse tillers, and limited regeneration capacity. They have the potential to produce significant grain; however, considerable variation exists among forage type sorghums for grain yield (ranges from negligible to 40 per cent of dry matter yield as grain). Tall forage type sorghums are best utilized for silage production (Aruna *et al.*, 2011).

Sudan Grass (*Sorghum sudanense*)

The value of Sudan grass was recognized only in 1909, though it was present in Egypt from early times. A handful of seeds were introduced in United States to replace the Johnson grass (*Sorghum halepense*) and it proved so successful that it has spread to other states of US. Sudan grass was introduced in India in 1920 and now it is valuable fodder sorghum in the country. It is a quick growing, drought tolerant annual plant, which is very useful for hay, silage and pasture. It can be grazed or cut many times without damage. Sudan grass has thin stems, it tillers profusely, it is very leafy, it produces little seed and has rapid growth potential.

Sorgum-Sudan Grass Hybrid

It is intermediate in texture but has high fodder yield potential. Leaf : Stem ratio is less than 50 per cent. It is useful for green chop or silage but is frequently utilized for production of coarse hay (cane) for over wintering of the cattle (Pedersen and Fritz, 2000).

Johnson Grass (*Sorghum halepense*)

Johnson grass is a native of Mediterranean region but grows throughout Europe and Middle East. It is named after an Alabama plantation owner, Colonel William Johnson, who sowed its seeds on his farm land on the bank of Alabama river in 1840. It thrives in open, disturbed, rich, bottom ground, particularly in cultivated fields. Presently it is considered as one of the ten worst weeds in the world (Holm *et al.*, 1977).

Grain Sorghum Stover

After removing the panicles from grain sorghum, it stems are dried in sun (dry sorghum stems are called 'stover') and chaffed off as '*kutti*' which is a major source of animal feed in dry areas during summer in southern parts of the country.

Crop Improvement

Development of improved varieties/hybrids and production technology has led to an average yield of 50 t/ha in single cut forage sorghum and up to 70 t/ha in multi-cut hybrids. A number of forage sorghum varieties have been released in our country. The list of single, multi-cut and dual purpose sorghum genotypes is presented in Tables 16.3, 16.4 and 16.5, respectively.

Climate and Soil

The forage sorghum can be successfully grown in areas with 500-750 mm average rainfall with proper distribution. The relative humidity during *kharif* season ranges between 80 per cent – 85 per cent. The optimum soil temperature for germination should be 18-21°C and for vegetative growth, 33-35°C. However, during *rabi*, temperature above 25°C is considered optimum. Sandy loams, medium-deep black soils with proper drainage are most suitable for forage sorghum. Soil pH 6.5-7.5 is considered to be optimum.

Production Technology

The suitable cultural practices for forage sorghum production are:

Field Preparation

In general one summer plough followed by 2-3 harrowing and planking are required for most of the soil types to prepare the field for sowing of forage sorghum. In un-irrigated areas, sorghum for fodder should be sown immediately after onset of monsoon.

Sowing Time

The single-cut varieties may be planted between 15 June to 30 June, with onset of monsoon. In *Tarai* region of Uttar Pradesh, the best time of sowing is from last week of May to first fortnight of June. This helps in avoidance of major pests. The multi-cut varieties/hybrids can be planted early (March-April) under irrigation as a summer crop.

Seed Rate and Method of Sowing

In single-cut sorghum, depending on seed size, 25 kg seed/ha in small-seeded varieties and 40 kg/ha in bold seeded varieties is recommended, however for multi-cut, a seed rate of 10 kg is most favourable. The row to row spacing of 30 cm is optimum for higher fodder yield and better quality in case of single-cut and for multi-cut, 45 cm row spacing is best.

Nutrient Management

Sorghum being a cereal and high biomass crop requires balanced fertilizer application to get high yields. In case of single-cut varieties 80 kg N + 40 kg P_2O_5 per ha is recommended. N should be applied in two split doses under irrigated condition. First half as basal with full dose of P_2O_5 at the time of last ploughing or at the time of sowing and remaining half after 35-40 days after sowing when there is adequate moisture in the soil. In rainfed areas, 40 kg N/ha as basal is preferred. Use of micronutrients especially Zn has been found to increase the fodder yields. Experiments conducted under All India Coordinated Sorghum Improvement Project (AICSIP, 2010) revealed that application of $ZnSO_4$ at 15 kg/ha in soil followed by foliar sprays (0.20 per cent) twice produced 11.6 per cent higher green fodder yield (61.99 t/ha) as compared to unsprayed control (55.45 t/ha) (Table 16.1).

In multi-cut varieties, 100-120 kg N + 60 kg P_2O_5 per ha is recommended. Nitrogen should be applied in three splits. First, one-third of N along with full dose of P_2O_5 should be applied at the time of sowing. The second dose of 1/3 N should be applied after the first cut and remaining 1/3 after the second cut. These split doses should be applied when there is adequate moisture in the soil.

Irrigation

Crop sown in summer season (March-April) should be irrigated 3-4 times. First irrigation should be given after 15-20 days of sowing and subsequent irrigations at an interval of 10-15 days to get better fodder yields. During *kharif* season, irrigation is

Table 16.1: Effect of Micronutrients on Green and Dry Fodder Yields of Forage Sorghum

Treatment	Green Fodder Yield (t/ha)				Dry Fodder Yield (t/ha)			
	Pantnagar	Udaipur	Ludhiana	Mean	Pantnagar	Udaipur	Ludhiana	Mean
RDF + ZnSO$_4$ 25 kg (Soil appl.)	79.01	42.59	54.60	58.73	16.6	13.6	14.2	14.8
RDF + FeSO$_4$ 25 kg (Soil appl.)	79.01	41.85	51.11	57.32	17.2	12.6	13.3	14.4
RDF + 0.2 per cent ZnSO$_4$ Foliar spray at 15 and 30 DAS	72.84	39.81	47.85	53.50	17.8	12.8	12.4	14.3
RDF + 0.5 per cent FeSO$_4$ Foliar spray at 15 and 30 DAS	71.60	39.25	44.92	51.92	18.6	11.8	11.6	14.0
RDF + ZnSO$_4$ 15 kg (Soil appl.) + 0.20 per cent as foliar spray at 15 and 30 DAS	86.42	45.74	53.81	61.99	21.4	14.1	14.0	16.5
RDF + FeSO$_4$ 15 kg (Soil appl.) + 0.50 per cent as foliar spray at 15 and 30 DAS	80.98	40.74	47.93	56.55	16.3	13.2	12.4	13.9
RDF + Soil application of 15 kg ZnSO$_4$ + 15 kg FeSO$_4$	72.84	42.22	42.69	52.58	15.3	13.5	11.3	13.4
RDF + Foliar application of 0.20 per cent ZnSO$_4$ + 0.50 per cent FeSO$_4$	85.18	36.66	51.42	57.76	17.0	12.0	13.3	14.1
RDF alone	77.77	35.74	52.85	55.45	19.2	11.6	13.8	14.9
Control (Native fertility)	70.37	24.63	44.52	46.50	14.8	7.7	11.7	11.4
Location mean	77.60	38.92	49.17	55.23	17.4	12.3	12.8	14.2
C.D. (P = 0.05)	11.61	6.73	14.56	6.30	3.0	2.2	3.7	2.2

adjusted according to rainfall distribution and 1-2 irrigation (if required), might be given during long dry spells. Water stagnation should be avoided.

Weed Control

Weeds are a major problem in initial stage of crop growth and they compete for water and nutrients. Summer ploughing to keep field weed free, 1-2 hand weeding after 15-20 days of crop sowing, reduce weeds considerably. The per-emergence spray of atrazine @ 0.5 kg a.i/ha effectively control the weeds. The soil surface needs to be moist. Spray of weedicide should be applied immediately after sorghum sowing.

Mixed Cropping

The planting of fodder legumes like cowpea and guar along with sowing in 2:1 ratio increases fodder yield and quality. In low rainfall or less irrigated areas intercropping of sorghum and cluster bean is desirable. In irrigated or high rainfall areas, intercropping with cowpea gives high greed fodder yield. The erect variety of fodder cowpea is preferred.

Crop Rotation

The yield of sorghum is high when planted after taking the leguminous crop like berseem, senji and metha. It saves nitrogen application to sorghum crop. The crop rotation of fodder sorghum – wheat; fodder sorghum - chickpea or pea are popular. Thus, early flowering variety or early planting is useful to get higher yields of forage sorghum as well as *rabi* corp.

Table 16.2: HCN Content of CSH 5 Sorghum Hybrid (Muthuswamy *et al.*, 1976)

Days from Sowing	HCN Content (ppm; fresh weight basis)	
	Shoot	Root
18	650	375
20	600	425
23	575	500
27	300	575
30	200	575
34	150	500
40	75	325
45	43	400
49	7	350
53	15	300

Harvesting

Single-Cut

Such varieties are harvested from 50 per cent flowering to full flowering. At this stage, the HCN content in sorghum plants is reduced to safer limits and the quality of fodder is also good.

Table 16.3: Single-Cut Varieties of Forage Sorghum

Cultivars	Fodder Yield (t/ha)		Characteristics
	Green	Dry	
Pusa Chari-6	44	16.5	It flowers in 85-90 days. Stem is medium thick, non-sweet, pithy and nonjuicy. Leaves are medium long and broad with white midrib. Pancile is semi-compact. Seeds are medium bold and white. It matures for seed in 135-140 days and gives 8-9 q/ha seed.
HC-136	55	17.5	It is tall, sweet, juicy and moderately thick stemmed. The leaves are very broad and long with green midrib and remain green upto maturity. It has high protein, low toxic constituents and better digestibility. It is also good in regeneration and yields 800-850 q green fodder and 260-280q dry matter per ha in two cuts. It matures for seed in 140 days.
Jawahar Chari-6 (JC-6)	41.2	12.0	Its stem is tall, thick juicy and non-sweet. Leaves are broad and long with white midrib. It is tolerant to leaf spot diseases. Panicle is semi-laxed. It flowers in 80 days and matures in 130-135 days. Grains are bold, pearly white with reddish brown glumes.
U.P. Chari-1	35-40	9-10	Released in 1983 from Pantnagar. It flowers in 75-80 days and thus becomes ready for fodder. Its stem is moderately thick, sweet and juicy. Leaves are dark green, long and broad with green midrib. Panicle is medium in size, flat and chalky white. It matures in 115-120 days for seed and yields 8-10 q/ha seed.
U.P. Chari - 2	40-45	12-13	Released in 1984 from Pantnagar. It flowers in 75-80 days. It is moderately thick stemmed with tan colour and is juicy. Leaves are very broad and long having light green colour. Panicle oval-shaped, medium in size and compact. Grains are medium bold, round and pearly white in colour. It matures for seed in 110 days and gives 10-12 q/ha seed yield.
Pant Chari-3	38-42	8-10	Released in 1989 from Pantnagar. It is tall (275-300 cm), thick juicy stems with long and broad leaves. Can be used as dual purpose with 15-20 q/ha seed yield/ha. Suitable for early sowing. Tolerant to foliar diseases.
Pant Chari-4	43-48	12-15	Released in 1995 from Pantnagar. It is tall (300-325 cm), juicy, moderately thick and very sweet stem with dark green foliage; high digestibility and high protein content; tolerant to shoot fly and stem borer. Tolerant to bird damage during seed production due to glume coverage.
Pant Chari-5	47-48	13-14	Released in 1999 from Pantnagar. Dual purpose variety with 18-22 q/ha grain yield, very tall (325-350 cm), thick, juicy and sweet stem. Highly tolerant to foliar diseases.
Pant Chari-7	50-57	18-22	Released in 2010 from Pantnagar. Can be used as dual purpose variety with 18-19 q/ha grain yield, semi-erect stem with high protein content and digestibility, tolerant to major foliar diseases.

Contd...

Table 16.3–*Contd...*

Cultivars	Fodder Yield (t/ha)		Characteristics
	Green	Dry	
K1	–	4.0	Released in 1942 from Kovilpatti for Tamil Nadu state. Crop duration is 115 days. Drought tolerant with pithy and non-juicy stem. Grain yield 1 q/ha
K3	–	6.0	Released from Kovilpatti for southern Tamil Nadu state. Crop duration is 120 days. Stem is non-juicy and pithy. Grain yield 2.5 q/ha.
K7	–	14-15	Released in 1980 from Kovilpatti for Tamil Nadu state. Early with 105 days duration. Stem is juicy and non-pithy with 10.5 per cent TSS content. Grain yield 8-8.5 q/ha.
K10	–	16-17	Released in 1991 from Kovilpatti for Tamil Nadu state. Crop duration is 90 days. Juicy stem, non pithy with a TSS content of 12.5 per cent. Grain yield 10-11 q/ha.
K11	–	18-20	Released during 2001 from Kovilpatti for Tamil Nadu state. Crop duration is 115 days, juicy stem with stay-green traits, non pithy with high TSS content of 16.8 per cent. Grain yield 16 q/ha.
Improved Ramkel	40-50	–	Released during 1998 from Akola for Maharashtra State. Ready for cutting in 75-80 days. Best for *kharif* as well as summer seasons. Grain yield 20-22 q/ha.
GJ 39	–	11-12	Released in 1993 from Surat for Gujarat. It is a dual purpose variety, flowers in 75-80 days, Grain yield 35-40 q/ha
GFS-4	30-35	13-14	Released in 1989 from Surat for Gujarat state. Very early, flowers in 45-50 days, plant height 160-220 cm, low incidence of shoot fly, grain yield 5-6 q/ha.
GFS-5	30-40	14-15	Released in 1999 from Surat for Gujarat state. Early, flowers in 55-57 days, tan plants with juicy stem, grain yield 25-30 q/ha.
CSV 21F	38-41	11-13	Released in 2006 from Surat at national level. Tall (220 cm), flowers in 76 days, leaves are broad and long, tolerant to leaf diseases, shoot fly and stem borer.
Pusa Chari -9	42.5	13.5	Released from IARI, New Delhi. It flowers in 80-85 days. It is medium thick stemmed, non-sweet and pithy. Leaves are long and medium broad with midrib. Panicles are semi-loose, straight but sometimes goose necked. It matures in 120 days and yields 8 q/ha.
Pusa Chari -615	65-70	18-20	Released from IARI, New Delhi in 2005. It flowers in 70 days. Tall plants (300-320 cm). Stems are juicy and sweet with 8.1 per cent protein and 55.3 per cent digestibility.

Contd...

Table 16.3–Contd...

Cultivars	Fodder Yield (t/ha) Green	Dry	Characteristics
Rajasthan Chari-1 (RC-1)	45.0	12.5	Released in 1984 from Udaipur for all India cultivation. It flowers in 80-85 days. Its stem is moderately thick, leaves long and dark green with white midrib. Earheads oblong fully exerted from the flag leaf. Grains are bold and chalky white. It matures for seed in 110-115 day.
Rajasthan Chari - 2 (RC-2)	33.0	10.0	Released from Udaipur for all India cultivation. It flowers in 65-70 days. Plant height 200-260 cm, stem is medium thick, leaves light green having 60-70 cm length and 5-6 cm breadth with white midrib. Plants have 11-13 leaves with drooping habit. Earheads are fully exerted from the leaf. Grains are bold, flat and chalky white. It matures for seed in 100-150 days.
HC 171	45-50	15-16	Released in 1987 from Hisar for all India cultivation. Its stem is sweet and juicy and leaves have green midrib. Panicles are semi compact with small and creamy white seeds. It is highly resistant to most of the foliar diseases being tan pigmented. It is highly resistant to mites. Seed yield 11-12 q/ha.
HC 260	45-50	15-16	Released in 1987 from Hisar for all India cultivation. It becomes ready for fodder in 55-60 days and matures for seed in about 85-90 days. It is non-sweet and juicy. Best suited for 'kadvi' making. Leaves are medium broad and long with white midrib. Its panicles are semi-compact with white seeds. It is resistant to foliar diseases. It gives good seed (13 q/ha).
Haryana Chari-6 (HC-308)	50-55	17-18	Released in 1996 from Hisar for all India cultivation Tall, leafy and medium maturity, stem is sweet and juicy, midrib green, panicle semi compact. Grain yield 14-15 q/ha. highly resistant to all foliar diseases,
HJ 513	50-55	17-18	Released in 2005 from Hisar for Haryana State. Low HCN and high digestibility. Tolerant to gray leaf spot, zonate leaf spot and shooty stripe. Grain yield 16-18 q/ha.
HJ 541	53-55	16-18	Released during 2010 from Hisar for Haryana State. Tolerant to stem borer and shootfly. Stem tall, sweet, leafy and juicy. Low HCN content and high digestibility. Grain yield 14-15 q/ha.
Phule Amruta	45-50	–	Released in 2003 from Rahuri for Maharashtra State. Flowers in 76-80 days, tall leafy plant with long and broad leaves, moderately thick, sweet and juicy stem. High protein and digestibility with low HCN. Tolerant to shoot fly and foliar diseases.

Table 16.4: Multi-Cut Cultivars of Forage Sorghum

Variety/Hybrid	Fodder Yield (t/ha)		Characteristics
	Green	Dry	
M.P. Chari (Variety)	30.0	9.5	Tall, thin stemmed, leaves are moderately long and narrow with white midrib. Non-sweet, non tan, non-juicy and pithy. Takes 65-70 days to become ready for fodder. Panicles are erect and lax with purple or black glumes. Brown coloured grains. Better generation and for two cuttings. Crop matures for seed in about 110 days. Leaf spot disease susceptible.
Meethi Sudan SSG 59-3	75	20	Released at national level in 1978. A popular multi-cut sudan grass, suitable for 4 cuts. It is thin stemmed, sweet with profuse tillering early flower in 55-60 days. Tolerant to drought and water logging. Panicle is laxed with profuse lateral spikes. Seeds purple red coloured with glumes adhered to them. Matures in 95-100 days and yields 10-12 q/ha seed.
Pant Chari 6	60-75	–	Released in 2004 from Pantnagar for Uttarakhand. Plant height 225-250 cm, stem-medium thick, juicy and sweet with 3-4 basal tillers. 2-3 cuts if planted during summer under irrigated conditions. Tolerant to foliar diseases, high digestibility, high protein and low HCN (90-100 ppm). Grain yield 15-18 q/ha.
Pant Chari 8	75-85	25-30	Released in 2010 from Pantnagar for Uttarakhand. Suitable for cultivation during summer under irrigated conditions. Tolerant to major foliar diseases, high digestibility, high protein and low HCN (98 ppm).
COFS 29	170/year	–	Released for Tamil Nadu state. Fast growing multi-cut (5 cuts in a year) variety, with high ratoonability and profuse tillering (10-15 tillers/plant), suitable for ratoon cultivation for 1-2 years in well managed conditions
HC 136	55-60	17-18	Released in 1982 from Hisar for all India cultivation. Suitable for 2 cuts. Good palatibility, sweet, tall, medium thick stem with broad leaves. Remains green till maturity, high protein content with better digestibility, grain yield 12 q/ha.
SL-44	60	–	Released in 1974 from Ludhiana for Punjab state for cultivation during summer and rainy seasons. Stem is sweet, juicy and thin; high digestibility.
Pusa Chari 23	55	16	Released in 1984 from IARI, New Delhi for all India cultivation. Tall (170-175 cm), profuse leaves with lateral branching, thin stem, sudan type, non-sweet and non-juicy. Grain yield 14 q/ha under North Indian conditions.
Jawahar Chari - 69 (JC-69)	50.0	16.5	A multicut sudan type having high regeneration, and faster growth and multicut ability. Its stem is thin and non-sweet and leaves are narrow and long with white midrib. Its panicle is highly laxed with small seeds covered with black or brown glumes.

Contd...

Table 16.4–*Contd...*

Variety/Hybrid	Fodder Yield (t/ha)		Characteristics
	Green	Dry	
Hara Sona (855F) (Hybrid)	60-70	14-15	Released in 1995 for national level cultivation by Proagro Seeds, suitable for 3 cuts, 5-6 tillers, takes 60-65 days to flower, quick in regeneration, stem thins and juicy, plant height 205-220 cm. Resistant to major foliar diseases.
Proagro Chari (SSG 988)	45-50	–	Released in 1991 by Proagro Seeds. Plant height 200-250 cm with 4-6 tillers. Resistant to major foliar diseases and insects.
Safed Moti (FSH 92079)	60-65	–	Released in 1999 by Proagro Seeds for all India cultivation. Plant height 225-230 cm with broad leaves, awned and thick stem.
Punjab Sudex Chari 1 (Hybrid)	115-120	20-22	Released in 1994 for cultivation in Punjab state. Tall plants with long and broad leaves, stem juicy and sweet, suitable for 3-4 cuts, 8-10 tillers under irrigation, takes 60-64 days for flowering, profuse tillering habit, quick regeneration. Resistant to red-leaf spot disease.
Pusa Chari Hybrid (PCH) 106	68-70	18-20	Released from IARI New Delhi in 1996 for all India cultivation. Suitable for 3-4 cuts, profuse tillering, quick regeneration, thin stem, non-tan, plant height 235 cm, flowers in 60-65 days. Has high protein (8.2 per cent) and digestibility (52.7 per cent).
PCH 109	72-75	15-17	Released from IARI New Delhi in 2003 for all India cultivation. Suitable for 3-4 cuts, profuse tillering, quick regeneration, thin stem, non-tan, plant height 235 cm, flowers in 60-65 days. Has high protein (8.6 per cent) and digestibility (52.7 per cent).
GFSH 1	58-65	14-15	Released in 1983 from Anand for cultivation in Gujarat State, Plants are 240-260 cm tall with thick and juicy stem, tolerant to foliar diseases.
CSH 20MF	80-85	24-25	Released in 2005 from Pantnagar for all India cultivation. Tan, dark green heavy foliage with green midrib. Medium thick juicy stem, resistant to foliar diseases, high digestibility 48-55 per cent), protein (7.5-8.5 per cent) and low in HCN content (100-110 ppm).
CSH 24MF	90-92	23-24	Released in 2009 from Pantnagar for all India cultivation. Plant height 200-210 cm, digestibility (55-58 per cent IVDMD), protein (7.5-8.0 per cent) and low HCN (80-95 ppm); thick, juicy and semi-sweet stem with 2-3 tillers, resistant to foliar diseases.
MFSH 3	54-55	14-15	Released in 1989 by MAHYCO for all India cultivation. Plant height 220-240 cm, resistant to major foliar diseases.
MFSH 4	58-64	–	Released by MAHYCO
MFSH 5	61-64	–	Released by MAHYCO
GK 905	64-65	–	Released by Ganga Kaveri Sedds

Table 16.5: Dual Purpose Cultivars for Forage Production

Variety/Hybrid	Fodder Yield (t/ha)		Characteristics
	Green	Dry	
CSV 15 (as fodder variety)	44-45	12-13	It is a dual purpose variety but can be grown as single cut forage variety in North Western India. It is tall, juicy with sweet stem, flowering in 68-70 days, tan, stays green, resistant to leaf spot diseases. Tolerant to grain mold and drought. Its seed can be multiplied in Bundelkhand and Northern MP as a dual purpose variety and sold for fodder purpose.
CSH 13 (as fodder hybrid)	48-50	15-16	Green forage yield as single cut, 10 per cent higher than HC 6, Tan, resistant to leaf spot diseases, juicy stem, early vigour, stays green as multicut, gives more yield in first cut, flowering in 68-70 days.

Multi-Cut

In multi-cut varieties first cut taken 55-60 days after sowing produces higher yield of green fodder. Subsequent cuts may be done at 35-40 days interval. Harvesting of multi-cut forage sorghum should be done, 5-8 cm above ground level to obtain good regeneration after cutting. Harvesting of sudan grass, 5 cm above the ground level produces significantly higher forage yield over 10 cm stubble height. The variety 'HC 136' may give two cuts where first cut can be taken at 75 days and second cut after 90 days of the first cut.

Management of HCN Poisoning

The value of sorghum fodder has increased over the years compared to that of grain. However, one of the major factors limiting the utilization of sorghum fodder is the production of cyanogenic (HCN-producing) glycoside 'dhurrin' that lowers the nutritive value of fodder due to its toxic effects on the feeding livestock (Haskin *et al.*, 1987). Leaves and stems of all sorghum species contain hydrocyanic acid or prussic acid (HCN) glycoside 'dhurrin'. The dhurrin is hydrolyzed in the rumen liberating the toxic HCN. HCN can build up to toxic levels (200 µg/g dry weight is the threshold limit, McBee *et al.*, 1980) in the leaves of forage sorghum. HCN causes death of animals by interfering with the ability of red corpuscles in the blood to transfer oxygen. Muthuswamy *et al.* (1976) estimated the HCN content of CSH 5 sorghum hybrid at different growth stages (Table 16.2). They reported that HCN content was more at the early stage of crop (35 - 40 days stage of crop growth, 8-leaf stage) and decreases gradually with the growth of the crop. Young plants, young branches and tillers contain high levels of HCN. Prussic acid content decreases to non-harmful levels when forage is cut and dried. The HCN in excess of 250 ppm is toxic to livestock. HCN content increases under moisture stress. In most of sorghum varieties, HCN decreases below toxic level after 40 days of the crop growth. If sorghum suffers from drought stress or early frost or if there is a re-growth after frost, the HCN contents may reach to toxic levels for livestock. Under severe moisture stress conditions, nitrate toxicity (Accumulation of nitrate in sorghum plants) may be hazardous to livestock. In summers, the crop should be irrigated 2-3 days before harvesting or else it is safer to harvest crop after flowering. The permissible/safe threshold limit for HCN in sorghum fodder is 200 mg/kg on dry weight basis and 500 mg/kg on fresh weight basis (McBee and Miller, 1980).

Chapter 17

Sorghum Grain Quality and Plant Composition

Grain Quality

Sorghum has been an important staple in the semi-arid tropics of Africa and Asia for centuries. In addition to human consumption, sorghum is also used as an animal feed, particularly in developed countries like the United States, Japan, and Australia. Currently, the demand of sorghum for animal feed is the driving force for sorghum production around the world (FAO, 1995a). Sorghum kernels are generally spherical in shape and come in different sizes and colours.

The basic anatomical components are pericarp (outer layer), germ (embryo), and endosperm (storage tissue). The distribution of these components differs among varieties and environment, with an average of 8 per cent, 82 per cent, and 10 per cent for pericarp, endosperm, and germ, respectively (Hubbard *et al.*, 1950). The pericarp has thickness from 8 to 160 µm and is divided into three layers: epicarp, mesocarp, and endocarp. Endosperm, the major storage tissue, is composed of the aleurone layer, peripheral endosperm, vitreous (hard) endosperm, and floury (soft) endosperm. The aleurone layer is a single layer of cells. Indian sorghum genotypes includes 160 germplasm lines, 200 elite SPV genotypes and 60 released parents, hybrids and many other varieties. These genotypes were analyzed for both physical, and biochemical characters. The physical characters include; a) grain size, b) 100 grains weight c) endosperm texture. The proposed biochemical characters to be evaluated are: per cent starch, per cent protein, per cent fat, per cent *in vitro* protein digestibility, phytic acid content, amylase, starch digestibility, and dietary fiber. The proposed biochemical characters to be evaluated are: a) per cent protein, b) per cent starch, c) per cent fat, d) per cent *in vitro* protein digestibility, e) phytic acid content, f) amylase, g) starch digestibility, and h) dietary fiber.

Protein Body and Protein Matrix Characteristics of Sorghum

Sorghum storage proteins are accumulated inside organelles known as protein bodies. Sorghum protein bodies are circular in shape with diameter of 0.3 to 3.0 μm depending on their location within the kernel (Rooney and Miller, 1982; Taylor *et al.*, 1985). The protein bodies in the peripheral and vitreous- endosperm average 0.3 to 3.0 μm in diameter whereas the ones in the floury endosperm range from 0.3 to 1.5 μm in diameter (Rooney and Miller, 1982). The typical structure of protein bodies is showed in Figure 17.1. It has been observed that the protein bodies are encapsulated by protein matrix. This matrix protein consists mainly of glutelins and small amounts of albumins or globulins (Seckinger and Wolf, 1973). Kafirins by far comprise the majority of the protein inside protein bodies accompanied by a small amount of glutelins and minute amounts of albumins and globulins (Taylor *et al.*, 1984). Using immunocytochemistry and transmission electron microscopy, it was shown that β- and γ- kafirins are located on the core and the periphery of the protein bodies, while the α-kafirin, which makes up about 80 per cent of the total kafirin, is located in the interior (Shull *et al.*, 1992). This distribution is similar to that of zein distribution in corn protein bodies.

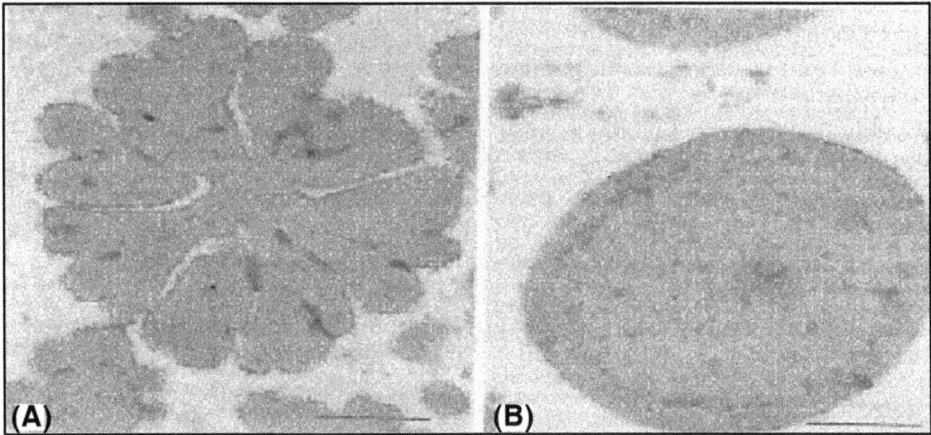

Figure 17.1: Protein Body Structure of Sorghum from Mutant Genotype (A) and Normal Genotype (B) (Oria *et al.*, 2000). Note the folded structure of the mutant protein bodies (A) as compared to the round structure of the normal protein bodies (B).

Recently, Oria *et al.* (2000) identified a unique structure of protein bodies from a high protein digestibility sorghum mutant genotype. These protein bodies were irregular in shape and had crevices that reached the center of the structure forming lobes (Figure 17.1A). In the mutant, α-kafirin was still the major protein of the protein bodies, with β-kafirin mainly found distributed in the lobes and γ-kafirin concentrated at the base of the crevices. This structure resulted in the rapidly digesting α-kafirin protein exposed to proteases and is the basis for the high protein digestibility of this genotype.

Digestibility of Uncooked Sorghum Proteins

It is well accepted that sorghum has lower protein digestibility compared to other cereal grains (MacLean et al., 1981; Hamaker et al., 1987). The low protein digestibility characteristic is more prominent in cooked than uncooked sorghum (Axtell et al., 1981; Hamaker et al., 1987). Although protein digestibility of uncooked sorghum is only slightly lower than corn, it is still considered to affect its feed grain value especially for non-ruminant animals. Ruminants, likes cattle and sheep, have micro floras in their rumen that have the ability to convert poor quality protein and non-protein nitrogen into quality protein. As for non-ruminants, like pigs and poultry, the quality and quantity of the protein from cereal-based diets is important because it contributes approximately 30-50 per cent of the dietary protein required by the animals (Bramel-Cox et al., 1995).

One of the first factors identified as a cause of low protein digestibility in sorghum were polyphenolic compounds known as tannins. Tannins can bind proteins and render them indigestible by proteases (Butler et al., 1984). Tannins also interact with protein digesting enzymes (proteases) and inhibit their activity (Butler et al., 1981, 1996; Weaver et al., 1998), indicating that tannin is not the only factor that affects protein digestibility of sorghum. Hamaker et al. (1987) proposed that the comparably low protein digestibility of low tannin sorghum genotypes is due to the composition and structure of protein bodies and accessibility to interior proteins by digestive proteases. Additional detailed studies on protein bodies indicated that the γ- and possibly β-kafirins, which are high in cysteine, form disulfide bonded polymers around the periphery of the protein body, thus limiting the access of the enzyme to the α-kafirin in the interior of the protein bodies (Oria et al., 1995a,b; Weaver et al., 1998). This theory is supported by recent findings by Oria et al. (2000) for the mutant genotype with high protein digestibility. In this mutant genotype, the exposed α-kafirin - the major storage protein, and the position of the β- and γ- kafirins at the base of the highly folded structure allowed proteases to reach and hydrolyze α-kafirin directly, thus giving higher protein digestibility value.

Starch

Starch is the storage form of energy in cereals and usually makes up 60 per cent to 75 per cent of the total weight of cereal grains. It is found in plants in the form of granules. Starch granules are made up of two distinct components of glucose polymers: amylose and amylopectin.

Amylose

Before 1950, amylose was believed to be a completely linear polymer of D-glucopyranosyl units. However, in the early 50's a study (Peat et al., 1952) showed that amylose is not completely hydrolyzed into maltose when treated with crystalline β-amylase, indicating that amylose is not entirely linear. In 1966, Banks and Greenwood concluded the presence of α- (1→6) side-chains with considerable length using bacterial pullulanase as the debranching enzyme. In a more recent study, Cura et al. (1995) confirmed that the branching linkages in amylose are indeed that of α - (1→6). Takeda et al. (1987) found, depending on the source, 3 to 10 branch points per amylose molecule. It is now widely accepted that amylose consists of the linear polymer of (1→4) linked α-D-glucopyranosyl units with lightly branched side chains joined by (1→6)-α-linkage.

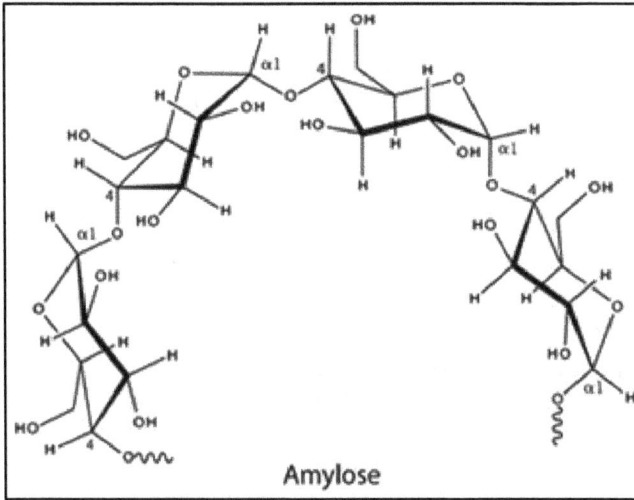

Figure 17.2: Segment of Amylose Chain. The glucopyranosyl units are connected by α-(1→4) linkages (printed with permission from Dr. Martin Chaplin. South Bank University, London).

Figure 17.2 illustrates the un-branched portion of the amylose molecule. The side chains are either very long or very short and are located far from one another. Since the building block of amylose is the chair (4C1) conformer of the glucose molecule, a helical twist is imparted on amylose. In the interior of the helix, starch hydroxyl groups are hydrogen bound to each other which both stabilizes the helix and makes it relatively hydrophobic. The molecular weight of amylose depends on the botanical source of the starch and the extraction methods (Ong *et al.*, 1994). The average molecular weight of amylose is about 1.3 × 106 to 9 × 106 Daltons (Ong *et al.*, 1994).

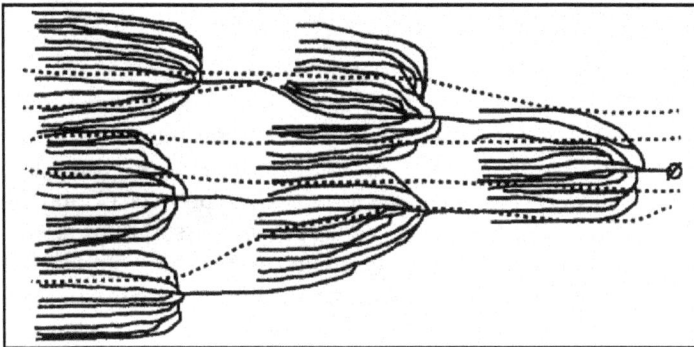

Figure 17.3: Proposed Location of Amylose in Starch Granules (adapted from Kemesuwan and Jane, 1994). Dotted line = Amylose and solid line = amylopectin.

By making several assumptions, Buléon *et al.* (1998) calculated the number of amylose chains inside a single granule to be approximately 1.8×109. Although the structure of amylose is well established, its location is still not well understood. Two theories have emerged: one states that amylose is found in bundles between amylopectin molecules (Nikuni, 1978; Blanshard, 1986; Zobel, 1992) while the other theory declares that amylose is arbitrarily scattered among amylopectin molecules (Jane *et al.*, 1992; Kamesuwan and Jane, 1994). Figure 17.3 (Kamesuwan and Jane, 1994) depicts the location of amylose based on the latter theory.

Amylopectin

Amylopectin, the counterpart of amylose, is the major component of starch by weight and one of the largest molecules found in nature. It too is composed of linear chains of $(1\rightarrow4)$ linked α-D-glucopyranosyl units but with a much greater extent of α-$(1\rightarrow6)$ branching than amylose.

These branch points make up approximately 4 per cent to 6 per cent of total linkages (Hood, 1982). Peat *et al.* (1952) proposed that amylopectin consists of three different types of chains. The A chains, also known as the un-branched chains, are the linear segments joined to other chains by a single $(1\rightarrow6)$ -α- linkage. The B chains are those connected to other chains via α- $(1\rightarrow6)$ linkages and also carry one or more A or B chains attached to them. The C chain is the single, central chain that carries the only reducing group of the amylopectin molecule.

Tannins and Phenols of Sorghum Grain

All sorghums contain phenols, which can affect the colour, appearance and nutritional quality of grain and sorghum products. The phenolic compounds can be divided in to three basic groups' phenolic acids, flavonoids and tannins. All sorghum contains phenolic acids and most contain flavonoids. Only the brown high tannin, bird resistant sorghums contain condensed tannins.

Many phenolic acids inhibit the growth of microorganisms and may impart resistance to grain moulds before and after grain maturity. Phenolic acids apparently do act adversely affect the nutritional quality of sorghum grain, but they may form undesirable colours under certain food processing conditions, such as alkaline conditions used in the making of tortillas.

Flavonoids are the largest group of phenols in the plant kingdom. Flavonoid compounds consist of two distinct units: A C6-C3 fragment from cinnamic acid forms the β-ring, and a C6 fragment from malonyl –CoA forms the α-ring the three major groups of flavonoids are the flavonols and flavans: the major group of flavonoids sorghum are the flavans. Flavan-3-en-3-ols (double bond between C5 and C4 hydroxyl at C3) are called anthocyanidins and are the major flavans in sorghum. Anthocyanidins are primarily in their ionized form (flavylium in sorghum on double bond between C5 and C4 hydroxyl at C3) are called anthocyanidins and are the major flavans in sorghum. Anthocyanidins are found primarily and in their ionized form flavylium on double bond between C2-C3 and C-O, hydroxyl at C3 positive charge at position 1. The flavylium ion is primarily responsible for the intense red pigmentation of anthocyanidins in acid medium. Flavan-3-ols (hydroxyl at C3) are called catechins or 4-deoxyleuco-anthocyanidinsflavan-3, 4-diols (hydroxyl at C3 and C4) are called leucoanthocyanidins. When treated with mineral acid, the colourless leucoanthocyanidins produced red anthocyanidins. In plants anthocyanidins and leucoanthocyanidins exist often as glucosides at the 3 or 7 position and are called anthocyanidins and leucoanthocyanidins respectively. Anthocyanidins are the major pigments in many flowers, stalks, and leaves. The colour depends on the pH and substitution on the β-ring. Many plant colours in the orange to blue region are caused by co-pigmentation of anthocyanidins with metal ion and other phenolic compounds.

Anthocyanidins are very unstable in acid medium and are readily converted to their corresponding anthocyanidin in even slightly acidic solvents. This makes it difficult to determine whether a pigment is the anthocyanin or anthocyanidin. Both types of pigments have been reported in sorghum. Luteolindine and apigeninidin are actually 3-deoxyanthocyanidins and would be produced from a flavan-4-ol rather than a flavan-3, 4-diol. The flavan-4-ol apiforol a precursor for apigeninidin has been found in sorghum leaf tissue and grains. The pericarp colour of sorghum appears to be due to a combination of primarily anthocyanin and anthocyanidins pigments and other flavonoidin compounds. There appears to be a good deal of variation between sorghum of the same genetic pericarp colour. The most abundant polyphenols are the condensed tannins, Lignins, Catechol melanins, Flavolans found in virtually all families of plants, and comprising up to 50 per cent of the dry weight of leaves.

Some polyphenols produced by plants in case of pathogens attacks are called phytoalexins. Such compounds can be implied in the hypersensitive response of plants. High levels of polyphenols in some woods can explain their natural preservation against rot.

Forage Composition

Forage quality is very important for palatability and acceptability or animal intake. Forage sorghums differ widely in chemical composition and nutritive value, both of which are genetically controlled. Plant morphology, anatomical components, digestibility, protein, mineral, cellulose and lignin contents, and anti-nutritional factors like hydrocyanic acid determine animal preference, milk and meat production (Hanna, 1993). Some of the characters for improving the fodder yield and quality include:

☆ Higher leaf-stem ratio (better digestibility)

☆ Juicy and sweet stalk (more cell soluble- nitrogen and sugars)

☆ Brown midrib (high digestibility of the vegetative material due to low lignin)

☆ Tan plant colour (low polyphenol content and greater resistance to foliar diseases)

☆ Bloomless (aid rumen degradation)

☆ Glossiness (to reduce wax load on leaf surface)

☆ Good leafiness

☆ Green leaf retention

☆ High IVDMD

☆ Good protein content

☆ Low tannin content (reduce interference with protein digestion)

☆ Low HCN-p (minimize prussic acid poisoning)

Although most forage quality parameters appear to be quantitatively inherited (Bramel-Cox *et al.*, 1995), several simply inherited qualitative characters have significant impact on forage quality such as juiciness, sweetness, plant colour, bloom and so on. However, the impact of one single-gene trait, brown mid-rib (bmr), is very great on quality. Generally good quality forage is high in protein and digestible nutrients, and low in fiber and lignin.

a. Chemical Composition (Per cent of dry matter) of Sorghum Fodder*

Protein per cent	:	6-8
Sugar per cent	:	8-17
Dry matter per cent (at flowering)	:	20-35
Dry matter digestibility per cent	:	45-60
Mineral content (per cent)	:	
Calcium	:	0.53
Phosphorous	:	0.24
Fiber content per cent	:	30-32
Neutral detergent fiber (NDF per cent)	:	65-72
Acid detergent fiber (ADF per cent)	:	40-45
Lignin	:	7.6
Cellulose	:	34.6
Silica	:	2.2
Hemicellulose	:	26.3
Cell content	:	29.3

Source: Singh *et al*. (1977)

The stage of crop growth is the most important factor that influences the quality and quantity of forage produced. Maximum green fodder with highest nutritive value is obtained at 50 per cent flowering stage. Advancing harvesting time lowers leaf/stem ratio and increases lignifications of forage. Crude protein concentrations, digestibility and intake would be significantly reduced with the maturity of the forage. Sweet sorghum with its high palatability for the animal can be used as forage. It can also be used in the silage preparation (Marco *et al.*, 2009; Mohammed and Mohammed, 2009).

b. Brown Midrib Sorghum

Grass midribs are typically whitish green in colour. Mutations of maize, sorghum and pearl millet have been identified that result in a brown midrib. Brown midrib trait is controlled by a single recessive gene. The significance of the mutation is that plant tissues have less lignin than normal tissues, and digestibility of bmr genotypes is higher than normal genotypes (Table 17.1). The extent of lignin reduction due to the presence of this gene is upto 51 per cent in the stem, and 25 per cent in leaves (Porter *et al.*, 1978). There are alleles (mutants) for this gene with variable effect on reduction of lignin quantity (Bout and Vermerris, 2003). Lignin inhibits fibre digestibility, which reduces milk production in dairy animals. Research revealed that brown midrib sorghum silage has 17 per cent less lignin than regular sorghum silage thereby making it more digestible.

Table 17.1: Forage Quality of Brown Midrib and Normal Sorghum

Component	Normal (g/kg)	Brown Midrib (g/kg)	Significance
Nitrogen	19	21	ns
IVDMD[1]	568	642	p<0.01
NDF[2]	704	678	p<0.01
Cellulose	311	307	p<0.01
Hemicellulose	337	325	ns
Lignin	55	43	p<0.01

Source: Cherney *et al.* (1991). 1= IVDMD, *in vitro* dry matter digestibility; 2-NDF= Neutral detergent fiber.

The breeding challenge for sorghum would be to introduce bmr trait into hybrids which are acceptable and competitive in the market place.

c. Antinutritional Factors

Sorghum is relatively an unique forage that can be acutely toxic to livestock under certain environmental or management conditions. Livestock deaths are known to occur due to lack of awareness of factors causing toxic compounds to accumulate in forage sorghum, or mismanagement of sorghum forage making it potentially toxic to livestock (Pedersen and Fritz 2000). Sorghum contains tannins, nitrates and HCN that affect forage quality adversely.

Tannin Content

Tannins cause bitterness and affect the palatability and digestibility in forage sorghum. It varies from 0.1 to 6.2 per cent as catechin equivalent on dry weight in sorghum grains, while in fodder plants from 0.3 to 2.9 per cent. In fodder plant, it decreased after 20 days of growth and again increased at 50 – 55 days of growth with concomitant increase of soluble sugars. Leaves contain higher amount of tannin than the stems. A significant negative relationship exists between tannin content and digestibility. The tannin content has also been found to increase with the severity of leaf spot disease in forage sorghum, resulting in marked decrease in digestibility of sorghum leaves.

Nitrate

Like other C4 forages (maize and pearl millet), sorghum is known to be a nitrate accumulator. Most of the soil nitrogen absorbed by plant roots is in nitrate form. Normally, nitrate in a plant is rapidly converted to amino acids by the enzyme nitrate reductase. This reduction requires energy from sunlight, adequate water, nutrients and favourable temperature. When plants are stressed, the nitrate to protein conversion is disrupted and nitrates begin to accumulate. Under certain environmental and managerial conditions sorghum can accumulate potentially toxic nitrate levels. Heavy nitrogen fertilization, especially late in the growing season, increases the likelihood of nitrate accumulation. Nitrates normally are highest in young plant growth; however concentrations remain high in mature sorghum and sudan grass. Ruminant livestock convert nitrate to nitrite then to ammonia, which is then synthesized into protein by microbes present in the rumen. Excess nitrite enters the bloodstream and changes haemoglobin to methemoglobin, which is incapable of carrying oxygen (Rasby *et al.*, 1996). Generally if forages contain more than 6,000 ppm nitrate, they should be considered potentially toxic (Table 17.2).

Table 17.2: Levels of Nitrate in Forage (Dry matter basis) and Potential Effect on Animals

Nitrate (ppm)	Effects on Animals
0 – 3,000	Virtually safe
3,000 – 6,000	Moderately safe in most situations; limit use for stressed animals to 50 per cent of the total ration.
6,000 – 9,000	Potentially toxic to cattle depending on the situation; should not be the only source of feed.
9,000 and above	Dangerous to cattle and often will cause death.

HCN (Prussic Acid) Poisoning

Prussic acid is also known as hydrocyanic acid or hydrogen cyanide (HCN). Prussic acid poisoning is caused by cyanide production in all types of sorghum and its closely related species, under certain growing conditions. It is found in sorghum at early stage of 30-35 days of crop growth and decreases gradually with the crop growth. HCN levels exceeding 500 ppm on a wet weight basis are dangerous (Table 17.3). On a dry weight basis, forages with more than 200 ppm HCN should be considered potentially toxic. The hydrogen cyanide potential (HCNp; mg HCN/kg plant dry matter) of forage sorghums typically ranges from 100 to 800 ppm.

Factors affecting HCNp in forage sorghums include genotype, plant age, plant morphology, environmental stress (such as drought, frost, and light intensity), and soil fertility (Fjell *et al.*, 1991). HCN content increases under moistures stress. After 45 days of crop growth, the HCN content reduces below the toxic level. Strategies to avoid HCN poisoning include:

☆ Select a cultivar that is low in HCNp

☆ Avoid grazing on sudan grasses or sorghum sudan grass hybrids until they reach 38 to 46 cm in height or forage sorghums until they reach 61 cm in height

☆ Avoid grazing forage sorghum pastures that have been damaged by frost or drought.

☆ In summer season, crop should be irrigated 2-3 days before harvesting or else it is safer to harvest crop after flowering.

Table 17.3: Levels of Prussic Acid in Sorghum (Wet matter basis) and Potential Effect on Animals

HCN (ppm)	Effects on Animals
0 – 500	Generally safe, should not cause toxicity
600 – 1000	Potentially toxic, should not be the only source of feed.
Above 1000	Dangerous to cattle and usually will cause death.

Leaving the green fodder 3-4 hours in sun after harvest also helps to reduce HCN content.

Chapter 18

Sorghum as Bioenergy Crop (Sweet Sorghum)

Sorghum has great potential as an annual bioenergy crop. Sorghum is morphologically diverse, with grain sorghum being of relatively short stature and grown for grain, while forage and sweet sorghums are tall and grown primarily for their biomass. Sweet sorghum was first introduced into the United States in 1852. With the increase in global fuel process in the past few years and also the environmental pollution, there has been growing interest in supplementing fossil fuel supplies with biofuels (fuels that come from plants). By blending petrol (gasoline) with ethanol from sweet sorghum, developing countries can save on valuable foreign exchange spent on importing petrol and also benefit the environment. In India, the replacement of just 20 per cent of the grain sorghum crop with sweet sorghum would meet the nation's target for ethanol for a 10 per cent blend of ethanol in petrol. Sweet sorghum is the same species (*Sorghum bicolor* L. Moench.) as grain sorghum, but has high sugar content (10-15 per cent) in the stalks similar to sugarcane. Although sweet sorghum is primarily grown to produce sorghum syrup, but being a water-use efficient crop, it has the potential to be a good alternative feedstock for ethanol production. It is a multi-purpose crop which can be cultivated for simultaneous production, of grain from its ear head as food and feed ingredients, sugary juice from its stalk for making syrup, jaggery, or ethanol, and bagasse and green foliage as an excellent fodder for animals, as organic fertilizer, or for paper manufacturing.

Government of India's decision to blend 10 per cent ethanol in petrol and 5 per cent ethanol in diesel requires about 1.0 billion litres and 2.80 billion litres of ethanol, respectively. Thus, the country's ethanol deficit is about 3 billion litres/year/annum. Hence, it is suggested that sweet sorghum is the best alternative feedstock for bioethanol production.

In favourable environments, sweet sorghum varieties can grow 3 meter tall and produce 50-125 tons of biomass (fresh weight) per hectare. Like grain sorghum, sweet sorghum is also grown during rainy and post-rainy seasons. The productivity of sweet sorghum in post-rainy (*rabi*) (October-November planted) season is 30-35 per cent less than that in rainy (*kharif*) and summer seasons because of short day length and low night temperatures. In order to meet the industry demand for raw materials especially during lean periods of sugar cane crushing, there is a need to develop sweet sorghum cultivars that are photoperiod and thermo-insensitive with high stalk and sugar yields. The production technologies are similar to that of grain sorghum.

Adaptation and Growing Conditions

Sweet sorghum can be grown under dryland conditions with annual rainfall ranging from 550 to 800 mm. Air temperatures suitable for its growth vary between 15 and 37°C. Sorghum being a C_4 tropical grass adapted to latitudes ranging from 40°N to 40°S of equator.

Planting Time and Method

Planting time significantly affects sweet sorghum cane yield and quality parameters. Sweet sorghum can be grown during *kharif, rabi* and summer seasons depending upon the availability of soil moisture/irrigation sources and with suitable temperature regimes.

Kharif Season Crop (June–October)

Sowing should be taken immediately after the onset of monsoon, preferably from first week of June to first week of July, (depending on the onset of monsoon). Delay in sowing reduces cane yield, juice yield and ethanol production (Rao *et al.*, 2013) (Table 18.1). Seeds (two to three) should be sown in a furrow, opened by the bullock drawn plough or locally available implement. In the ridges and furrow method, planting is done on the top or side of the ridge at 5 cm depth at a distance of 10-15 cm by hand dibbling. In this method, the rainwater is conserved in the furrow and avoids runoff. It should be made sure that soil is fully charged with rainwater or irrigation at least in the top 0-15 cm soil (plough layer) in order to ensure good and uniform germination and seedling emergence.

Rabi Season Crop (October–February)

Planting should be done from last week of September to first week of November. The night temperatures should be above 15°C at the time of sowing. Irrigate the crop if there is no rainfall at the time of sowing to ensure uniform germination and establishment. The planting method followed is ridges and furrow method to conserve irrigation water is similar to kharif season crop.

Summer Season Crop

Planting is done from mid-January to mid-March under supplemental irrigated conditions. The night temperatures should be above 15°C at the time of sowing. Summer planting will enable to realize excellent cane yield, provided irrigation water is available. The planting method followed is ridges and furrow method to conserve irrigation water as similar to *kharif* season crop.

Table 18.1: Influence of Planting Dates on Various Traits of Rainy Season Sweet Sorghum

Traits	Planting Dates					
	1 June	16 June	1 July	16 July	1 August	LSD (P=0.05)
Plant height (cm)	363	378	303	268	240	106
Fresh total biomass (t/ha)	80.5	70.6	50.6	29.4	28.3	18.5
Fresh stalk yield (t/ha)	58.1	44.0	30.7	21.5	18.0	16.7
Juice yield (t/ha)	27.8	19.4	15.6	10.2	7.9	12.3
Juice extraction (per cent)	48.5	46.8	51.2	50.0	43.3	NS
Juice brix (per cent)	14.9	16.5	16.2	15.3	15.0	NS
Total soluble sugar (per cent)	12.6	13.4	13.1	10.8	11.1	NS
Reducing sugar (per cent)	1.47	1.50	1.58	2.05	1.68	NS
Sucrose content (per cent)	109	11.8	11.2	8.5	9.3	NS
Sugar yield (t/ha)	3.30	2.61	2.01	1.17	0.83	0.80
Ethanol yield (t/ha)	1758	1373	1070	624	495	423

Source: Rao *et al.* (2013).

Soil Type and Depth

Deep black soil (Vertisol) or deep red loamy soil (Alfisol), with a soil depth of ≥1.0 m deep are most suitable. Planting on light shallow soils should be avoided. The ideal pH range is 5.5-8.5.

Seed Rate and Seed Treatment

A seed rate of 8-10 kg/ha. Seeds should be treated with carbendazim or thirum @ 2 g/kg seed and with azospirillum @ 100 g/10 kg seed. Seeds should also be treated with 2 per cent KH_2PO_4 for 6 hours as pre sowing treatment under rainfed condition. If a planter is used for sowing, then the existing seed rate can be further reduced.

Spacing

Row to row distance should be: 45-60 cm and plant to plant distance should be 12-15 cm. Sowing can be done on ridges and furrows. Three to four seeds are dibbled in each hill/planting hole and the seedlings are to be finally thinned to one per hill.

Plant Population

The optimum plant population for sweet sorghum is 1.10 to 1.20 lakh plants/ha (40000 to 48000 plants/acre). Excessive plant population leads to lodging during heavy winds or rains due to thiner and weaker stem.

Thinning

Thinning operation is very essential in sweet sorghum for uniform stand establishment and growth of plants. Improper thinning results in very thin stalks of uneven size leading to crop lodging and low stalk yields. Lack of crop uniformity will also pose problem in harvesting. First thinning should be done in about 15 days after planting (DAP) and retain two seedlings per hill at 15 cm apart and second and final thinning in about 20-25 DAP, retaining single plant per hill.

De-tillering

Tillers are produced mainly due to planting in late Rabi (Octo-Dec) coupled with low temperature during the early vegetative stage. Basal tillers should be removed manually within 20-25 days from planting.

Intercultivation or Hoeing

Intercultivation should be done, with blade harrow or cultivator once or twice between 20 to 35 days after sowing. The second interculturing should be followed by earthling up of crop rows with bullock or tractor drawn implements to prevent crop lodging.

Irrigation and Nutrient Management

Irrigation should be based on available soil moisture, which depends on the type of soil and the rainfall distribution. During rainy season the areas receiving 550-800 mm rainfall with proper distribution do not require irrigation. Irrigation is required if the dry spell continues for more than two weeks especially at critical crop growth stages such as panicle initiation (35-40 DAS) and boot stages (55-65 DAS). In winter season, 2-3 irrigations, each at 30-35 DAS, 50-55 DAS and at 65-70 DAS are required for realizing good stalk yield. However in summer season, a minimum of 6 to 7 irrigations are required with an interval of 7-10 days.

Recommended dose of fertilizer for soils with normal fertility level is 100-120 kg nitrogen, 40kg phosphorus and 40 kg potassium. Half of N and whole of P and K are applied as basal. Remaining N is to be top-dressed during 30-35 days after manual weeding or intercultivation. Miri *et al*. (2012) reported that stalk yield and fodder yield increased significantly only up to 100 kg N/ha, while fermentable sugar, estimated ethanol, and grain yields responded up to 150 kg N/ha (Table 18.2). There was a significant interaction between N levels and sweet sorghum cultivars for juice, ethanol and grain yields.

Weed Management

Similar to grain sorghum.

Improved Cultivars

Currently available crop cultivars in India are CSH 22SS, SSV84, SSV74, and CSV 19SS from public sector and Madhura, SPSSV 11 (PAC 52093) and SPSSV 30 (Urja) from private sector. A list of promising hybrids and varieties of sweet sorghum with their yield and quality parameters is given in Table 18.3.

Table 18.2: Interaction Effects of Nitrogen × Genotypes on Juice Yield, Estimated Ethanol Yield and Grain Yield of Sweet Sorghum (Miri *et al.*, 2012)

Genotype	Nitrogen Levels (kg/ha)			
	0	50	100	150
Juice yield (KL/ha)				
RSSV 9	17.2	18.6	23.7	26.2
SSV 84	106	1302	15.6	17.8
CSH 22SS	19.7	24.5	36.0	39.8
CD (P = 0.05) = 3.18				
Estimated ethanol yield (KL/ha)				
RSSV 9	1.52	1.68	2.21	2.39
SSV 84	0.90	1.13	1.36	1.54
CSH 22SS	1.67	2.12	3.17	3.47
CD (P = 0.05) = 0.30				
Grain yield (t/ha)				
RSSV 9	1.13	1.70	2.20	2.51
SSV 84	1.01	1.51	1.91	2.10
CSH 22SS	1.32	2.12	2.92	3.31

Harvesting Management

Crop should be harvested in about 35-40 days after flowering of the plants *i.e.*, at physiological maturity of grain where black spot appears on lower end (hylar end) of the grain. Alternately, the brix of standing crop can be measured using hand Refractometer as similar to sugarcane crop. The methodology of pre-harvest crop quality survey and assessment as followed for sugarcane (*i.e.* use of Refractometer) is recommended for sweet sorghum also. Crop should be harvested if stalk brix reaches to about 16-18 per cent at physiological maturity of the grain. Influence of stage of harvesting on changes in stalk yield, quality, bioethanol yields and biomass indicated that fresh stalk yield increased from flowering to soft-dough stage and then declined until maturity. Harvesting at soft-dough stage gave maximum stalk yields, and CSH22SS yielded highest (39.0 t/ha) than others. There was 10 per cent increase in bioethanol yields when sweet sorghum was harvested at hard-dough stage than when it was at physiological maturity (Table 18.4) and cv CSH22SS recorded highest bioethanol yield (AICSIP 2006 and 2007).

For cost-effective harvesting, it is advantageous to have an extended harvest season or, in the case of an area which is also growing sugar cane, to have the sorghum harvest season offset from the sugar cane harvest season and thereby be able to utilize sugar cane harvesters that would otherwise be idle. Sweet sorghum is similar to sugar cane and thus, the juice (sugar) in the stalk needs to be processed fairly rapidly otherwise, the sugars in the stalk are lost. Reddy *et al.* (2008) show data on how the amount of sugar decreases over the course of four days (Table 18.5).

Table 18.3: Performance of Released Hybrids and Varieties of Sweet Sorghum

Cultivars	Year of Release	Plant Height (m)	Grain Yield (t/ha)	Cane Yield (t/ha)	Ethanol Yield (Litre/ha)	Duration (Days)	Juice (per cent)	Brix (per cent)	Adoptation (Season)
(A) HYBRIDS									
CSH22SS	2005	3.5	1.5-2.0	42-45	1100	115-125	35-40	16-17	Irrigated areas of *Kharif* season
(B) VARIETIES									
SSV 84	1992	2.8	2.2-2.5	35-40	1000	120-125	40-45	17-18	Suitable for *Kharif* season
SSV 74	1999	3.6	2.0-2.1	40-42	1100	125-130	40-45	17-18	Suitable for *Kharif* season
CSV 19 SS	2004	3.6	0.8-1.0	40-45	1000	115-120	32-36	16-17	Suitable for *Kharif* season
PAC52093	2005	3.6	1.5-2.0	40-45	1000	115-120	35-36	16-17	Suitable for *Kharif* season

Table 18.4: Influence of stage of harvesting on calculated bioethanol yield in sweet sorghum.

Cultivar/ Stage of Harvest	At 50 per cent Flowering	At Soft-dough (15DAF)	At Hard-dough (30DAF)	At Physiological Maturity	Cultivar Mean
		Calculated bioethanol yield (L ha⁻¹)			
SSV84	457	613	674	642	596
CSH22SS	715	850	948	864	844
CSV19SS	461	635	661	563	580
PAC52093	554	835	872	816	769
Treat. mean	547	733	789	721	697
CD (P = 0.05)					
Stage of harvest	215				
Cultivar	215				
Interaction	NS				

DAF: Days After Flowering.

Table 18.5: Effect of Crushing Time on Juice Extraction, Brix and Sugar Yield in Sweet Sorghum (Reddy *et al.*, 2008)

Crushing (Days after harvest)	Juice Extraction (L x 10³ ha⁻¹)	Brix Reading	Sugar Yield (Mg ha⁻¹)	Sugar Reduction from Harvest Day (per cent)
0	42.4	18.5	2.62	–
1	40.6	19.2	2.47	5.7
2	35.0	20.9	2.18	16.8
3	37.6	21.4	2.20	16.0

De-trashing

After harvesting the plants, leaves should be removed manually similar to that of sugarcane crop.

Chapter 19
Sorghum in Rice-Fallows

In recent years, sorghum cultivation in rice-fallows during late-*rabi* is gaining popularity in coastal Andhra Pradesh, especially in Guntur and adjoining Krishna and Prakasham districts due to insufficient water for second crop of rice. The farmers are planting sorghum after harvest of rice in mid-December under zero-tillage to utilize the residual soil moisture. The crop is harvested during first week of April. Usually, farmers grow pulses (greengram and blackgram) in rice-fallows of the Krishna-Godavari zone of Andhra Pradesh as *utera* cropping (broadcasting of seeds in standing crop of rice). This practice helps the farmers to harness the residual moisture (Singh, 2007), and at the same time increasing nitrogen content in soil by biological nitrogen fixation. However, in the recent times, the area under pulses has declined due to late planting of rice and severe attack of viral diseases and parasitic weed *Cuscuta* (Mishra *et al.*, 2009). The farmers of the coastal area with assured irrigation facilities have now shifted to maize and those with limited irrigation, to sorghum. The area under sorghum in rice-fallows has increased from 2000 ha in 2005-06 to more than 24000 ha during 2012-13 (Figure 19.1), with an average productivity of 6.5 t/ha, which is, highest in the country. Sorghum also requires fewer inputs such as nutrients and plant protection measures as compared to maize. Farmers of the area are harvesting up to 6-7 t/ha sorghum grains depending upon management practices. Keeping in view the scarcity of water for irrigation in future, the area under sorghum cultivation is expected to increase.

Production Technology

Cultivars

In rice-fallows of coastal Andhra Pradesh, sorghum is grown for grain purpose. The hybrids are preferred over varieties due to their high yields. Mishra *et al.* (2009) evaluated thirteen sorghum cultivars including hybrids and varieties in rice-fallows under zero tillage at farmer's field in Guntur district of Andhra Pradesh and reported

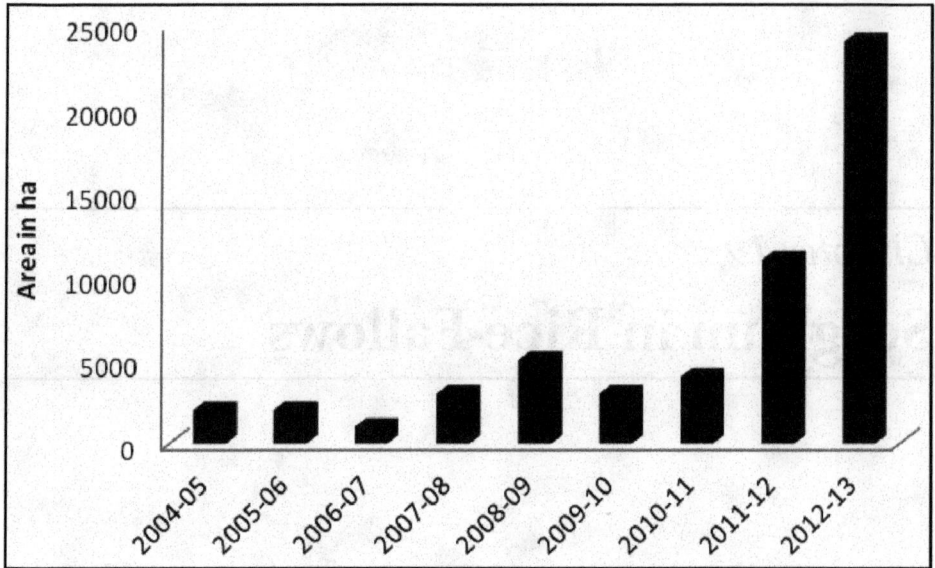

Figure 19.1: Sorghum Area in Rice-Fallows in Guntur District of Coastal Andhra Pradesh.

that, sorghum hybrids, 'Sudama 333' (8.44 tonnes/ha), 'CSH 16' (7.80 tonnes/ha), 'MJ 4334' (7.37 tonnes/ha) and 'MRS 4094' (7.14 tonnes/ha) were promising. Chapke *et al.* (2011) demonstrated the performance of sorghum hybrids in rice-fallows at farmer's fields in Guntur district and found that hybrids NSH 27 (7.57 t/ha), CSH 16 (7.43 t/ha), Kaveri 6363 (7.4 t/ha), Mahalaxmi (7.11 t/ha), and SBSH 151 (6.97 t/ha) registered higher grain yield (Table 19.1).

Table 19.1: Plant Height, Yield and Yield Attributes of Sorghum Hybrids in Rice-Fallows in the Farmers' Fields in Guntur District

Hybrid	Plant Height (cm)	Panicles/ m²	Panicle Length (cm)	Grains/ Panicle	Grain Weight/ Panicle (g)	100-grain Weight (g)	Grain Yield (t/ha)
NSH 27	163	15.1	29.6	2951	54.7	2.58	7.57
CSH 16	174	18.4	30.7	2471	50.1	2.66	7.43
Kaveri 6363	163	17.4	28.4	2780	52.8	2.46	7.40
Mahalaxmi	146	17.2	28.9	2352	46.9	2.55	7.11
SBSH 151	171	15.8	28.5	2446	49.5	2.88	6.97
CSH 15R	251	16.2	26.7	1948	41.4	2.86	5.95
CSH 23	155	17.9	25.4	2498	36.8	2.41	5.39
CD (P=0.05)	19	3.6	1.9	611.63	8.3	0.36	0.92

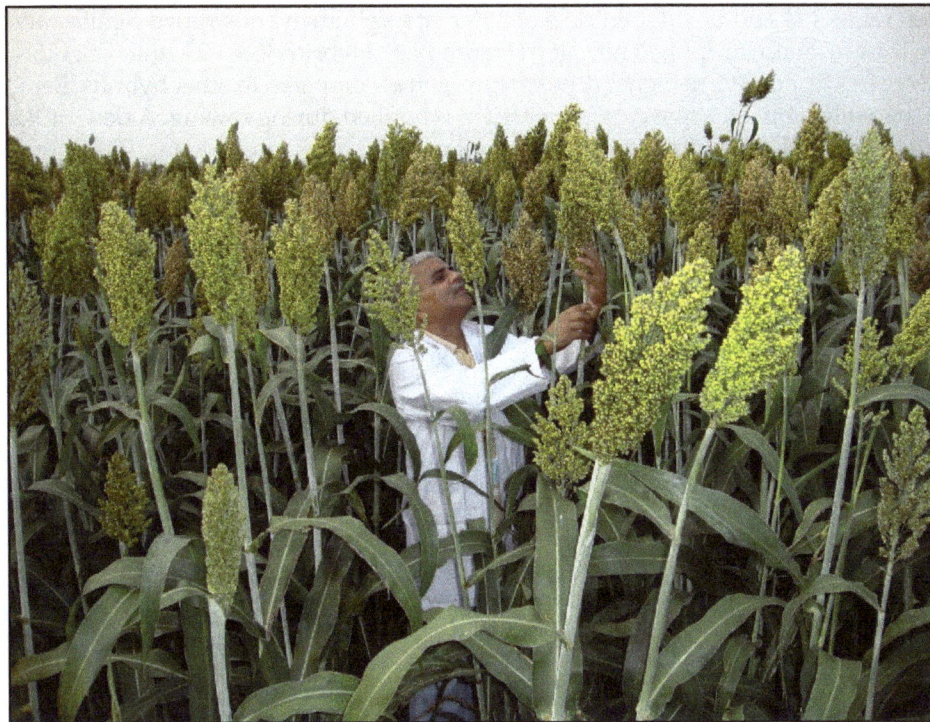

Figure 19.2: Performance of Sorghum Hybrid CSH 16 in Rice-Fallows.

Time of Sowing

The time of sowing sorghum in rice-fallows depends solely on the time of *kharif* paddy harvesting as the crop is sown on the residual soil moisture. In general, 2nd to 3rd week of December is an ideal time. Delayed sowing in January affects the seed setting and grain filling due to high temperature in March and April. Sometimes unusual rains in coastal areas during the month of April cause heavy damage in sorghum.

Method of Sowing and Seed Rate

The crop is sown in zero tillage after harvesting paddy. The sowing is done manually in rows (40 × 15cm apart) at 4-6 cm depth by making a hole with wooden stick and putting 2-3 seeds in each hole (Figure 19.2). However making holes manually for sowing is, time consuming, back breaking and costly. Therefore manually operated small implement (Figure 19.2) and tractor operated hole maker (Figure 19.3) have been developed for easy and timely sowing. Around 8-10 kg seed/ha is required for optimum plant population.

Nutrient Management

For obtaining high yield of sorghum, 200 kg N, 60 kg phosphorus and 60 kg potassium per hectare is recommended. Mishra *et al*. (2013) obtained maximum sorghum grain yield (8.04 t/ha), nutrient uptake and income benefits with 225 kg N/

ha (Tables 19.2 and 19.3). Grain yield of different sorghum hybrids varied significantly in their response to applied nitrogen (Figure 19.4). Hybrids 'CSH 23' and 'CSH 15R' were less responsive to higher doses of nitrogen as compared to other hybrids. Being a zero till manually sown crop, no nutrient is applied during sowing. A dose of 100 kg N and full dose of phosphorus is applied at 30 days after sowing (DAS) (just before 1st irrigation). Remaining 100 kg N and 60 kg potassium is applied at 60 DAS (just before 2nd irrigation). Nutrients are applied manually to individual plants by mixing different fertilizers (Figure 19.5). In the event of using seed-cum-fertilizer drill, 50 per cent of N and total P and K should be applied while sowing and remaining 50 per cent of N should be applied at 30 DAS.

Figure 19.3: Progress in Sowing Machinery of Sorghum in Rice-Fallows.

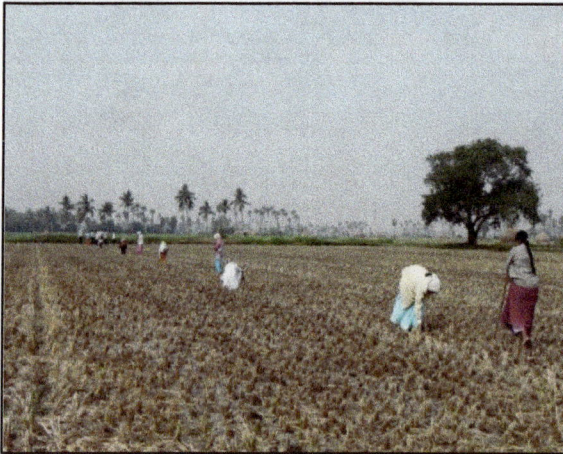

Seeding with wooden stick

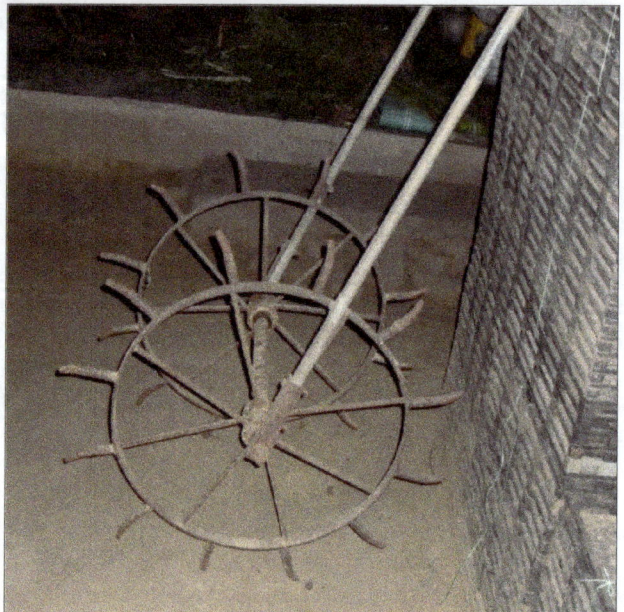

Twine wheel hole maker

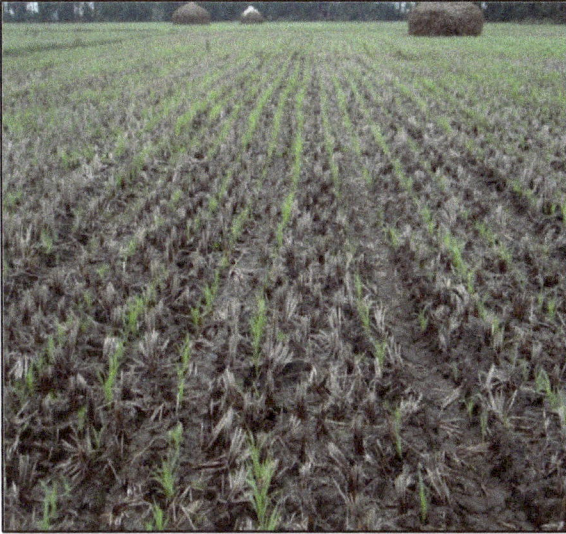

Crop sown by tractor drawn hole maker

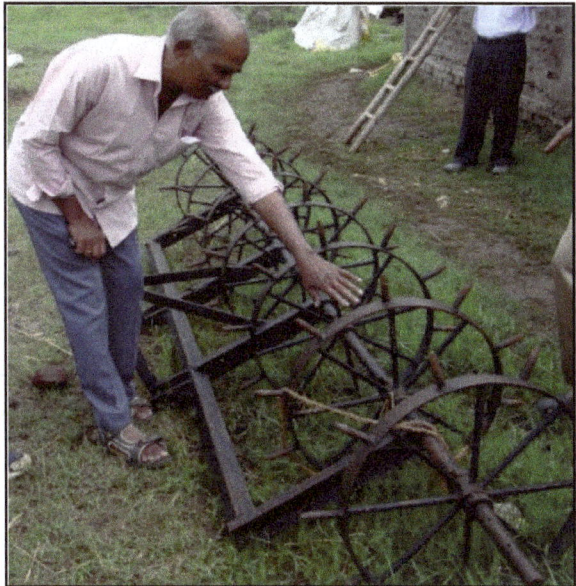

Tractor-drawn hole maker

Weed Management

Weeds are major problem in rice-fallows sorghum. As the crop is grown under zero tillage weeds infest the crop heavily due to adequate soil moisture. Moreover, due to moisture and favourable weather conditions, large number of rice ratoons and new rice plants also germinate and compete with sorghum crop for resources. For effective weed control, tank mixed application of paraquat + atrazine (0.50+0.75 kg/ha) should be done one day after sowing. Paraquat controls the rice rations and

Table 19.2: Effect of Nitrogen Levels and Genotypes on Growth, Yield Attributes and Yields of Sorghum Cultivars in Rice-fallows

Treatment	Plant Height at Harvest (cm)	Leaf Area Index	Panicles/ m²	Panicle Length (cm)	Grains/ Panicle	Grain Weight/ Panicle (g)	100-grain Weight (g)	Grain Yield (t/ha)
				Nitrogen levels (kg/ha)				
25	159	2.19	13.1	26.24	1401	38.39	2.63	4.81
75	170	2.29	13.3	26.33	1851	48.10	2.69	5.96
125	177	2.91	12.9	28.19	2225	58.81	2.74	7.38
175	187	3.26	12.4	29.10	2391	65.81	2.78	7.82
225	188	3.94	13.2	29.05	2249	66.35	2.96	8.04
LSD (P=0.05)	12	0.36	1.7	0.85	93	2.79	0.09	0.89

Table 19.3: Effect of Nitrogen Levels and Genotypes on Nutrient Content and Uptake in Sorghum Grains

Treatment	Nutrient Content (per cent) in Grain			Nutrient Uptake (kg/ha) by grain			Protein Content (per cent)	Net Returns (/ha)	B:C Ratio
	N	P	K	N	P	K			
				Nitrogen levels (kg/ha)					
25	1.49	0.46	0.33	72.6	22.1	16.0	9.31	24625	2.05
75	1.54	0.48	0.34	96.1	29.9	21.1	9.61	35589	2.48
125	1.55	0.49	0.34	112.3	35.5	24.6	9.69	49254	3.00
175	1.57	0.49	0.34	120.2	37.6	26.1	9.81	53060	3.11
225	1.58	0.49	0.35	129.4	40.0	28.8	9.86	54782	3.13
LSD (P=0.05)	0.03	0.01	0.01	5.3	3.4	2.3	0.26	2127	0.15

already emerged vegetations and atrazine checks the emergence of new weeds (Figure 19.6).

Irrigation

Sorghum in rice-fallows is grown on residual soil moisture, which supports the germination and early establishment of crop. Two irrigations are sufficient to harvest good yield in this area. First irrigation should be applied at 30 days after sowing (DAS) and 2nd irrigation at 60 DAS. Irrigation frequency however, depends on the seasonal rains.

Harvesting and Threshing

Crop is harvested manually at 105-110 days after sowing depending upon the genotypes duration. The harvested panicles are left in the field for about a week for drying and thereafter the grains are separated from panicles manually. The panicles are harvested first and remaining plants latter.

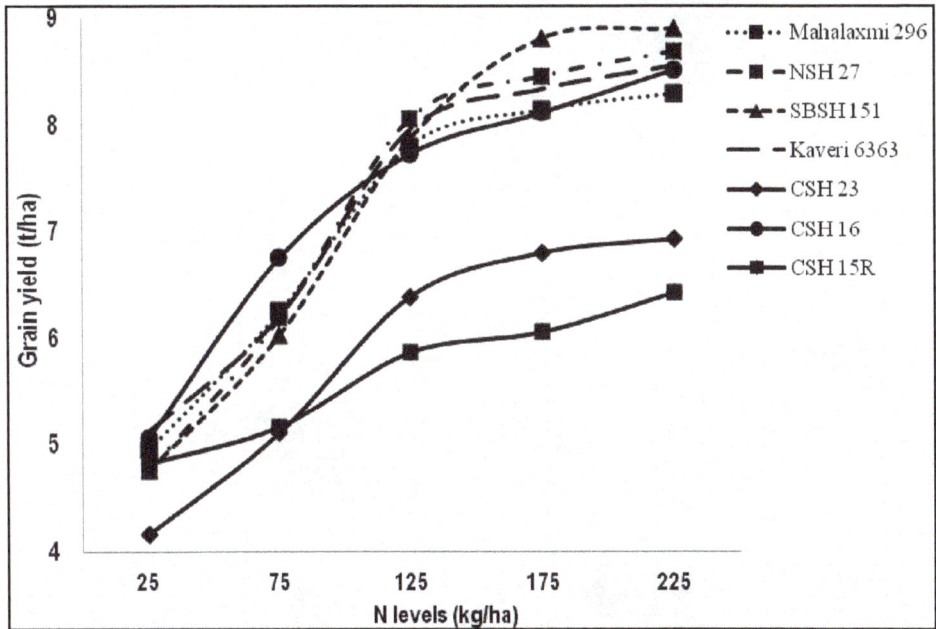

Figure 19.4: Response of Sorghum Hybrids to Nitrogen in Rice-Fallows.

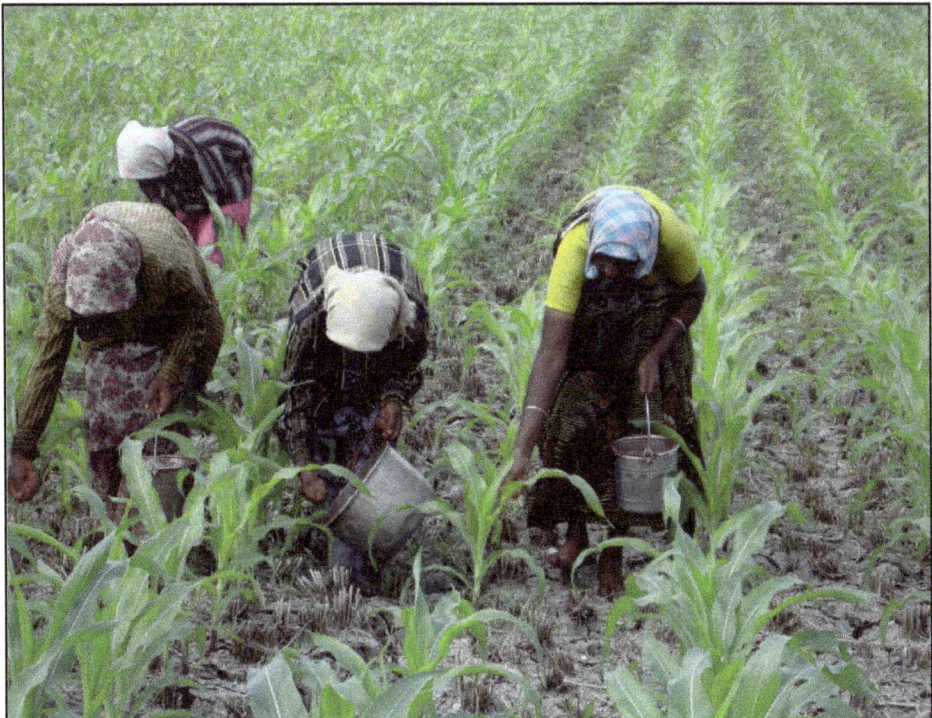

Figure 19.5: Nutrient Application at 30 DAS (just before 1ˢᵗ irrigation).

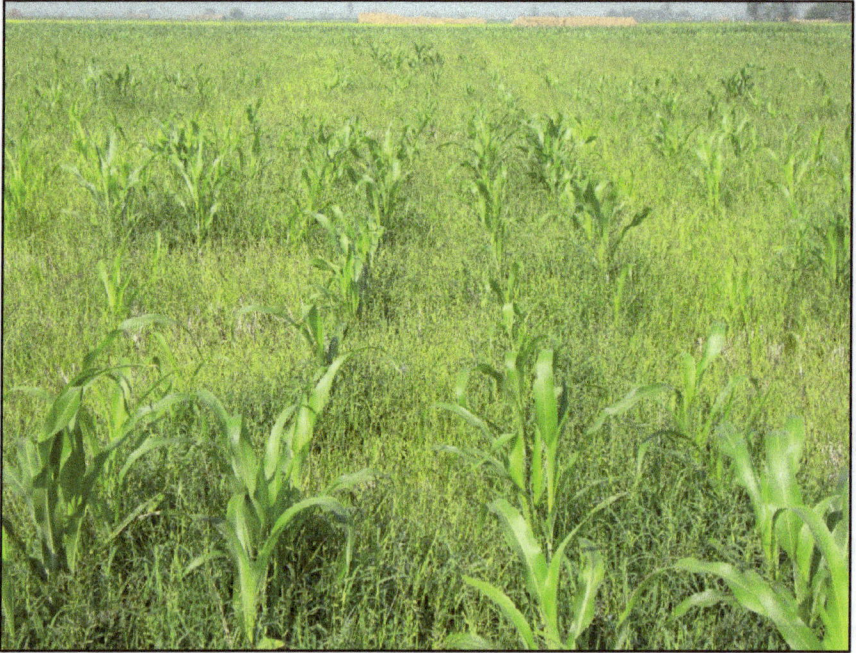

Severe infestation of weeds

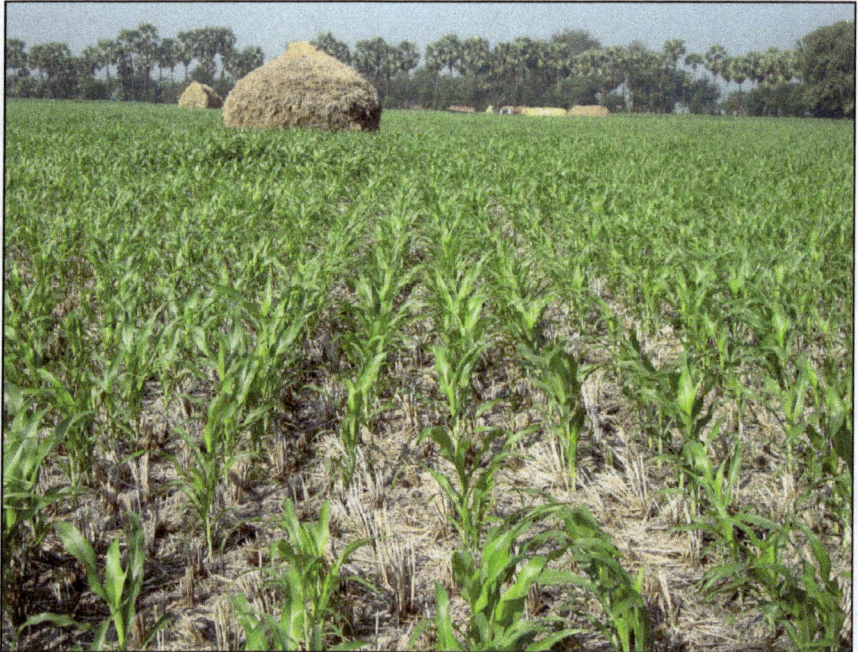

Atrazine + paraquat used as pre-emergence

Figure 19.6: Weed Management with Herbicides.

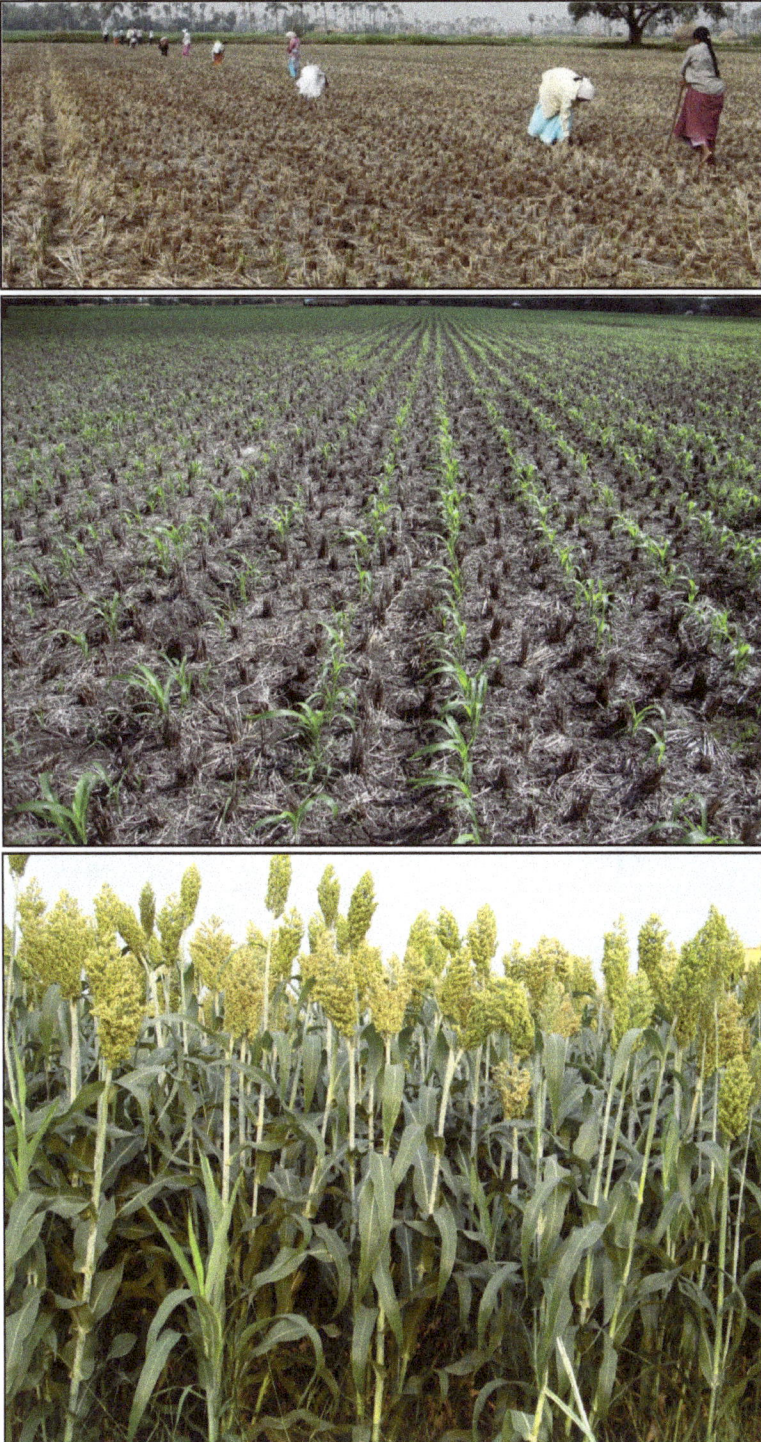

Figure 19.7: Sorghum Cultivation in Rice-Fallows.

Economic Analysis

On an average, farmers' expenditure incurred on sorghum cultivation was Rs. 28,000 – 30,000 per ha with net profit of around Rs.35000/ha. Component-wise cost and benefits are highlighted in Table 19.4. However, the cost of stover was not included in the net benefit as it is either burnt or incorporated in the soil.

Table 19.4: Economics of Sorghum Cultivation in Rice-Fallows as per the Farmer's Experience

Sl.No.	Particular	Cost (Rs./ha)
1.	Sowing and seed cost	3,500
2.	Fertilizers' cost + its application	6,000
3.	Herbicide cost + its application	1,500
4.	Pesticides cost + its application	4,500
5.	Irrigation water and labour charges	5,000
6.	Harvesting	3,000
7.	Threshing	3,000
8.	Drying/Bagging	1,500
10.	Total cost of production	28,000
11.	Gross returns*	63,000
12.	Net returns	35,000
13.	Benefit: Cost ratio	2.25:1

*Excluding fodder's price, selling price of sorghum grain @Rs. 10000/- per tonne.

Broad-Leaved Weeds

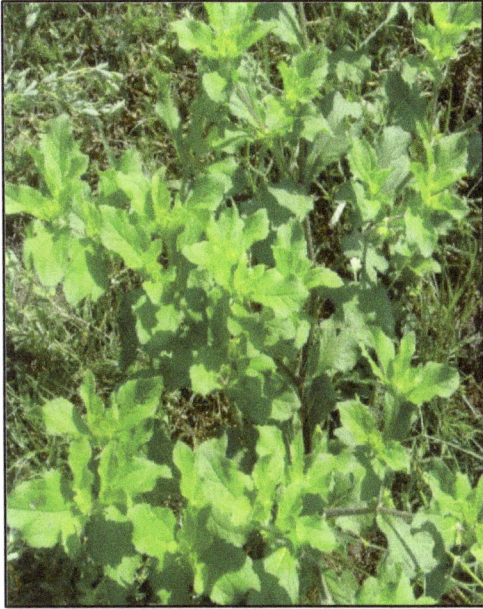

Acanthospermum hispidum

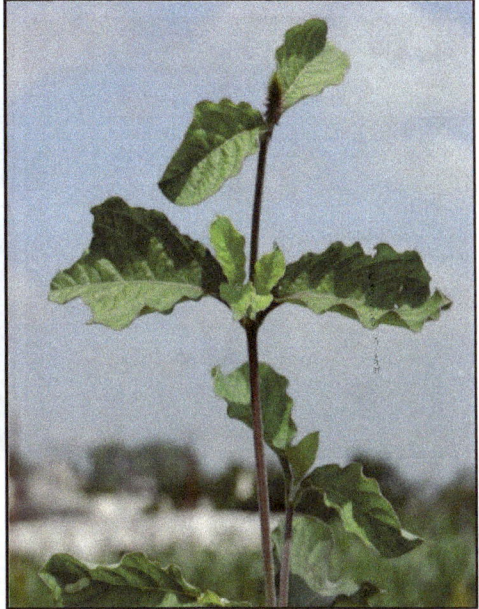

Achyranthes aspera

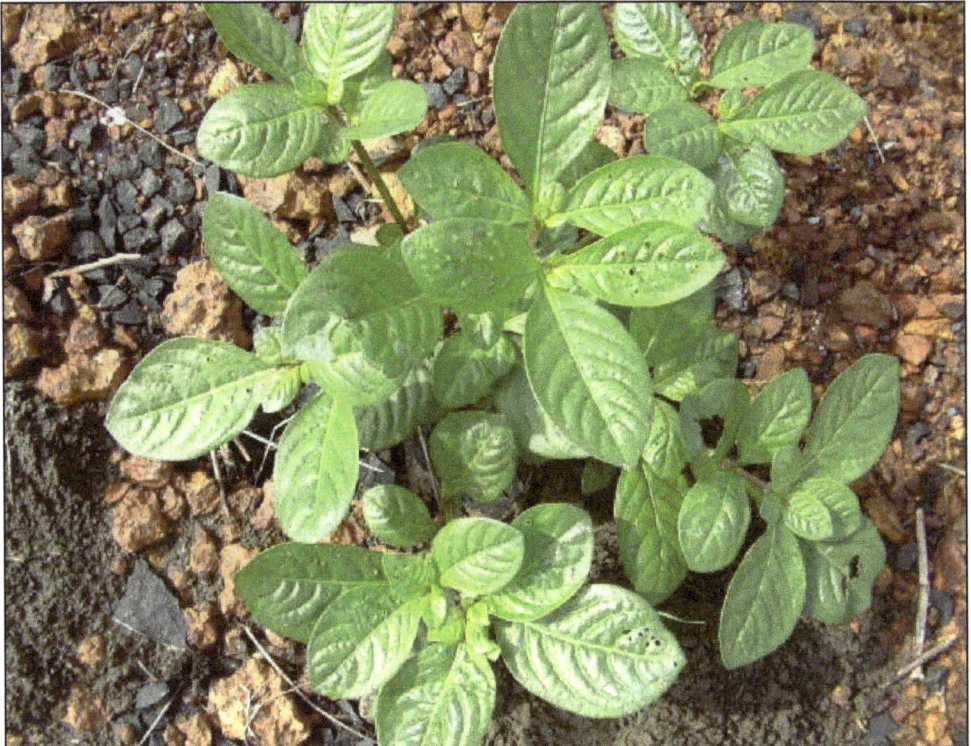

Alternanthera sessilis

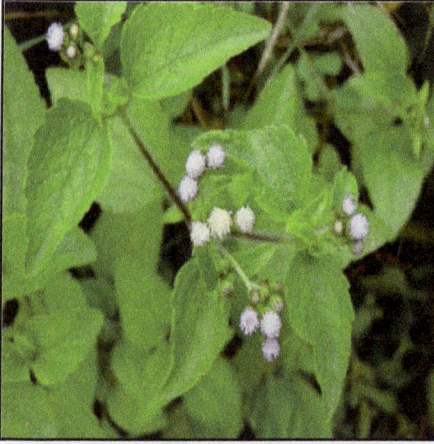

Ageratum conyzoides

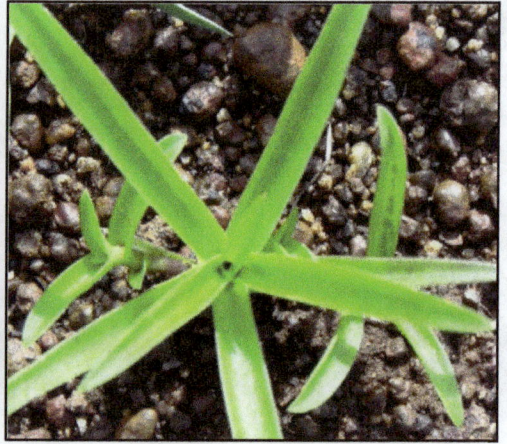

Cyanotis axillaris

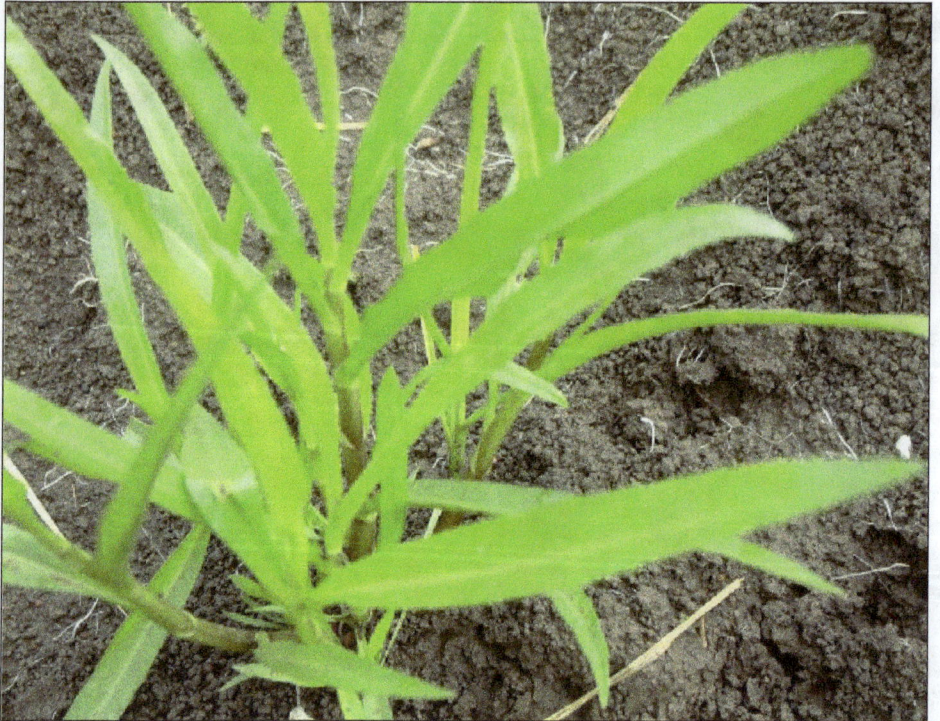

Caesulia axillaris

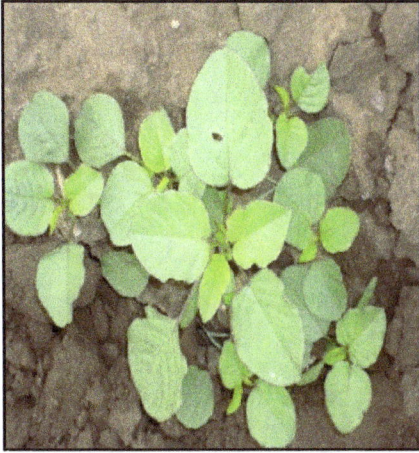

Digera arvensis

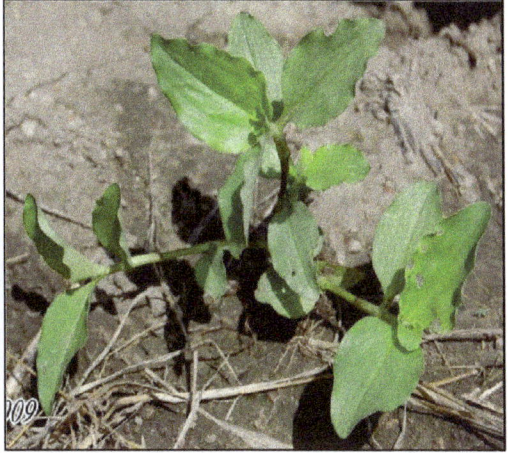

Commelina benghalensis

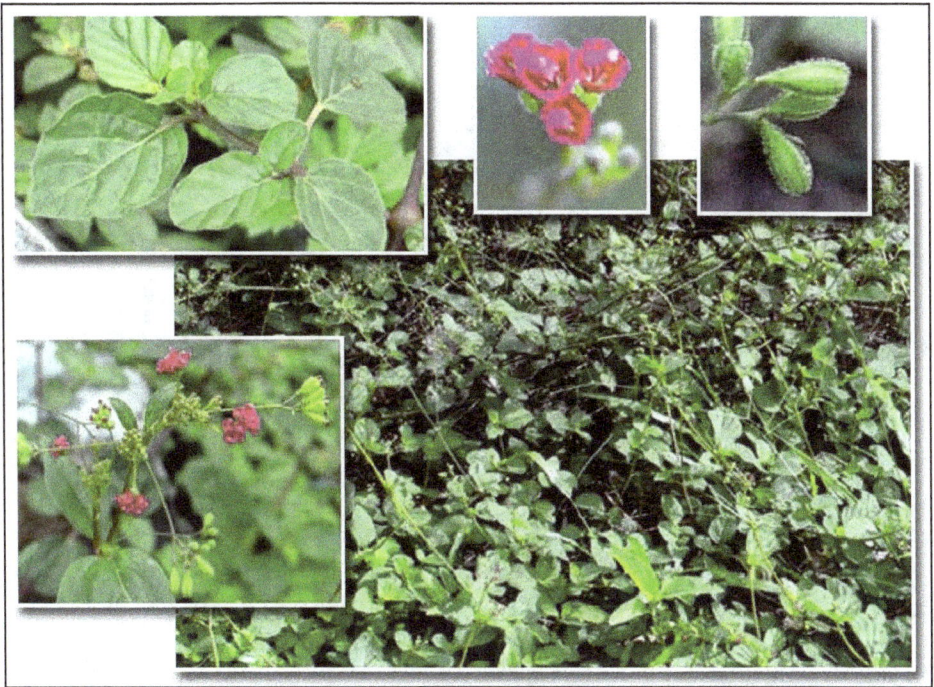

Boerhavia diffusa

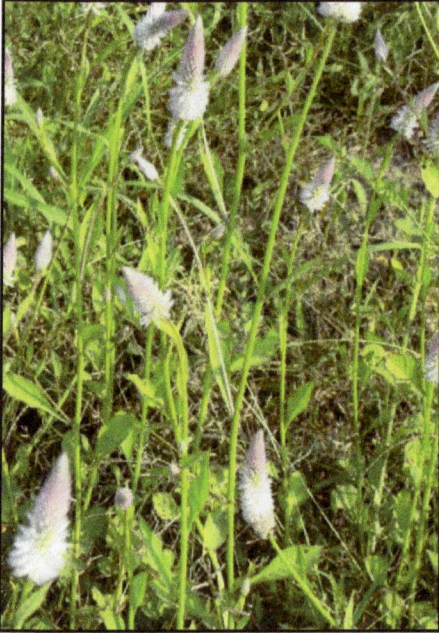
Celosia argentea

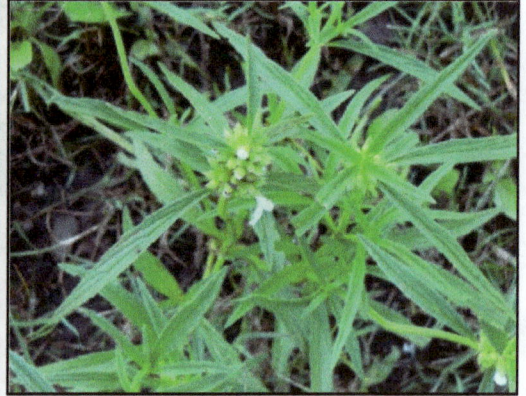
Leucas aspera

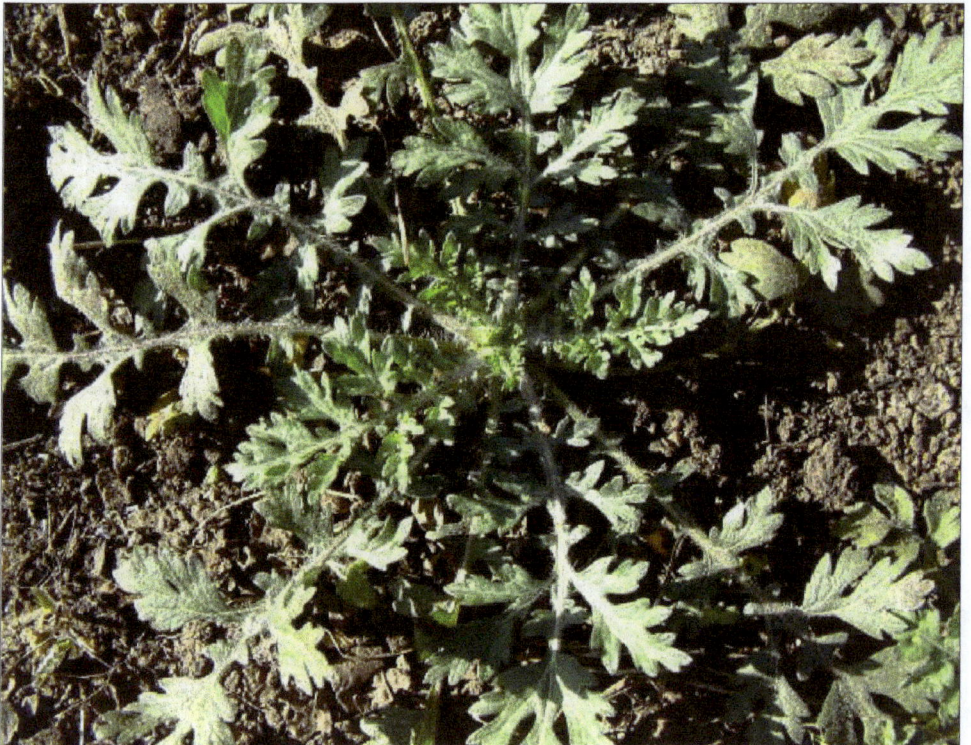
Parthenium hysterophorus

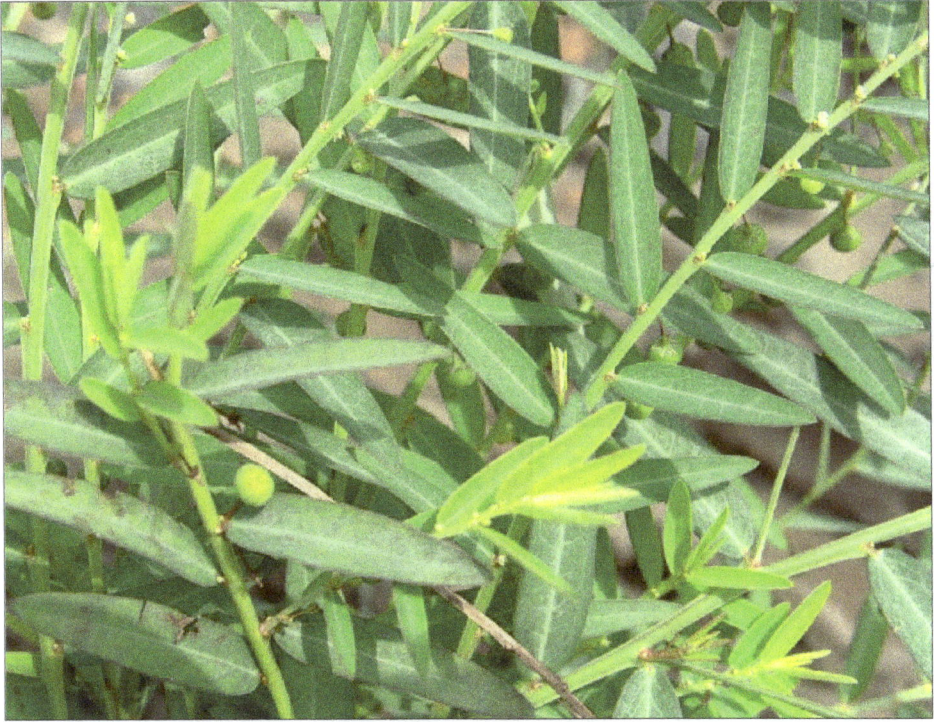

Phyllanthus urinaria

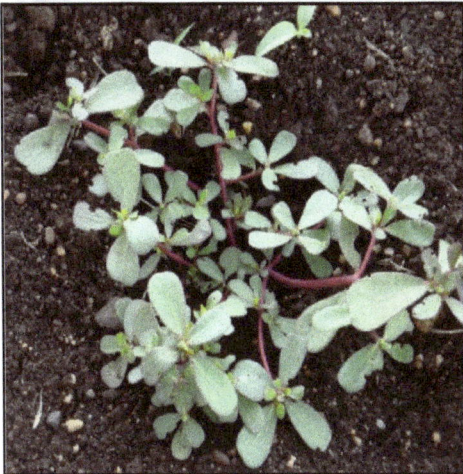

Portulaca oleracea

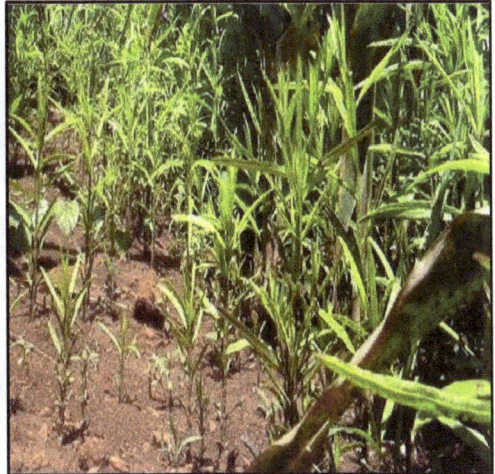

Striga lutea

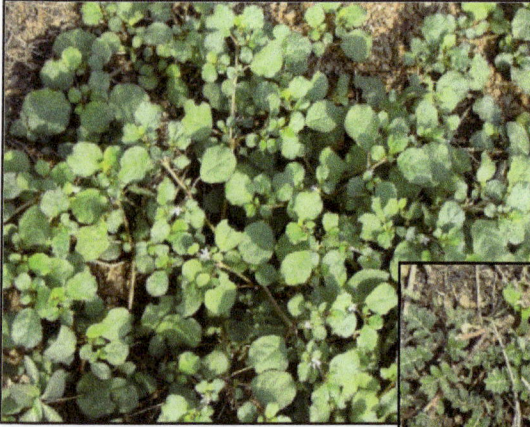

Trianthema portulacastrum

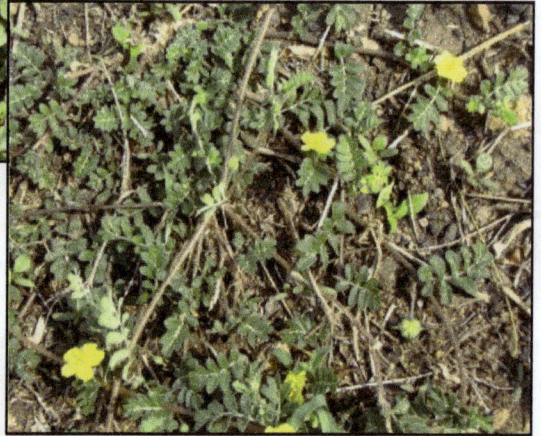

Tribulus terrestris

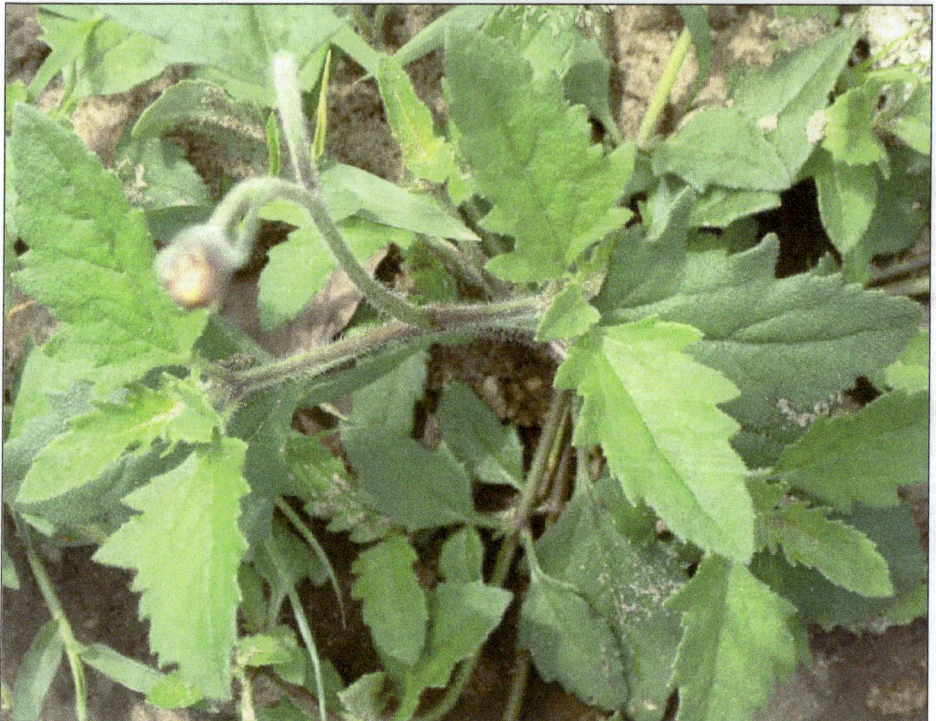

Tridax procumbens

Grasses and Sedges

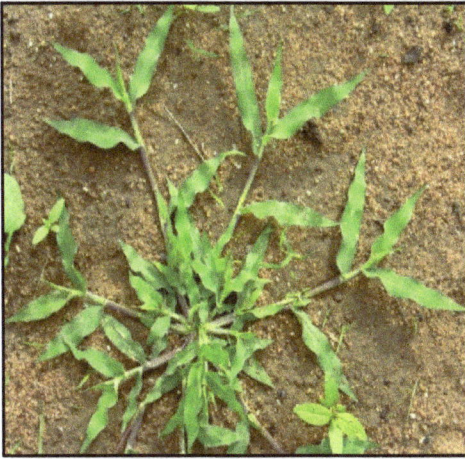
Brachiaria ramosa

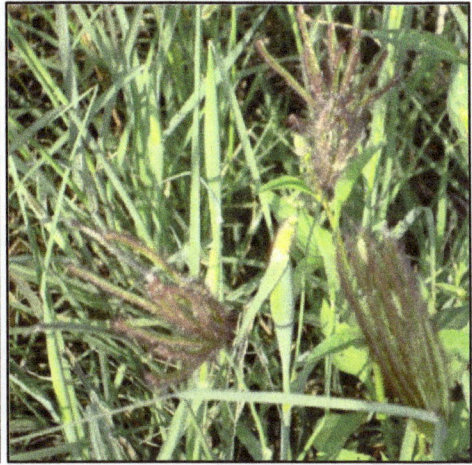
Chloris barbata

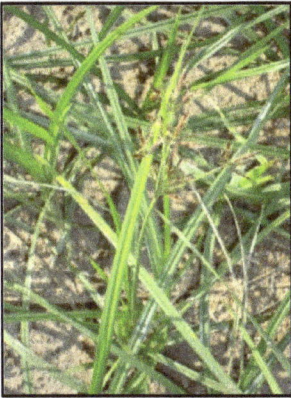
Cyperus rotundus

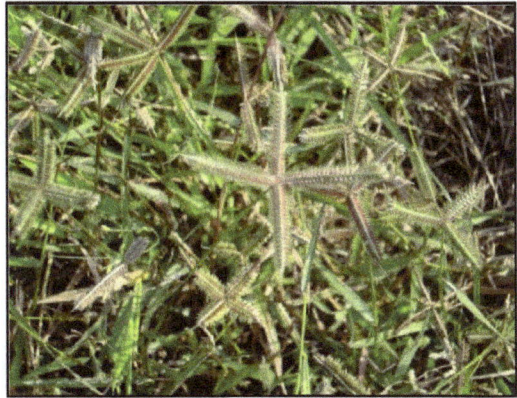
Dactyloctenium aegyptium

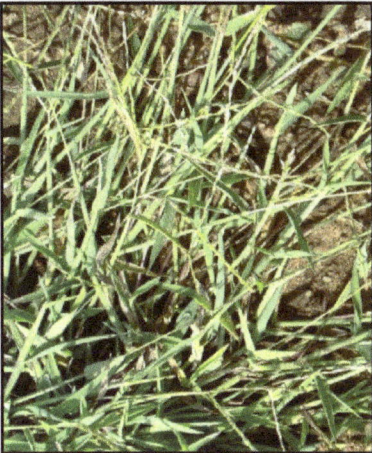
Digitaria sanguinalis

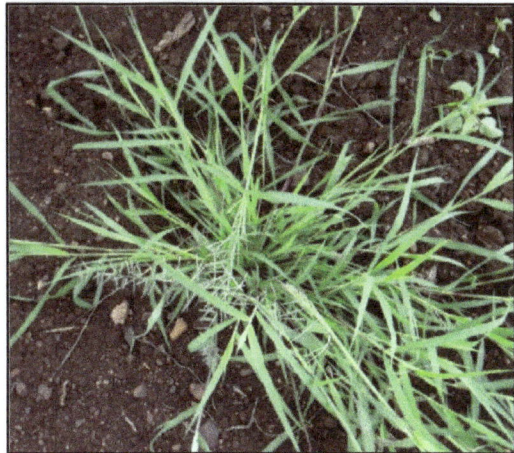
Dinebra retroflexa

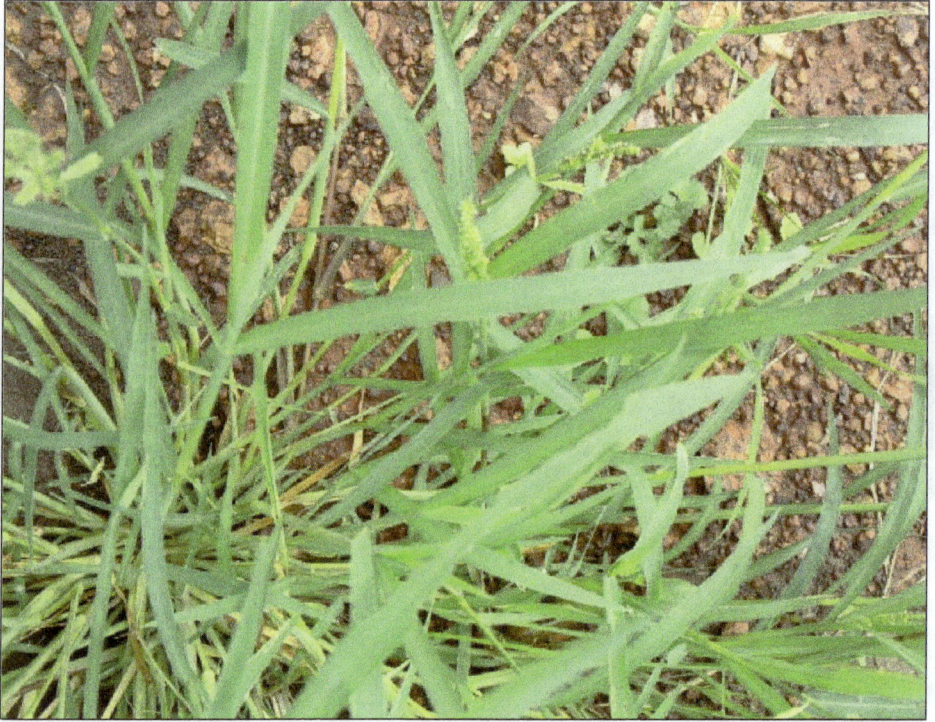

Echinochoa colona

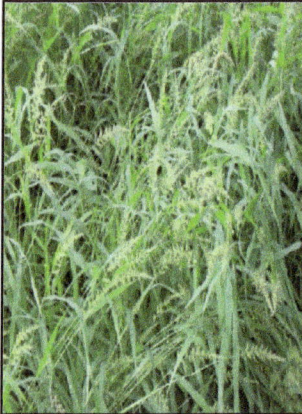

Setaria glauca

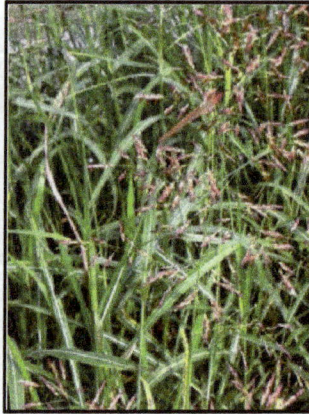

Sorghum halepense

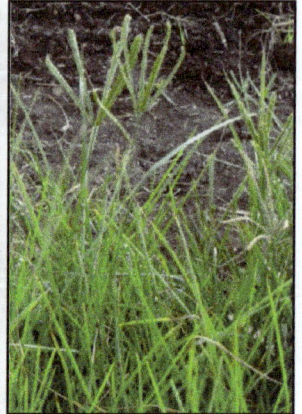

Eleusine indica

References

Abunyewa, A., Richard, F., Charles, W., Drew, L. and Steve, M. 2008. Sorghum yield and yield components under different skip-row configuration and plant density in Nebraska. *Proceedings of the Great Plains Soil Fertility Conference.* Denver, CO. Vol. 12. pp. 94-100.

Ackley, J.A., Wilson, H.P. and Hines, T.E. 1996. Yellow nutsedge (*Cyperus esculentus*) control POST with acetolactate synthase-inhibiting herbicides. *Weed Technology* 10: 576-580.

Agrama H, Widle G, Reese J, Campbell L, Tuinstra M (2002) Genetic mapping of QTLs associated with greenbug resistance and tolerance in Sorghum bicolor. *Theoretical and Applied Genetics* 104: 1373-1378.

AICSIP, 2007. All India Coordinated Sorghum Improvement Project, *Annual Progress Report* 2006-07. Directorate of Sorghum Research, Hyderabad, AP, India.

AICSIP, 2009. All India Coordinated Sorghum Improvement Project, *Annual Progress Report* 2008-09. Directorate of Sorghum Research, Hyderabad, AP, India.

AICSIP, 2010. All India Coordinated Sorghum Improvement Project, *Sorghum Agronomy Kharif 2009*. Directorate of Sorghum Research, Hyderabad, India.

AICSIP, 2012. All India Coordinated Sorghum Improvement Project, *Sorghum Agronomy Kharif 2011*. Directorate of Sorghum Research, Hyderabad, India.

AICSIP, 2013. All India Coordinated Sorghum Improvement Project, *Sorghum Agronomy Kharif 2012*. Directorate of Sorghum Research, Hyderabad, India.

Akwasi, A. A., Richard, B. F., Charles, S. W., Drew, J. L., Stephen, C. M., Suat, I. and Robert, N. K. 2011. Grain sorghum water use with skip-row configuration in the Central Great Plains of the USA. *African Journal of Agricultural Research*, 6 (23): 5328-5338.

Ali, S.Z., Meera, M.S., Malleshi, N.G. Processing of sorghum and pearl millet for promoting wider utilization for food. Alternative uses of sorghum and pearl millet in Asia. Proceedings of an expert meeting, ICRISAT, Patancheru, Andhra Pradesh, India, 1-4 July, 2003. 2004; 169-187.

Almodares A and Hadi MR (2009). Production of bioethanol from sweet sorghum: A review. *African Journal of Agricultural Research* vol. 4 (9), pp. 772 – 780.

Anda, A. and Pinter, L.1994. Sorghum germination and development as influenced by soil temperature and water content. *Agronomy Journal* 86: 621-24.

Anglani, C. 1998. Sorghum for human food – A review. *Plant Foods for Human Nutrition* 52: 85–95.

Anonymous, 2006. Ratnavathi, CV, 2006 Annual Report, National Research Centre for Sorghum, Rajendranagar, Hyderabad.

Apotikar D, Venkateswarlu D, Ghorade R, Wadaskar R, Patil J, Kulwal P (2011) Mapping of shoot fly tolerance loci in sorghum using SSR markers. *Journal of Genetics* 90: 59-66.

Archangelo, E.R., Silva, A.A. da, Silva, J.B. da, Karam, D. and Cardoso, A.A. 2002. Selectivity and efficacy of post emergence herbicide on forage sorghum. *Revista Brasileria de Milho-e-Sorgo* 1: 107-115.

Arri. BK. 1989. Problems associated with the use of Sorghum for Lager beer production. Proceedings of a symposium on the current status and potential of Industrial Uses of sorghum in Nigeria. 4-6Dec, Kano, Nigeria. Pp 29.

Arriola, P.E. and Ellstrand, N.C. 1996. Crop- to- gene flow in the genus Sorghum (Poaceae): spontaneous interspecific hybridization between Johnsongrass, *Sorghum halepense*, and crop sorghum, *S. bicolor*. *American Journal of Botany* 83: 1153-1160.

Arumuganathan K, Earle E (1991) Nuclear DNA content of some important plant species. *Plant Molecular Biology Reporter* 9: 208-218.

Aruna C, Bhagwat V, Madhusudhana R, Sharma V, Hussain T, Ghorade R, Khandalkar H, Audilakshmi S, Seetharama N (2011) Identification and validation of genomic regions that affect shoot fly resistance in sorghum [*Sorghum bicolor* (L.) Moench]. *Theoretical and Applied Genetics* 122: 1617-1630.

Aruna, C., Bhat, B.V.,Umakanth, A.V., Shyam Prasad, G., Das, I.K. and Patil, J.V. 2011. In. *Forage Sorghum*. Directorate of Sorghum Research, Hyderabad, India, 52pp.

Ashok Kumar A, Reddy BVS and Sahrawat KL. 2013b. Biofortification for combating micronutrient malnutrition: Identification of commercial sorghum cultivars with high grain iron and zinc contents. *Indian Journal of Dryland Agricultural Research and Development* 28(1): 95–100.

Assefa, Y. and Staggenborg, S.A. 2010. Grain sorghum yield with hybrid advancement and changes in agronomic practices from 1957 through 2008. *Agronomy Journal* 102: 703-706.

Attalla, S.I. 2002. Effect of weed control treatments and two sowing mwthods on weeds and sorghum (*Sorghum bicolor*). *Bulletin of faculty of Agriculture*, Cairo University 53: 539-551.

Axtell JD and Ejeta G. 1990. Improving sorghum grain protein quality by breeding. P. 117-125. In Ejeta G. (ed.) Proceedings of the international conference on sorghum nutritional quality. Purdue University. West Lafayette. IN.

Axtell JD, Kirleis AW, Hassen MM, Mason ND, Mertz ET and Munck L (1981). Digestibility of sorghum proteins. *Proc. Natl. Acad. Sci.* 78: 1333-1335.

Axtell JD, Mohan D and Cummings D. 1974. Genetic improvement of biological efficiency and protein quality in sorghum. In Proceedings, 29th annual corn and sorghum research conference, Chicago. American Seed Trade Association. Washington. D.C. pp. 29-39.

Ayyanagouda P, Bashasab F, Salimath PM, Rajkumar (2012) Genome-wide molecular mapping and QTL analysis, validated across locations and years for charcoal rot disease incidence traits in Sorghum bicolor (L.) Moench. *Indian Journal of Genetics and Plant Breeding* 72: 296-302.

Ayyangar, G.N.R. and Ayyer, 1942. Mixed cropping: a review. *Madras Agricultural Journal* 30: 3-13.

Babaria, C.J. and Patel, C.L. 1981. Response and uptake of Fe by sorghum to application of iron, farm yard manure and sulphur in calcarious soils. *GAU Research Journal* 6(2): 121-124.

Badi S, Pedersen B, Monowar L, Eggum BO. 1990. The nutritive value of new and traditional sorghum and millet foods from Sudan. *Plant Foods Hum Nutr* 40: 5–19.

Balasubramanian N and Subramanian S, 1989. Studies in integrated weed management in irrigated sorghum based cropping system. *Indian Journal of Agronomy* 34: 436-438.

Balasubramanian, C.R. *etal.* 1966. *Madras Agric. J.*, 53: 150-157.

Bandaru Varaprasad, Stewart B A, Baumhardt RL, Ambati S, Robinson CA, Schlegel A 2006. Growing dryland grain sorghum in clumps to reduce vegetative growth and increase yield. *Agronomy Journal*, 98: 1109-1120.

Bandopadhyay, S.K. 1992. Measurement of symbiotic nitrogen fixation by legumes in sorghum (*Sorghum bicolor*) + legume intercropping. *Indian Journal of Agronomy*, 37: 211-213.

Baumhardt, R. L., Tolk, J. A. and Winter, S. R. 2005. Seeding practices and cultivar maturity effects on simulated dryland grain sorghum yield. *Agronomy Journal*, 97: 935-42.

Bebawi, F.F. and Farah, A.F. 1981. Effect of parasitic and non-parasitic weeds on sorghum. *Experimental Agriculture* 17: 415-418.

Beil G, Atkins R (1967) Estimates of general and specific combining ability in F1 hybrids for grain yield and its components in grain sorghum, *Sorghum vulgare* Pers. *Crop Science* 7: 225-228.

Bekker, R.M., Forcella, F., Grundy, A.C., Jones, N.E., Marshall, E.J.P. and Murdoch, A.J. 2003. Depletion of natural soil seed banks of *Striga hermonthica* in West Africa under different integrated management regimes. Seedbanks: Determination, dynamics and management. Papers from meeting of the Association of Applied Biolologists, Reading, UK, 17-18 September, 2003 *Aspects Applied Biology* 69: 261-268.

Bennett, W. F., Tucker, B. B. and Maunder, A. B. 1990. *Modern Grain Sorghum Production*. Iowa State Univ. Press, Ames, IA.

Bhat BV, Krishna DB, Sateesh K, Srinivas G, Seetharama N (2004). Molecular marker-aided approaches for sorghum improvement. *AgBiotechNet* 6: 1-13.

Bhattramakki D, Dong J, Chhabra AK, Hart GE (2000). An integrated SSR and RFLP linkage map of Sorghum bicolor (L.) Moench. *Genome* 43: 988-1002.

Bhonde, M.B. and Bhakare, B.D. 2008. Influence of integrated nutrient management on soil properties of vertisol under sorghum (*Sorghum bicolor*)-wheat (*Triticum aestivum*) cropping sequence. *Journal of Research ANGRAU* 36: 1-8.

Bilbro, J. D. 2008. Grain sorghum producers contends with many insect pests. Southwest farm Press, September 4, 2008, www.southwestfarmpress.com.

Blanshard JMV (1986). The significance of structure and function of the starch granule in baked products. Pages 1-13 in: Chemistry and physics of baking. Blanshard, J.M.V. [Eds.] Royal society of chemistry. London.

Bodade, V.N. 1964. Agronomic trials on jowar (*Sorghum vulgare*). *Indian Journal of Agronomy*, 9: 184-195.

Bodade, V.N. 1966. Effect of foliar application of nitrogen and phosphorus on yield of jowar (*Sorghum vulgare*). *Indian Journal of Agronomy*, 11: 267-269.

Bond, J. J., Army, T. J., and Lehman, O. R. 1964. Row Spacing, Plant Populations and Moisture Supply as Factors in Dryland Grain Sorghum Production. *Agronomy Journal* 56: 3-6.

Boora K, Frederiksen R, Magill C (1999).1 A molecular marker that segregates with sorghum leaf blight resistance in one cross is maternally inherited in another. *Molecular and General Genetics* MGG 261: 317-322.

Bramel-Cox PJ, Hancock JD, Kumar KA and Andrews DJ (1995). Sorghum and millets for forage and feed. Pages 325 – 364 in: Sorghum and millets chemistry and technology. Dendy, D.A.V. [Eds.] Amer. Assoc.*Cereal Chem*. St.Paul, Mn, USA.

Brandon, J. F., Curtis, J. J. and Robertson, D. W. Harvesting Sorghums in Colorado. Fort Collins: Colorado State College, Agricultural Experiment Station, 18-20.

Brown, D.W., Al-Khatib, K., Regehr, D.L., Stahlman, P.W. and Loughin, T.M. 2004. Safening grain sorghum injury from metsulfuron with growth regulator herbicides. *Weed Science* 52: 319-325.

Buleon A, Colonna P, Planchot V and Ball S 1998. Starch Granule: structure and biosynthesis. *Int. J. Biol. Macromol*. 23: 85-112.

Burnside, O.C. and Wicks, G.A. 1969. Influence of weed competition on sorghum growth. *Weed Science* 17: 332-334.

Burnside, O.C. and Wicks, G.A. 1972. Competitiveness and herbicide tolerance of sorghum hybrids. *Weed Science* 20: 314-316.

Burnside, O.C., Wicks, G.A. and Fenster, C.R. 1964. Influence of tillage, row spacing and atrazine on sorghum and weed yields from non-irrigated sorghum cross Nebrasks. *Weeds* 12: 211-215.

Burow G, Burke JJ, Xin Z, Franks CD (2011) Genetic dissection of early-season cold tolerance in sorghum (*Sorghum bicolor* (L.) Moench). *Molecular Breeding* 28: 391-402.

Butler LG, Riedl DJ, Lebryk DG and Blytt HJ 1984. Interaction of proteins with sorghum tannin: mechanism, specificity and significance. *J. Am. Oil Che. Soc*. 61: 916-920.

Capinera, J.L. 2005. Relationship between insect pests and weeds: an evolutionary perspective. *Weed Science* 53: 892-901.

Carson-LC. and Sun-XS. 2000. Breads from white grain sorghum: rheological properties and baking volume with exogenous gluten protein *Applied-Engineering-in-Agriculture*. 2000, 16: 4, 423-429.

Carter PR, Hicks DR, Oplinger ES, Doll JD, Bundy LG, Schuler RT and Holmes BJ. 1989. Grain Sorghum (Milo). Alternative Field Crops Manual. University of Wisconsin and University of Minnesota (http: //www.hort.purdue.edu/newcrop/afcm/index.html).

Chamberlain, E.W., Becton, A.J. and LeBaron, H.M. 1970. Tolerance of sorghum to post-emergence application of atrazine. *Weed Science* 18: 410-412.

Chandramohan, J. 1970. *Madras Agric. J., 57*: 251-263.

Chapman, S.R., and Carter, L.P. 1976. *Crop production, Principle and Practices*. San Francisco: W.H. Freeman. 566 pp.

Cheema, Z.A. and Khaliq A., 2000. Use of sorghum allelopathic properties to control weeds in irrigated wheat in a semi-arid region of Punjab. *Agricultural Ecosystems and Environment* 79: 105-112.

Cheema, Z.A., Khaliq, A. and Saeed, S. 2007. Weed control in maize (*Zea mays*) through sorghum allelopathy. *Journal of Sustainable Agriculture* 23: 73-86.

Childs KL, Miller FR, Cordonnier-Pratt M-M, Pratt LH, Morgan PW, Mullet JE 1997. The sorghum photoperiod sensitivity gene, Ma3, encodes a phytochrome B. *Plant Physiology* 113: 611-619.

Choudhary, S.D. 1978. Efficiency of nitrogen applied through soil and foliar on grain sorghum. *Journal of Maharashtra Agricultural University*, 3: 26-27.

Clark, R.B. 1982a. Mineral nutritional factors reducing sorghum yields; micronutrients and acidity. Sorghum in the Eighties. *Proceedings of the International Symposium on sorghum*, ICRISAT, 2-7 November, 1981, Patancheru, AP, India, 179-190.

Clark, R.B. 1982d. Plant response to mineral element toxicity and deficiency. In: Christiansen, M.N. and Lewis, C.F. eds., Breeding plants for less favourable environments, New York, USA, John Wiley and Son, 71-142.

Cothren JT, Matocha JE and Clark LE. 2000. Integrated crop management for sorghum. *Sorghum: Origin, History, Technology, and Production*. Ed. C. Wayne Smith and Richard A. Frederiksen. New York: Wiley, pp.409-441.

Crasta O, Xu W, Rosenow D, Mullet J, Nguyen H (1999). Mapping of post-flowering drought resistance traits in grain sorghum: association between QTLs influencing premature senescence and maturity. *Molecular and General Genetics* MGG 262: 579-588.

Crawford, P.W., Flower, D.J. and Peacock, J.M. 1993. Effect of heat and drought stress on sorghum (*Sorghum bicolor*). I. Panicle development and leaf appearance. *Experimental Agriculture*, 29: 61-76.

Croissant, R. L. 1969. *Environmental Effects on Crop Maturity*. Thesis. Colorado State University, 1969. Fort Collins: Colorado State University, p23.

Cura JA, Jansson PE and Krisman CR (1995). Amylose is not strictly linear. Starch Stärke 47: 207-209.

Dahlberg, J. A. 2000. Classification and Characterization of Sorghum. *Sorghum: Origin, History, Technology, and Production*. Ed. C. Wayne Smith and Richard A. Frederiksen. New York: Wiley, pp. 99-130.

Dalby A and Tsai Y. 1976. Lysine and tryptophan increases during germination of cereal grains. *Cereal Chemistry* 53: 221–226.

Dastane NG. 1974. Economic and efficient use of irrigation water *In: Proceedings, 1st FAO/SIDA Seminar on Improvement and Production of Field Crops*, FAO, Rome. Pp 388-398.

Dastane, N.G. *et al.*, 1970. *Water Requirements of Crops in India*. Navbharat Prakasham. Poona. P: 106.

de Wet JMJ and Harlan JR. 1971. The Origin and Domestication of Sorghum Bicolor. *Economic Botany* 25(2): 128-35.

de Wet, J. M. J. 1978. Systematics and Evolution of Sorghum Sect. Sorghum (Gramineae). *American Journal of Botany* 65: 477-84.

de Wet, J.M.J. and Harlan, J.R. 1971. The origin and domestication of *Sorghum bicolor*. *Economic Botany*, 25: 128-135.

de Wit, C.T. 1960. On competition. Verslag Landbouwkundige, *Onderzoek* 66(8): 1-82.

de Wit, C.T. and Van Den Bergh, J.P. 1965. Competition among herbage plants. *Netherlands Journal of Agricultural Science*, 13: 212-221.

Deshpande SP, ST Borikar, S Ismail and SS Ambekar. 2003. Genetic Studies for Improvement of Quality Characters in *Rabi* Sorghum using Landraces. *International sorghum and Millets Newsletter* 44: 6-8.

Dhanapal, G.N., Reddy, B.M.V. and Bomme, Gowda A. 1989. Screening of herbicides for dryland crops under Bangalore condition. *Mysore Journal of Agricultural Sciences* 23: 159-163.

Dhonde. P.W. *et al.* (1986). *Sorghum Newsletter*, 29: 50-51.

Dhruvanarayan, V.V. and Rambabu, B. 1983. Estimation of soil erosion in India. *Journal of Irrigation and Drainage Engineering* 109: 419-433.

Dicko, M.H., Gruppen, H., Traore, A.S. Voragen, A.G.J. and van Berkel, W.J.H. 2006. "Review: Sorghum grain as human food in Africa: relevance of starch content and amylase activities." *African Journal of Biotechnology* 5: 384-395.

Dillon, S. L., Frances M. S., Robert J. H., Giovanni C., Liz I. and L. Slade Lee. Domestication to crop improvement: genetic resources for Sorghum and Saccharum (Andropogoneae). *Annals of Botany* 100: 5: 975-89.

Dogget, H. 1976. *Sorghum*. In: Simmonds, N.W. (ed.), Evolution of Crop Plants, Logmans, pp. 112-117.

Doggett, H. 1970. Morphology and Reproduction. *Sorghum*. London: Longmans. pp. 49-71.

Doggett, H. 1970. Physiology and Agronomy. *Sorghum*. London: Longmans, 1970. 180-211.

Doggett, H. 1970. The History, Origins and Classification of Sorghum. *Sorghum*. London: Longmans, pp.1-48.

Doggett, H. 1988. Utilization of grain sorghum. *In. Sorghum*. Longman Scientific and Technical.John Wiley and Sons., Inc., New York.

Done, A.A. *et al.* (1984). *Australian. Journal of Agricultural Research*, 35: 17-29.

Downes, R. W. 1972. Effect of temperature on the phenology and grain yield of *Sorghum bicolor*. *Australian Journal of Agricultural Research* 23: 585-94.

Dudal, R. 1976. Inventory of the major soils of the world with special reference to mineral stress hazards. In: Wright, M.J. ed., Plant adaptation to mineral stress in problem soils. Ithaca, New York, USA, Coronell University Agricultural Experiment Station, 3-13.

Duncan RR, Bockholt AJ and Miller FR. 1981. Descriptive comparison of senescent and non-senescent sorghum genotypes. *Agron. J.* 73: 849–853.

Eastin, J.D. 1983. Sorghum. In. IRRI (ed). *Potential Productivity of Field Crops under different Environments.*, IRRI, Los Banos, Philippines, pp. 181-204.

Eastin, J.D., Joe, Hultquist, H. and Sullivan, C. Y. 1973. Physiological maturity in grain sorghum. *Crop Science* 13: 2: 175-78.

Edwards D, Forster JW, Chagné D, Batley J 2007. What Are SNPs? Association mapping in plants. Springer, pp. 41-52.

Emechebe, A.M., Ellis Jones, J., Schulz, S., Chikoye, D., Douthwaite, B., Kureh, I., Tarawali, G., Hussaini, M.A., Kormawa, P. and Sanni, A. 2004. Farmers perception of the Striga problem and its control in Northern Nigeria. *Experimental Agriculture* 40: 215-232.

Enrique, R. R., Ricardo S-de-la-cruz, Jaime, S.G. and Victor, P.Q. 2005. Broadleaf weed management in grain sorghum with reduced rates of post-emergence herbicides, *Weed Technology* 19: 385-390.

EtokAkpan,-O-U, 2004a Preliminary study of the enzymolysis of sorghum and barley pentosans and their levels in worts. *World Journal of Microbiology and Biotechnology*. 20(6): 575-578.

EtokAkpan,-O-U, 2004b Changes in sorghum malt during storage. *J. Inst. Brew.* 110 (3), 189–192.

Fakrudin B, Kavil S, Girma Y, Arun S, Dadakhalandar D, Gurusiddesh B, Patil A, Thudi M, Bhairappanavar S, Narayana Y (2013) Molecular mapping of genomic regions harbouring QTLs for root and yield traits in sorghum (*Sorghum bicolor* L. Moench). *Physiology and Molecular Biology of Plants*: 1-11.

FAO, 1989. *Fertilizers and Food Production*, FAO, Rome, 111p.

FAO, 2005. *Fertilizer use by crops in India*. Land and Plant Nutrition Management Service, Land and Water Development Division, Food and Agricultural Organizations of the United Nations, Rome.

FAO, 2005. *Fertilizer use by crops in India*. Land and Plant Nutrition Management Service, Land and Water Development Division, Food and Agricultural Organizations of the United Nations, Rome.

FAO, 2011. http: //faostat.fao.org/site/567/DesktopDefault.aspx?PageID=567# ancor verified on December 5, 2011.

FAO. 1995a. Production and utilization. Ch. 2 in Sorghum and millets in human nutrition, p 13-30. FAO, Rome.

Farre, I., Faci, J.M. 2004.Comparative response of maize (*Zea mays*) and sorghum (*Sorghum bicolor*) to irrigation deficit in a Mediterranean climate. http: // www.cropscience.org.au/icsc2004.

Feltner, K.C., Hurst, H.R. and Anderson, L.E. 1969a. Yellow foxtail competition in grain sorghum. *Weed Science* 17: 211-213.

Feltus F, Hart G, Schertz K, Casa A, Kresovich S, Abraham S, Klein P, Brown P, Paterson A (2006) Alignment of genetic maps and QTLs between inter-and intra-specific sorghum populations. *Theoretical and Applied Genetics* 112: 1295-1305.

Fischer RA and Hagan RM. 1965. *Exptl. Agric.*, 1: 161-177.

Fisher, N.M. 1984. Crop growth and development: The vegetative phase. In.P.R. Goldsworthy and N.M Fisher (eds.). *The Physiology of Tropical Field Crops*. Wiley, New York, pp. 119-261.

Francois, L.E., Donovan, T. and Maas, E.V. 1984. Salinity effects on seed yield, growth and germination of grain sorghum. *Agronomy Journal*, 76: 741-744.

Frederiksen, R.A. 1984. Anthracnose stalk rot. In L.K. Mughogho (ed.), Sorghum root and stalk rots: A critical review. International Crop Research Institute for the Semi-Arid Tropics, Patencheru, A.P., India, pp. 37-42.

Gawai, P.P. and Pawar, V.S. 2006. Integrated nutrient management in sorghum (*Sorghum bicolor*)–chickpea (*Cicer arietinum*) cropping sequence under irrigated conditions. *Indian Journal of Agronomy*, **51**: 17-20.

Gbehounou, G. Adango, E., Hinvi, J.C. and Nonfon, R. 2004. Sowing date or transplanting as components for integrated *Striga hermonthica* control in grain-cereal crops. *Crop Protection* 23: 379-386.

Gerik, T. J., and Neely, C. L. 1987. Plant density effects on main culm and tiller development of grain sorghum. *Crop Science* 27: 1225-230.

Gerik, T. J., Bean, B. and Vanderlip, R. L. 2003. *Sorghum Growth and Development*. College Station, Texas: Texas Cooperative Extension, Texas A and M University System.

Gill, A.S. and Abichandani, C.T. 1972. A note on response of hybrid jowar to micronutrients. *Indian Journal of Agronomy*, 17: 231-232.

Giri, A.N. and Bhosle, R.H. 1997. Weed management in sorghum (*Sorghum bicolor*)-safflower (*Carthamus tinctorius*) sequence. *Indian Journal of Agronomy* 42: 214-219.

Gode, D.B. and Bobde, G.N. 1993. Intercropping of soybean in sorghum. *P.K.V. Research Journal*, 17: 128-129.

Gomez MH, Mcdonough, CM., Waniska, RD., and Rooney LW. 1989. Changes in corn and sorghum during nixtamalization and tortilla baking. *J. food Science*. 54: 330.

Gomez. MH., Rooney, LW., Waniska, RD and Pflugfelder, RL 1987. Dry corn masa flours for tortilla and sanck food production. *Cereal Foods World* 32: 372.

Gopalkrishna Rao, M., Kulkarni, M.V., Havanagi, G.V., Venkat Rao, B.V. and Patil, S.V. 1975. Studies on problems of Dry farming at Hagari, University of Agricultural Sciences, Bangalore, UAS Station Series-1 pp. 63.

Gopalkrishnan, S. 1960b. Copper nutrition of millets. Part II. *Madras Agric Journal*, 47: 95-108.

Gorz HJ, Haskins FA, Pedersen JF and Ross WM. 1987. Combining ability effects for mineral elements in forage sorghum hybrids. *Crop Science* 27: 216-219.

Gowda PB, Frederiksen RA, Magill CW, Xu G-W (1995). DNA markers for downy mildew resistance genes in sorghum. *Genome* 38: 823-826.

Graham, P.L., Steiner, J.L. and Wiese, A.F. 1988. Light absorption and competition in mixed sorghum-pigweed communities. *Agronomy Journal* 80: 415-418.

Grichar, W.J. 2006. Weed control in grain sorghum tolerant to flumioxazin. *Crop Protection* 25: 174-177.

Grichar, W.J., Besler, B.A. and Brewer, K.D. 2004. Effect of row spacing and herbicide dose on weed control and grain sorghum yield. *Crop Protection* 23: 263-267.

Grichar, W.J., Besler, B.A. and Brewer, K.D., 2005. Weed control and grain sorghum response to post-emergence application of atrazine/pendimethalin and trifluralin. *Weed Technology* 19: 999-1003.

Grundon, N.J., Edwards, D.G., Takkar, P.N., Asher, C.J. and Clark, R.B. 1987. Nutritional disorders of grain sorghum. *ACIAR Monograph* No.2, 99p.

Guneyli, E., Burnside, O.C. and Nordquist, P.T. 1969. Influence of seedling characteristics on weed competitive ability of sorghum hybrids and inbred lines. *Crop Science* 9: 713-716.

Gworgwor, N. A, Weber, H. C., Ransom, J. K. (ed.); Musselman, L.J.(ed.); Worsham, A.D. (ed.), Parker, C., 1991. Effect of nitrogen fertilization and resistant variety on *Striga hermonthica* infestation in sorghum. In: *Proceedings of the 5ᵗʰ International Symposium of Parasitic Weeds*, Nairobi, Kenya, 24-30 June 1991, pp. 96-103.

Gworgwor, N.A. and Lagoke, S.T.O. 1992. Weed control in sorghum-groundnut mixture in the simultaneous system of farming in Northern Guinea savanna zone of Nigeria. *Tropical Pest Management* 38: 131-135.

Gworgwor, N.A., Hudu, A.I. and Joshua, S.D. 2002. Seed treatment of sorghum varieties with brine (NaCl) solution for control of *Striga hermonthica* in sorghum. *Crop Protection* 21: 1015-1021.

Gworgwor, N.A., Hudu, A.I., Bidliya, B.S., Lale, N.E.S. (ed.), Molta, N.B. (ed.), Donli, P.O. (ed.), Dike, M.C. (ed.), Aminu, K.M., 1998. Herbivore of *Striga hermonthica* in the semi-arid zone of Nigeria and its potential as bio-control agent. Entomology in the Nigerian economy, Research focus in 21ˢᵗ century, pp.183-186.

Hamakar BR, Mohamed AA, Habben JE, Huang CP and Larkins BA. 1995. Efficient procedure for extracting maize and sorghum kernel proteins reveals higher prolamin contents than the conventional method. *Cereal Chemistry* 72: 583-588.

Hamaker BR, Kirleis AW, Butler LG, Axtell JD and Mertz ET (1987). Improving the in vitro protein digestibility of sorghum with reducing agents. *Proc. Natl. Acad. Sci.* 84: 626 – 628.

Hariprakash, M. 1979. Soil testing and plant analysis studies on hybrid sorghum CSH 1. *Mysore Journal of Agricultural Sciences*, 13: 178-181.

Harlan, J. R. 1982. Relationship between crops and weeds. Madison, WI, *American Society of Agronomy*, pp. 295.

Harlan, J. R., and de Wet, J. M. J. 1972. A simplified classification of cultivated sorghum. *Crop Science* 12: 172-76.

Harris K, Subudhi P, Borrell A, Jordan D, Rosenow D, Nguyen H, Klein P, Klein R, Mullet J (2007) Sorghum stay-green QTL individually reduce post-flowering drought-induced leaf senescence. *Journal of Experimental Botany* 58: 327-338.

Hart G, Schertz K, Peng Y, Syed N 2001. Genetic mapping of *Sorghum bicolor* (L.) Moench QTLs that control variation in tillering and other morphological characters. *Theoretical and Applied Genetics* 103: 1232-1242.

Hash C, Bhasker Raj A, Lindup S, Sharma A, Beniwal C, Folkertsma R, Mahalakshmi V, Zerbini E, Blümmel M 2003. Opportunities for marker-assisted selection (MAS) to improve the feed quality of crop residues in pearl millet and sorghum. *Field Crops Research* 84: 79-88.

Haskin, F.A., Gorz, H.J. and Johnson, B.F. 1987. Seasonal variation in leaf hydrocyanic acid potential of low and high Dhurrin sorghum. *Crop Science* 27: 903-906.

Haussmann B, Mahalakshmi V, Reddy B, Seetharama N, Hash C, Geiger H (2002) QTL mapping of stay-green in two sorghum recombinant inbred populations. *Theoretical and Applied Genetics* 106: 133-142.

Hegedus M, Pedersen B, Eggum BO. 1985. The influence of milling on the nutritive value of flour from cereal grains, 7: Vitamins and tryptophan. *Qual Plant Plant Foods Hum Nutr* 35: 175–180.

Hiebsch, C.K. and R.E. McCollum. 1987. Area x time equivalency ratio. A method for evaluating the productivity of intercrops. *Agronomy Journal* 79: 15-22.

Hiremath, S.M., Hebbi, B.S. and Halikatti, S.I. 2003. Performance of *rabi* sorghum as influenced by nitrogen and in situ soil moisture conservation practices in *kharif* sunnhemp for green manuring. *Karnataka Journal of Agricultural Sciences* 16: 216–219.

Hoffmann, G., Marnotte, P. and Dembele, D. 1997. The use of herbicides to control *Striga hermonthica*. *Agriculture-et-Development* 13: 58-62.

Holm, L.G., Plucknett, D., Pancho, J.V. and Harberger, J.P. 1977. *The World's Worst Weeds*. University press of Hawaii, Honolulu.

Hood L.F. (1982). Current concepts of starch structure. Pages 217-236 in: Food Carbohydrates. Lineback DR [Eds.] The AVI publishing Company, Inc. Westport, Connecticut.

Hoseney, R. C.; Varriano-Marston, E.; Dendy,D. A. V. Sorghum and millets. In *AdVances in Cereal Science and Technology*; Pomeranz, Y., Ed.; AACC, Inc.: St Paul, MN, 1981; Vol. IV, pp S70-144.

House LR. 1985. *A guide to sorghum breeding*. 2nd Edn., ICRISAT, Patancheru, Andhra Pradesh, India. 206 p.

House, L. R. 1980. A Guide to Sorghum Breeding, ICRISAT, Patancheru, A.P. India.

House, L.R. 1985. *A Guide to Sorghum Breeding*. Patancheru 502 324, Andhra Pradesh, India: International Crops Research Institute for the Semi-Aird Tropics. 216 pp. http://info.ornl.gov/sites/publications/files/Pub22854.pdf.

Hubbard JE, Hall HH and Earle FR(1950). Composition of the component parts of the sorghum kernel. *Cereal Chem.* 27: 415-420.

Hukkeri, S.B. *et al.*, 1977. In: Water requirement and irrigation management of crops in India. IARI monograph No.4, Caxton Press, New Delhi. P: 402.

ICRISAT, 1984. A Review of fertilizer use research on sorghum in India. International Crop Research Institute for the Semi-Arid Tropics. *Research Bulletin* No.8, pp. 1-59.

ICRISAT, 1986. Annual Report, 1985. International Crop Research Institute for the Semi-Arid Tropics. Patancheru, AP, India pp 489.

ICRISAT, 1988. Plant Material Description no.17. International Crops Research Institute for the Semi-Arid Tropics Patancheru, Andhra Pradesh 502 324, India.

ICRISAT, 2005. Long-term effect of legume-based rotations. Global theme on agro-ecosystems. International Crop Research Institute for the Semi-Arid Tropics. Patancheru, AP, India. http: //www.icrisat.org/gt-aes/researchbreifs21-htm.pp 1-4.

Idowu. A. 1989. Bread from composite Flours. Proceedings of a symposium on the current status and potential of Industrial Uses of sorghum in Nigeria. 4-6Dec, Kano, Nigeria. pp 22.

Ikediobi. CO. 1989. Industrial production of Sorghum malt in Nigeria. Proceedings of a symposium on the current status and potential of Industrial Uses of sorghum in Nigeria. 4-6, December, Kano, Nigeria. pp 32.

Ishaya, D.B., Dadari, S.A. and Shebayan, J.A.Y. 2007. Evaluation of herbicides for weed control in sorghum (*Sorghum bicolor*) in Nigeria. *Crop Protection* 26: 1697-1701.

Jane J, Xu A, Radosavljevic M and Seib PA (1992). Location of amylose in normal starch granules. I. Susceptibility of amylose and amylopectin to cross-linking reagents. *Cereal Chem.* 69: 405-409.

Jen-Hshuan Chen, 2006. The combined use of chemical and organic fertilizers and or biofertilizer for crop growth and soil fertility. In: *International Workshop on Sustained Management of the Soil-Rhizosphere System for Efficient Crop Production and Fertilizer Use.* Land Development Department, Bankok-10900, Thailand. October, 16-20, 125-130.

Jones, C.A.1983. A survey of the variability in tissue nitrogen and phosphorus concentration in maize and green sorghum. *Field Crops Research,* 6: 133-147.

Jones, O. R., and Johnson, G. L. 1991. Row width and plant density effects on Texas High Plains Sorghum. *Journal of Production Agriculture* 4: 613-19.

Jordan D, Hunt C, Cruickshank A, Borrell A, Henzell R (2012) The relationship between the stay-green trait and grain yield in elite sorghum hybrids grown in a range of environments. *Crop Science* 52: 1153-1161.

Jordan WR, Clark RB and Seetharama N. 1984. The role of edaphic factors in disease development. In: Mughogho LK, Rosenberg G (eds) Sorghum Root and Stalk Rots: A Critical Review. Proceedings of the Consultative GroupDiscussion on Research Needs and Strategies for Control of Sorghum Root and Stalk Rot Diseases, 27 Nov.–2 Dec. 1983, Bellagio, Italy, pp. 81–97. ICRISAT, Patancheru, India.

Joshi, S.G. 1956. An examination of the results of the factorial design field experiment for the response of jowar crop to the application of different micronutrients. *Journal of Indian Society of Soil Science*, 4: 147-159.

Jost, A. 1997. Integrated cereal cropping in north Ghana with special attention for *Striga* problems. *Plits* 15: 10.

Kalyansundaram D and Kuppuswamy G, 1999. Effect of different weed control methods on the performance of sorghum and soil health. In: *Abstracts, 8ᵗʰ Biennial Conference, Indian Society of Weed Science*, February, 5-7, 1999. Varanasi, India, pp. 37.

Kandasamy, O.S. and Subramanian, S. 1980. *Madras Agric. Journal*, 67: 552-553.

Kandasamy, O.S., Raja, D. and Chandrashekhar, C.N. 1999. Evaluation of herbicides for selectivity and weed control in rainfed sorghum + pigeonpea intercropping system. In: *Abstracts, 8ᵗʰ Biennial Conference, Indian Society of Weed Science*, February, 5-7, 1999. Varanasi, India, pp. 106.

Kanwar, J.S. 1978. Fertilization of sorghum, millets and other food crops for optimum yield under dry farming conditions. Pages AGR II 3/1-16, *Proceedings of Annual Seminar*, Dec. 1977. Fertilizer Association of India (FAI), New Delhi.

Kanwar, J.S. and Randhawa, N.S. 1967. Micronutrient research in soil and plants in India-A Review, Indian Council of Agricultural Research, New Delhi.

Kasemsuwan T and Jane J 1994. Location of amylose in normal starch granules. II. Locations of phosphodiester cross-linking revealed by phosphorus-31 nuclear magnetic resonance. *Cereal Chem.* 71: 282-287.

Kassahun B, Bidinger F, Hash C, Kuruvinashetti M (2010). Stay-green expression in early generation sorghum [*Sorghum bicolor* (L.) Moench] QTL introgression lines. *Euphytica* 172: 351-362.

Katsar CS, Paterson AH, Teetes GL, Peterson GC (2002). Molecular analysis of sorghum resistance to the greenbug (Homoptera: Aphididae). *Journal of Economic Entomology* 95: 448-457.

Katyal, J.C. 2000. Organic matter maintenance. *Journal of Indian Society of Soil Science* 48: 704-716.

Kebede H, Subudhi P, Rosenow D, Nguyen H (2001). Quantitative trait loci influencing drought tolerance in grain sorghum (*Sorghum bicolor* L. Moench). *Theoretical and Applied Genetics* 103: 266-276.

Kempuchetty, N. and Sankaran, S. 1990. Soil moisture and herbicide interaction studies for weed control in rainfed sorghum intercropped with cowpea. In: *Abstracts, Biennial Conference, Indian Society of Weed Science*, March 4-5 1990. Jabalpur, India, pp. 112.

Khan, Z.R., Midega, C.A.O., Hassanali, A., Pickett, J.A. and Wadhams, L.J. 2007. Assement of different legumes for the control of *Striga hermonthica* in maize and sorghum. *Agronomy Journal* 47: 730-734.

Khune, N.N., Shiwankar, S.K. and Wangikar, P.D. 1980. Food, *Farming and Agriculture* 12: 192-193.

Klein R, Klein P, Chhabra A, Dong J, Pammi S, Childs K, Mullet J, Rooney W, Schertz K (2001a). Molecular mapping of the rf1 gene for pollen fertility restoration in sorghum (*Sorghum bicolor* L.). *Theoretical and Applied Genetics* 102: 1206-1212.

Klein R, Rodriguez-Herrera R, Schlueter J, Klein P, Yu Z, Rooney W (2001b). Identification of genomic regions that affect grain-mould incidence and other traits of agronomic importance in sorghum. *Theoretical and Applied Genetics* 102: 307-319.

Klein R, Rodriguez-Herrera R, Schlueter J, Klein P, Yu Z, Rooney W (2001c). Identification of genomic regions that affect grain-mould incidence and other traits of agronomic importance in sorghum. *Theoretical and Applied Genetics* 102: 307-319.

Klocke, N. L. and Hergert, G.W. 1990. How soil holds water. G 90-964. www.ianr.unl.edu/pub/fieldcrops/g964.htm.

Knezevic, S.A., Horak, M.J. and Vanderlip, R.L. 1997. Relative time of redroot pigweed (*Amaranthus retroflexux* L.) emergence is critical in pigweed-sorghum (*Sorghum bicolor*) competition. *Weed Science* 45: 502-508.

Knoll J, Gunaratna N, Ejeta G (2008). QTL analysis of early-season cold tolerance in sorghum. Theoretical and applied genetics Genetik 116: 577-587.

Kondap, S.M. and Bathkal, B.G. 1981.Crop-weed competition studies in sorghum under different management practices. In: *Proceedings of 8th Asian-Pacific Weed Science Society Conference*, Bangalore, India, Vol.II, pp. 117-122.

Kondap, S.M., Ramoji, G.V.N.S., Bucha Reddy, B. and Rao, A.N. 1985. Influence of nitrogen fertilization and weed growth on weed control efficiency of certain herbicides in sorghum crop. In: *Abstracts of Annual Conference of Indian Society of Weed Science*, 4-5 April, 1985, Gujarat Agricultural University, Anand (India), pp. 31-32.

Kondap, S.M., Rao, A.R. and Reddy, G.V. 1990. Studies on the effect of planting patterns and weeding intervals in sorghum based intercropping system on weed infestation and yield. *Madras Agricultural Journal* 77: 64-69.

Koraddi, U.R., Kulkarni, R.Y. and Kajjar, N.B. 1969. Lime induced iron chlorosis in hybrid sorghum. *Mysore Journal of Agricultural Sciences*, 3: 116-117.

Kramer NW and Ross WM. 1970. Cultivation of Grain Sorghum in the United States. *Sorghum Production and Utilization*. Ed. Joseph S. Wall and William M. Ross. Westport, CT: Avi Pub., pp.167-99.

Krishna, K.R. 2010. *Agroecosystems of South India: Nutrient Dynamics, Ecology and Productivity*. Brown Walker Press, Boca Raton, Florida, USA.

Krishna, K.R., Dart, P.J., Papavinasasundaram, K.G. and Shetty, K.G. 1985. Growth and phosphorus uptake responses of *Sorghum bicolor* to mycorrhyzal inoculations. *Proceedings of the 6th North America Conference on Mycorrhiza* (NACM), Bend, Oregon, USA, pp. 404.

Krishnasamy, S. and Krishnasamy, R. 1996. Integrated weed management for the premonsoon sown sorghum-cowpea intercropping system under rainfed vertisols. *Madras Agricultural Journal* 83: 300-302.

Kumar, A.A., Reddy, B.V.S., Sharma, H.C., Hash, T.C., Rao, P.S., Ramaiah, B. and Reddy, P.S., 2011. Recent advances in sorghum genetic enhancement research at ICRISAT. *American Journal of Plant Sciences* 2: 589-600.

Lafarge, T. A., Broad, I. J. and Hammer, G. L.2002. Tillering in grain sorghum over a wide range of population densities: identification of a common hierarchy for tiller emergence, leaf area development and fertility. *Annals of Botany* 90: 87-98.

Lagoke, S.T.O. 1987. Evaluation of sorghum varieties for resistance to *Striga*. *Cereals Research Programme Cropping Scheme Report* IAR, ABU, Zaria.

Larson, L. and Thompson, D. 2011. Dryland grain sorghum seeding rate and seed maturation, Brandon, 2010. *Plainsman Research Center 2010 Research Reports*: 14-18pp.

Latchanna, A., Boralkur, B.N. and Satyanarayana, V. 1989. Economics of chemical weed control in rainfed *rabi* sorghum. *Journal of Research, ANGRAU* 17: 309-311.

Leder I. 2004. Sorghum and millets. In: Fuleky, G. (Ed.), Cultivated Plants, Primarily as Food Sources, Encyclopedia of Life Support Systems (EOLSS), Eolss Publishers, Oxford, UK. p. 18.

Lima, G.S. de. 1998. Estudo comparativo da resistencia a' seca no sorgo forrageiro (*Sorghum bicolor* (L.) Moench) em differentes estadios de desenvolvimento. Recife: UFRPE.128 p.

Limon-Ortega, A., Mason, S.C. and Martin, A.R. 1998. Production practices improve grain sorghum and pearlmillet competitiveness with weeds. *Agronomy Journal* 90: 227-232.

Lin Y-R, Schertz KF, Paterson AH (1995). Comparative analysis of QTLs affecting plant height and maturity across the Poaceae, in reference to an interspecific sorghum population. *Genetics* 141: 391.

Lingegowda, B.K., Inamdar, S.S. and Krishnamoorthy, K. 1971. Studies on the split application of nitrogen to rainfed hybrid sorghum. *Indian Journal of Agronomy*, 16: 157-158.

Lomte, M.H., Kawarkhe, P.K. and Ateeque, M. 1992. Intercropping of safflower in post-rainy sorghum (*Sorghum bicolor*). *Indian Journal of Agricultural Sciences*, 62: 793-795.

Lugg, D. G. 1974. *Effect of Row Direction on Sorghum Production*. Thesis. Colorado State University, 1974. Fort Collins: Colorado State University.

Maas, E.V., Posss, J.A. and Hoffman, G.J. 1986. Salinity sensitive of sorghum at three growth stages. *Irrigation Science*, 7: 1-11.

Mace E, Jordan D (2010). Location of major effect genes in sorghum (*Sorghum bicolor* (L.) Moench). *Theoretical and Applied Genetics* 121: 1339-1356.

Mace E, Jordan D (2011). Integrating sorghum whole genome sequence information with a compendium of sorghum QTL studies reveals uneven distribution of QTL and of gene-rich regions with significant implications for crop improvement. *Theoretical and Applied Genetics* 123: 169-191.

Mace E, Xia L, Jordan D, Halloran K, Parh D, Huttner E, Wenzl P, Kilian A (2008). DArT markers: diversity analyses and mapping in *Sorghum bicolor*. *BMC Genomics* 9: 26.

MacLean WC, Lopez de Romana G, Placko RP, and Graham GG 1981. Protein quality and digestibility of sorghum in preschool children: Balance studies and plasma free amino acids. *J. Nutr.* 111: 1928-1936.

Maiti RK.1996. Panicle development and productivity. (*In*) *Sorghum Science*. Oxford and IBH Publishing Co. New Delhi, India. pp 140-181.

Maiti, R.K, Ramaiah KV, Bisen SS, Chidley, BL, 1984, A Comparative Study of the Haustorial Development of *Striga asiatica* (L.) Kuntze on Sorghum Cultivars, *Annals of Botany* 54: 447-457.

Maiti, R.K. 1996a. Panicle Development and Productivity. In. *Sorghum science*. Oxford IBH Publishing Co. Pvt. Ltd. New Delhi. pp. 139-180.

Maiti, R.K.1996. Panicle development and productivity. (*In*) *Sorghum Science*. Oxford and IBH Publishing Co. New Delhi, India. pp. 140-181.

Maman, N., Lyon, D.J., Mason, S.C., Galusha, T.D., Higgins, R. 2003. Pearl millet and grain sorghum yield response to water supply in Nebraska. *Agronomy Journal*, 95: 1618-1624.

Maqbool, S.B., Devi, P. and Sticklen, M.B. 2001.Biotechnology: Genetic improvement of sorghum (*Sorghum bicolor*). *In Vitro Cell Development Biology-Plant*, 37: 504-515.

Maraanville, J.W., Pandey, R.K., and Sirifi, S. 2002. Comparison of nitrogen use efficiency of a newly developed sorghum hybrid and two improved cultivars in the Sahel of west Africa. *Comm. in Soil Sci. Plant Anal.* 33: 1519-1536.

Marley, P.S. 1995. *Cynodon dactylon*: An alternate host for *Sporisorium sorghi*, the causal organism of sorghum covered smut. *Crop Protection* 14: 491-493.

Marley, P.S. Aba, D.A., Shebayan, J.A.Y., Musa, R. and Sanni, A. 2004. Integrated management of *Striga hermonthica* in sorghumusing a mycoherbicide and host plant resistance in the Nigerian Sudano-Sahelian savanna. *Weed Research* 44: 157-162.

Martin, J. H. 1970.History and Classification of Sorghum. *Sorghum Production and Utilization; Major Feed and Food Crops in Agriculture and Food Series.* Ed. Joseph S. Wall and William M. Ross. Westport, CT: Avi Pub., pp.1-27.

Martin, J. H., Waldren, R. P., and Stamp, D. L.2006. "Sorghum." *Principles of Field Crop Production*. 4th ed. Upper Saddle River, New Jersey: Pearson Education, pp.341-66.

Mastan, S.C. and Goud, D.V., 1980-83. Studies on intercropping of different crops in jowar. *Journal of Research, APAU*, VII-X: 127-129.

Maunder, A.B. 2000. History of Cultivar Development in the United States: From "Memoirs of A. B. Maunder-Sorghum Breeder. *Sorghum: Origin, History, Technology, and Production*. Ed. C. Wayne. Smith and Richard A. Frederiksen. New York: Wiley, pp.191-223.

Mboob, S.S. 1986. A regional progeamme for West and Central Africa. In: Proceedings of the FAO/OAU All African Government Consultation on *Striga* Control, Maroua, Cameroon, 20-24 October, pp. 183-186.

McBee, G.G. and Miller, F.R. 1980. *Hydrocyanic acid potential in several sorghum breeding lines as affected by nitrogen fertilization and variable harvests. Crop Science*, 20: 232-234.

McClure A, Stephen Ebelhar, Chad Lee, Emerson Nafziger and Terry Wyciskalla. 2010. High Plains Production Handbook. Ed. Jeff Dahlberg, Earl Roemer, Jeff Casten, Gary Kilgore, and James Vorderstrasse. Lubbock: United Sorghum Checkoff Program, 2010.

McClure, A., Stephen Ebelhar, Chad Lee, Emerson Nafziger, and Terry Wyciskalla. 2010. High Plains Production Handbook. Ed. Jeff Dahlberg, Earl Roemer, Jeff Casten, Gary Kilgore, and James Vorderstrasse. Lubbock: United Sorghum Checkoff Program, 2010.

McGillchrist, I.A. 1965. Analysis of competition experiments. *Biometrics* 21: 975-985.

McLean, G., Whish, J., Routley, R.A., Broad, I. and Hammer. G. 2003. The effect of row configuration on yield reliability in grain sorghum: II. Yield, water use efficiency and soil water extraction. *Proc. of 11ᵗʰ Aust.Agron. Conf.* Geelong, Victoria. 2–6 Feb. 2003. Australian Society of Agronomy. Gosford, Australia.

Miller FR. 1982. Genetic and environmental response characteristics of sorghum. ICRISAT, pp. 393-402.

Miller, F.R. and Bovey, R.W. 1969. Tolerance of *Sorghum bicolor* (L.) Moench to several herbicides. *Agronomy Journal* 61: 282-585.

Miri, Khaled, Rana, D.S., Rana, K.S, and Kumar Ashok. 2012. Productivity, nitrogen-use efficiency and economics of sweet sorghum (*Sorghum bicolor*) genotypes as influenced by different levels of nitrogen. *Indian Journal of Agronomy* 57: 49-54.

Mishra, J. S., Subbarayudu, B., Chapke, R. R. and Seetharama, N. 2009. Sorghum-a potential high yielder in rice-fallows of Andhra Pradesh. *ICAR NEWS* 15 (4): 8p.

Mishra, J.S. 1997. Critical period of weed competition and losses due to weeds in major field crops. *Farmers and Parliament* 33: 19-20.

Mishra, J.S. and Rao, S.S. 2011. Integrated weed management in sorghum. *Indian Farming* 61 (2): 7-11.

Mishra, J.S., Chapke, R.R., Subbarayudu, B., Hariprasanna, K. And Patil, J.V. 2013. Response of sorghum (*Sorghum bicolor*) hybrids to nitrogen under zero tillage in rice-fallows of Coastal Andhra Pradesh. *Indian Journal of Agricultural Sciences*, 83: 359-61.

Mishra, J.S., Talwar, H.S. and Patil, J.V. 2012. Conservation tillage and integrated nutrient management in *kharif* grain sorghum. *In. Summaries.* National Seminar on Indian Agriculture: Preparedness for Climate Change, March 24-25, 2012, New Delhi, 53-54pp.

Mishra, R.K., Choudhary, S.K. and Tripathi, A.K. 1997. Intercropping of cowpea (*Vigna unguiculata*) and horsegram (*Macrotyloma uniflorum*) with sorghum for fodder under rained conditions. *Indian Journal of Agronomy*, 43: 405-408.

Mittal M, Boora K (2005) Molecular tagging of gene conferring leaf blight resistance using microsatellites in sorghum [*Sorghum bicolor* (L.) Moench]. *Indian Journal of Experimental Biology* 43: 462-466.

Mohamed Ali and Sudhakar Rao, A. 1987. Effect of sublethal rates of phenoxy and triazine herbicides and nitrogen on sorghum. *Indian Journal of Agronomy* 32: 88-89.

Mohan D. 1975. Chemically induced high lysine mutants in *Sorghum bicolor* (L.) Moench. Thesis, Purdue University, West Lafayette, IN, 110 pp.

Mohandoss, M., Pannerselvam, P. and Kuppuswamy, G. 2002. Effect of intercropping on weed dynamics. *Agricultural Science Digest* 22: 138-139.

Mohmood, A. and Cheema, Z.A. 2004. Influence of sorghum mulch on purple nutsedge (*Cyperus rotundus* L.). *International Journal of Agriculture and Biology* 6: 86-88.

Monaghan, N. 1978. Problems caused by *Sorghum halepense* in Australia. *PANS* 24: 172-176.

Moody, K. 1978. Weed control in intercropping in tropical Asia. *Paper presented at the International Weed Science Conference*, 3-7 July 1978. IRRI, Los Banos, Philippines.

Moore, J.W. and Murray, D.S. 2002. Influence of palmer amaranth on grain sorghum yields, *Proceedings of Southern Weed Science Society* 53, pp. 143-144.

Moraghan, J.T., Rego, T.J., Buresh, R.J., Vlek, P.L. Burfora, J.R., Singh, S., and Sahrawat, K.L. 1983. Labelled nitrogen fertiliser studies on a Vertisol in the semi-arid tropics (in manuscript: ICRISAT).

Mughogho LK and Pande S. 1984. Charcoal rot of Sorghum. In: Mughogho LK, Rosenberg G (eds) Sorghum Root and Stalk Rots: A Critical Review. Proceedings of the Consultative Group Discussion on Research Needs and Strategies for Control of Sorghum Root and Stalk Rot Diseases, 27 Nov.–2 Dec. 1983, Bellagio, Italy, pp. 99–110. ICRISAT, Patancheru, India.

Mukherjee, A.K., Mandal, S.R., Mandal, Udita and Mandal., U. 2000. Comparative effect of different weed control measures on growth and forage yield of *jowar*. *Environmental Ecology* 18: 20-322.

Murali Mohan S, Madhusudhana R, Mathur K, Chakravarthi DVN, Rathore S, Nagaraja Reddy R, Satish K, Srinivas G, Sarada Mani N, Seetharama N (2010).

Identification of quantitative trait loci associated with resistance to foliar diseases in sorghum [*Sorghum bicolor (L.)* Moench]. *Euphytica* 176: 199-211.

Murty, M.V.R., Piara Singh, Wani, S.P, Khairwal, I.S. and Srinivas, K. 2007. Yield Gap Analysis of Sorghum and Pearl Millet in India Using Simulation Modeling. *Global Theme on Agro-ecosystems Report no. 37.* Patancheru 502 324, Andhra Pradesh, India: International Crops Research Institute for the Semi-Arid Tropics. 82 pp.

Muthama NL. 2001. Genetic analysis of nutritional quality traits in sorghum. PhD thesis submitted to Purdue University.ISBN 9780493576305, 0493576304.

Muthuswamy, P., Govindaswamy, M. and Krishnamurthy, K.K. 1976. Effect of stage of cutting on the crude protein and prussic acid content of CSH 5 sorghum. *Madras Agronomy Journal* 63: 200-201.

Muyanja, C.M.B.K; Kikafunda, J. K; Narvhus, J.A; Helgetun, K; Langsrud, T 2003. Production methods and composition of Bushera: a Ugandan traditional fermented cereal beverage. *African Journal of Food, Agriculture, Nutrition and Development.* 3(1): 10-19.

Myers, R.J.K. and Asher, C.J. 1982. Mineral nutrition of grain sorghum: Micronutrients. Sorghum in the Eighties. *Proceedings of the International Symposium on sorghum,* ICRISAT, 2-7 November, 1981, Patancheru, AP, India, 161-177.

Nagaraj N, Reese JC, Tuinstra MR, Smith CM, St. Amand P, Kirkham M, Kofoid KD, Campbell LR, Wilde G (2005). Molecular mapping of sorghum genes expressing tolerance to damage by greenbug (Homoptera: Aphididae). *Journal of Economic Entomology* 98: 595-602.

Narayana Reddy, S., Rangamannan, K.T., Reddy, S.R. and Shankara Reddy, G.S. 1972. A note on the foliar application of urea to jowar variety 'Swarna'. *Indian Journal of Agronomy,* 17: 363-367.

Natarajan, N., Subba Rao, P.V., and Gopal, S. 1991. Effect of intercropping of pulses in cereals on the incidence of major pests. *Madras Agric Journal,* 78: 59-67.

NCAER and FAI (National Council of Applied Economic Research and Fertilizer Association of India). 1974. Fertilizer use on selected crops in India. New Delhi, India, 52 pp.

New L. 2004. Grain sorghum irrigation. B-6152, 6-04. Texas Cooperative Extension.

Nikuni Z 1978. Studies on starch granules. *Starch Staerke* 30: 105-111.

Nimbal CI, Weston LA, Brown H (ed.); Cussans GW (ed.), Devine, MD (ed.), Duke SO (ed.), Fernandez Quintanilla C (ed.), Helweg A (ed.), Labrada RE (ed.), Landes M (ed.), Kudsk P (ed.), Streibig JC, 1996. *In: Proceedings of the Second International Weed Control Congress,* Copenhagen, Denmark, 25-28 June 1996, Volumes 1-4, pp. 863-868.

Nwilene FE, Nwanze KF and Reddy YVR, 1998. Effect of sorghum ecosystem diversification and sowing date on shoot fly, stem borer and associated parasitoids. *Crop Research* 16: 239-245.

Obizoba IC. 1988. Nutritive value of melted, dry or wet milled sorghum and corn. *Cereal Chem* 53: 222–226.

Ockerby, S.E., Midmore, D.J., Yule, D.F. 2001. Leaf modification delays panicle initiation and anthesis in grain sorghum. *Australian Journal of Agricultural Research*, 52: 127-135.

Ogundipe HO and O. Omasevwerha. 1989. Processing and acceptability studies of Soy- enriched Non wheat Biscuits. Proceedings of a symposium on the current status and potential of Industrial Uses of sorghum in Nigeria. 4-6, Dec, Kano, Nigeria. Pp 24.

Ogundiwin. JO, MO Ilori and A. Okelaye. 1989. Brewing of clear Beer from sorghum grains of SK 5912 variety without addition of external enzymes to achieve Saccharification: A case study. Proceedings of a symposium on the current status and potential of Industrial Uses of sorghum in Nigeria. 4-6 Dec, Kano, Nigeria. Pp 31.

Oh B, Gowda P, Magill C, Frederiksen R (1993). Tagging acremonium wilt, downy mildew and head smut resistance genes in sorghum using RFLP and RAPD markers. *Sorghum Newsl.* 35: 34.

Oizumi H. *et al.*, 1965. *Sorghum Newsletter*, 8: 43-44.

Okafor, L. I. and Zitta, C. 1991. The influence of nitrogen on sorghum weed competition in the tropics. *Tropical Pest Management* 37: 138-143.

Ong MH, Jumel K, Tokarczuk PF, Blanshard JMV and Harding SE (1994). Simultaneous determinations of the molecular weight distributions of amyloses and the fine structures of amylopectins of native starches. *Carbohydrate. Res.* 260: 99-117.

Oria MP, Hamaker BR, Axtell JD, Huang CP 2000. A Highly digestible sorghum mutant cultivar exhibits a unique folded structure of endosperm protein bodies. *Proc. Natl. Acad. Sci.* 97 (10): 5065-5070.

Oria MP, Hamaker BR, Schull JM 1995b. Resistance of sorghum α-, β-, and γ-kafirins to pepsin digestion. *J. Agric. Food Chem*. 43: 2148-2153.

Oria MP, Hamaker BR, Schull JM 1995a. *In vitro* protein digestibility of developing and mature sorghum grain in relation to α-, β-, and γ-kafirin disulfide crosslinking. *J. Cereal Sci.* 22: 85-93.

Pal, U.R., Upadhyay, U.C., Singh, S.P. and Umrani, M.K. 1982. Mineral nutrition and fertilizer response of grain sorghum in India-A review over the last 25 years. *Fertilizer Research*, 3: 141-159.

Palaniappan, S.P. and Ramaswamy, R. 1976. Residual effect of atrazine applied to sorghum on the succeeding crops. *Madras Agricultural Journal* 65: 230-232.

Palaniappan, S.P. *et al.* (1977). Annual Report, Tamil Nadu Agricultural University, Coimbatore.

Parh D, Jordan D, Aitken EAB, Mace E, Jun-Ai P, McIntyre C, Godwin I (2008). QTL analysis of ergot resistance in sorghum. *Theoretical and Applied Genetics* 117: 369-382.

Parh DK, Jordan DR, Aitken EAB, Gogel BJ, McIntyre CL, Godwin ID (2006). Genetic components of variance and the role of pollen traits in sorghum ergot resistance. *Crop Science* 46: 2387-2395.

Parker C, 2008. Observations on the current status of *Orobanche* and *Striga* Problems worldwide. *Pest Management Science* 65: 453-459.

Parkinson V, Kim SK, Efron Y, Bello L, and Dashiel, 1986. Potential trap crops for *Striga* Control. In: *Proceedings of the FAO/OAU All African Government Consultation on Striga Control,* Maroua, Cameroon, 20-24 October, pp. 136-140.

Paterson A H, Bowers J E, Bruggmann R, Dubchak I, Grimwood J, Gundlach H, Haberer G, Hellsten U, Mitros T, Poliakov A, Schmutz J, Spannagl M, Tang H, Wang X, Wicker T, Bharti A K, Chapman J, Feltus F A, Gowik U, Grigoriev I V, Lyons E, Maher C A, Martis M, Narechania A, Otillar R P, Penning B W, Salamov A A, Wang Y, Zhang L, Carpita N C, Freeling M, Gingle A R, Hash C T, Keller B, Klein P, Kresovich S, McCann M C, Ming R, Peterson D G, Mehboob ur R, Ware D, Westhoff P, Mayer K F X, Messing J and Rokhsar D S. 2009. The *Sorghum bicolor* genome and the diversification of grasses. *Nature,* 457, 551-556.

Paterson AH, Bowers JE, Bruggmann R, Dubchak I, Grimwood J, Gundlach H, Haberer G, Hellsten U, Mitros T, Poliakov A (2009). The *Sorghum bicolor* genome and the diversification of grasses. *Nature* 457: 551-556.

Patil, H.M., Tuwar, S.S and Wani, A.G. 2008. Integrated nutrient management in sorghum (*Sorghum bicolor*)-chickpea (*Cicer arietinum*) cropping sequence under irrigated conditions *International Journal of Agricultural Sciences* 4: 220-224.

Patil, J.V., Mishra, J.S., Chapke, R.R., Gadakh, S.R. and Chavan, U.D. 2013. Soil moisture conservation agro-techniques for rainfed *rabi* sorghum. *Indian Farming,* 62 (12): 04-07.

Patil, J.R. and Shah, S.R. 1979. Studies on weed control in sorghum. In: *Abstract of Papers, Annual Meet, Indian Society of Weed Science,* Marathwada Agricultural University, Parbhani, pp. 45.

Pawar, S.H. and Shelke, V.B. 1992. Intercropping of vegetables in *kharif* sorghum. *Journal of Maharashtra Agricultural University,* 17: 493.

Peacock, J. M. and Heinrich, G. M. 1984. "Light and Temperature Responses in Sorghum." *Agrometeorology of Sorghum and Millet in the Semi-Arid Tropics: Proceedings of the International Symposium, 15-20 Nov 1982, ICRISAT Center, India* . Patancheru. Ed. S. M. Virmani, M.V. K. Sivakumar, and Vrinda Kumble. Andhra Pradesh: ICRISAT (International Crops Research Institute for the Semi-Arid Tropics), pp. 143-58.

Peacock, J.M. 1980. The role of crop physiologists in a sorghum improvement programme. Institute Seminar, *ICRISAT, Internal Report.*

Peat S, Whelan WJ and Thomas GJ 1952. Evidence of multiple branching in waxy maize starch. *J. Chem. Soc.* 4546-4549.

Pedersen, J.F. and Fritz, J.O. 2000. Forages and fodder. In: Smith, C W and Federiksen, R A. (Eds). *Sorghum-Origin, History, Technology and Production*, John Wiley and Sons, Inc. New York. Pp, 798-810.

Peng Li En. 2013. Characterization of environmental and genetic effects on sorghum starch structure and functional properties PhD thesis submitted to The University of Queensland 146pp.

Pereira M, Lee M (1995) Identification of genomic regions affecting plant height in sorghum and maize. *Theoretical and Applied Genetics* 90: 380-388.

Pfeiffer WH and McClafferty B. 2007. Harvest Plus: Breeding crops for better nutrition. *Crop Science* 47: S88–S105.

Phillips, W.M. 1970. Weed control methods, losses and costs due to weeds, and benefits of weed control in grain sorghum. *In: Proceedings of First FAO International Conference on Weed Control*, Davis, CA. Weed Science Society of America, Urbana, IL, pp. 101-108.

Plessis Jean du. 2008. Sorghum Production. Department of Agriculture, Republic of South Africa, available on the web: *www.nda.agric.za/publications.*

Poehlman, J. M. 1987. Breeding Sorghum and Millet. *Breeding Field Crops*. 3rd ed. Westport, CT: AVI Publ., pp. 508-55.

Ponnuswami, K., Santhi, P. and Sankaran, N. 2003. Effect of intercrops and herbicides on weeds and productivity of rainfed sorghum. In: *Abstracts, Biennial Conference, Indian Society of Weed Science*, March, 12-14 2003, GBPUAT, Pantnagar, India, pp. 43.

Prasad, P.V.V., and Staggenborg, S.A. 2009. Growth and production of sorghum and millets. In. soils, plant growth and crop production –Volume II. In: Encyclopedia of life Support Systems, Eolss Publishers, Oxford, UK. http: //www.eolss.net.

Prasad, R. 2009. Efficient fertilizer use: The key to food security and better environment. *Journal of Tropical Agriculture*, 47: 1-17.

Priyolkar.VS. 1989. Use of Sorghum flour in biscuit and wafer production: The Nasco experience. Proceedings of a symposium on the current status and potential of Industrial Uses of sorghum in Nigeria. 4-6, Dec, Kano, Nigeria. pp. 22.

Purseglove JW. 1972. Trapical crops: monocotyledons, Vol. 1. Londres, Longman Group Limited. 334 p.

Quinby, J. R. and Schertz, K. F. 1970. Sorghum Genetics, Breeding, and Hybrid Seed Production. *Sorghum Production and Utilization*. Ed. Joseph S. Wall and William M. Ross. Westport, CT: Avi Pub., pp. 73-117.

Quinby, J.R. 1973. The genetic control of flowering and growth in sorghum. *In. Advances in Agronomy*. N.C. Brady (Ed.). Am. Soc. Agron., Madison.

Radder, G.D., Itnal, C.J., Surkod, V.S. and Biradar, B.M. 1991. Compartmental bunding- An effective in situ moisture conservation practice on medium deep black soil. *Indian Journal of Soil Conservation*, 19: 1-5.

Radder, G.D., Surakod, V.S., Biradar, B.M. and Patil, V.S. 1993. Border method of planting for etabilizing the yield of rainfed rabi crops. In. *Recent Advances in Dryland Agriculture*. Scientific Publishers, Jodhpur, 175-180 pp.

Raghuvanshi, R.K.S., Thakur, R.S., Unat, R. and Nema, M.L. 1990. Crop technology for optimum grain production in sorghum-wheat sequence under resource restraints. *Indian Journal of Agronomy* 35: 246-250.

Raheja. P.C. 1961. ICAR Res. Ser. No. 25, ICAR, New Delhi.

Ram, S.N. and Singh, B. 2001. Effect of nitrogen and harvesting time on yield and quality of sorghum (*Sorghum bicolor*) intercropped with legumes. *Indian Journal of Agronomy*, 46: 611-615.

Ramakrishna, A. 2003.Integrated weed management improves grain sorghum growth and yield on Vertisols. *Tropical Agriculture* 80: 48-53.

Ramakrishna, A. Ong, C.K. and Reddy, S.L.N. 1991. Studies on integrated weed management in sorghum. *Tropical Pest Management* 37: 159-161.

Ramamoorthy, K., Ali, A.M. and Prabhakaran, J. 1995. Integrated weed management in sorghum based intercropping system under rainfed conditions. *Mysore Journal of Agricultural Sciences* 29: 97-100.

Ramasamy P, Menz M, Mehta P, Katilé S, Gutierrez-Rojas L, Klein R, Klein P, Prom L, Schlueter J, Rooney W (2009) Molecular mapping of Cg1, a gene for resistance to anthracnose (*Colletotrichum sublineolum*) in sorghum. *Euphytica* 165: 597-606.

Rami JF, Dufour P, Trouche G, Fliedel G, Mestres C, Davrieux F, Blanchard P, Hamon P. 1998. Quantitative trait loci for grain quality, productivity, morphological and agronomical traits in sorghum (*Sorghum bicolor* L. Moench),*Theoretical and Applied Genetics* 97: 605-616.

Rami JF. 1999. Etude des facteurs génétiques impliqués dans la qualité technologique du grain chez le maïs et le sorgho. Ph. D. report. Université d'Orsay, France.

Ramu P, Kassahun B, Senthilvel S, Kumar CA, Jayashree B, Folkertsma R, Reddy LA, Kuruvinashetti M, Haussmann B, Hash C (2009). Exploiting rice–sorghum synteny for targeted development of EST-SSRs to enrich the sorghum genetic linkage map. *Theoretical and Applied Genetics* 119: 1193-1204.

Rana, B.S., Rao, M.H., Indira, S., Singh, B.U., Appaji, Chari and Tonapi, Vilas. 1999. Technology for increasing sorghum production and value addition. National Research Centre for Sorghum, Hyderabad.

Rao A.N. 1978. Ecophysiological responses of crops and weeds against herbicides and their residues. *Ph. D. Thesis*, Vikram University, Ujjain, Madhya Pradesh, India.

Rao SK, Gupta AK, Baghal and Singh SP. 1982. Combining ability analysis of grain quality sorghum. *Indian Journal of Agricultural Research* 16(1): 1-9.

Rao SS, Seetharama N, Kiran Kumar KA and Vanderlip RL. 2004. Characterisation of sorghum growth stages. NRCS Bulletin Series No. 14, National Research Centre for Sorghum, Rajendranagar, Hyderabad 500030. 20 p.

Rao, A.C.S. and Das, S.K. 1982. Soil fertility management and fertilizer use in dry land agriculture. Pages 120-139. *In. A Decade of Dry land Agriculture in India* 1971-80. AICRPDA, Hyderabad, India.

Rao, J.V., Khan, I.A. and Sujatha, S. 2003. Critical Review of Research on intercropping systems in rainfed regions of India. Agro-ecosystem Directorate (Rainfed), NATP, Central Research Institute for Dryland Agriculture, Hyderabad, AP, India.

Rao, M.R. and, Shetty, S.V.R. 1976. Some biological aspects of intercropping systems on crop-weed balance. *Indian Journal of Weed Science* 8: 32-43.

Rao, M.R., Shetty, S.V.R, Reddy, S.L.N. and Sharma, M.M. 1987. Weed management in improved rainfed cropping systems in semi-arid India. In: *Proceedings of International Workshop*, 7-11 Jan 1987. ICRISAT Sahelian Centre, Niamey, Niger, Patencheru, A.P., India, pp. 303-316.

Rao, N.G.P., Rao, J.V., Rana, B.S. and Rao, V.J.M. 1979. Responses to water availability and modifications for water-use efficiency in tropical dryland sorghums. *In. Proceedings, Symposium on Plant Responses to Water Availability*, Feb. 22-24, Indian Agricultural Research Institute, New Delhi, India.

Rao, R.V., Rao, R.M., Hosmani, S.A. and Ramchandram, M. 1973. Effect of sowing dates on incidence of shoot fly and varietal performance of *rabi* jowar in Mysore. *Indian Journal of Agronomy* 18: 314-322.

Rao, S. S., Seetharama, N., Kiran Kumar, K. A., and Vanderlip, R. L. 2004. Characterization of sorghum growth stages. *NRCS Bulletin* No. 14. National Research Centre for Sorghum, Rajendranagar, Hyderabad, Andhra Pradesh, India. 20 pp.

Rao, S.S., Patil J.V., Prasad, P.V.V., Reddy, D.C.S., Mishra, J.S., Umakanth, A.V., Reddy, B.V.S. and Kumar, A.A., 2013. Sweet Sorghum planting effects on stalk yield and sugar quality in semi-arid tropical environment. *Agronomy Journal*, 105: 1458-1465.

Ratnavathi C.V. and Ravi, S.B. 2000, Subramanian V, Rao, N.S. A study on the suitability of un-malted sorghum as a brewing adjunct. *Journal of the Institute of Brewing*. 106: 6, 383-387.

Ratnavathi, C.V., P.K. Biswas, M. Pallavi, M. Maheswari, B. S. Vijay Kumar and N. Seetharama, Alternative-uses of-sorghum-and-pearl-millet-in-Asia-Proceedings-of-an-expert-meeting,-ICRISAT,-Patancheru,-Andhra-Pradesh,-India,-1-4-July,-2003.2004; 188-200.

Ratnavathi, CV., Seetharama, N., and Chavan, UD. Dough and roti making qualities of sorghum genotypes (2008), *Jowar Samachhar*, Vol. 4, No.2.

Reddy PS, Fakrudin B, Punnuri S, Arun S, Kuruvinashetti M, Das I, Seetharama N (2008). Molecular mapping of genomic regions harboring QTLs for stalk rot resistance in sorghum. *Euphytica* 159: 191-198.

Reddy RN, Madhusudhana R, Mohan SM, Chakravarthi D, Mehtre S, Seetharama N, Patil J (2013). Mapping QTL for grain yield and other agronomic traits in post-rainy sorghum [*Sorghum bicolor* (L.) Moench]. *Theoretical and Applied Genetics*: 1-19.

Reddy, Belum V.S., Dar, W. D., Parthasarathy Rao, P., Srinivasa Rao, P., Ashok Kumar, A., and Sanjana Reddy, P. 2008. Sweet sorghum as a bioethanol feedstock: Challenges and opportunities. *International Conference on Sorghum for Biofuel*, 19-22 August 2008, Houston, TX. Accessed at: http://www.ars.usda.gov/meetings/Sorghum/presentations/Reddy.pdf.

Ribaut J, de Vicente M, Delannay X (2010) Molecular breeding in developing countries: challenges and perspectives. *Current Opinion in Plant Biology* 13: 213-218.

Robson, A.D. and Snowball, K. 1986. Nutrient deficiency and toxicity symptoms. In: Reuter, D.J. and Robinson, J,B., eds, *Plant Analysis: an Interpretation Manual*. Melbourne, Australia, Inkata Press Pty. Ltd., 13-19.

Rooney L.W., and Waniska R.D. Sorghum food and industrial utilization C.W. Smith, R.A. Frederiksen (Eds.), Sorghum: Origin, History, Technology, and Production, Wiley, New York (2000), pp. 689–729.

Rooney LW and Miller FR 1982. Variation in the structure and kernel characteristics of sorghum. Pages: 143-162 in Proc. Int. Symp. Sorghum Grain Quality(1981). Rooney LW and Murty DS, eds. ICRISAT, Pantacheru, A.P., India.

Rooney, W. L., and Aydin, S.1999. Genetic Control of a Photoperiod-Sensitive Response in *Sorghum bicolor* (L.) Moench. *Crop Science* 39: 397-400.

Rooney, W.L., 2000. Genetics and cytogenetics. In: C.W. Smith and R.A. Frederiksen (Eds.), Sorghum: Origin, History, Technology, and Production, pp. 261–308. JohnWiley and Sons., Inc. NewYork, NY.

Roozeboom, K. and Fjell, D. 1998. Selection of Grain Sorghum Hybrids. *Grain Sorghum Production Handbook*. Manhattan, Kansas: Kansas State University, pp.3-5.

Rosenow D, Clark L (1983). Use of post-flowering drought tolerance in a sorghum breeding program. Proceedings Thirteenth Biennial Grain Sorghum Res and Util Conf, Brownsville, TX.

Rosenow D, Clark L, Woodfin C (1981). Breeding for drought resistance in sorghum. Proceedings of the 12th Biennial Grain Sorghum Research and Utilization Conference, sponsored by the Grain Sorghum Producers' Association (GSPA) and the Sorghum Improvement Conference of North America Available from GSPA, Abernathy, Texas, USA, p. 11.

Rosenow DT and Clark LE. 1981. Drought tolerance in sorghum. In: Proceedings of the 36th Annual Corn and Sorghum Research Conference, pp. 18–30. American Seed Trade Association, Washington, DC (1981).

Routley, R., Broad, I., McLean, G., Whish, J., Hammer, G. 2003. The effect of row configuration on yield reliability in grain sorghum: 1. Yield,water use efficiency and soil water extraction. *Proc. 11th Aust. Agron.Conf.* Geelong, Victoria. 2–6 Feb. 2003. Australia Society of Agronomy. Gosford, Australia.

Roy, R.N. and Wright, B.C. 1974. Sorghum growth and nutrient uptake in relation to soil fertility, II. N,P and K uptake pattern by various plant parts. *Agronomy Journal*, 66: 5-10.

Saeed, M. and Francis, C. A.1983. Yield Stability in Relation to Maturity in Grain Sorghum1. *Crop Science* 23: 683-87.

Sahrawat, K.L., Pardhasaradhi, G., Rego, T.J. and Rahman, M.H. 2005. Relationship between extracted phosphorus and sorghum yield in a vertisol and an alfisol under rainfed cropping. *Fertilizer Research*, 44: 23-26.

Sajjanar G (2002) Genetic Analysis and Molecular Mapping of Components of Resistance to Shoot Fly (*Attorigota soccata* Rond) in Sorghum (*Sorghum bicolor* (L.) Moench). University of Agricultural Sciences.

Sang Y, Bean S, Seib PA, Pedersen J and Shi YC. 2008. Structural and functional properties of sorghum starches differing in amylose content. *J. Agric. Food Chem.* 56, 6680–6685.

Sankaranarayanan, K. 2000. *Ph.D. Thesis*, Tamil Nadu Agricultural University, Coimbatore.

Sarpe, N., Dradhici, I., Roibu, C. and Draghici, R. 1997. Selectivity and efficacy of herbicide pendimethalin compared with triazine herbicides applied on sorghum (*Sorghum vulgare* Pers.) for grains. *In*: *Proceedings of the 49th International Symposium on Crop Protection*, Gent, Belgium, 6 May, 1997, Part III, pp. 857-863.

Satao, R.N. and Nalamwar, R.V. 1993. Studies on uptake of nitrogen, phosphorus and potassium by weeds and sorghum as influenced by integrated weed control. Integrated weed management for sustainable agriculture. *In*: *Proceedings of an Indian Society of Weed Science International Symposium*, Hisar, India, 18-20 November 1993 Vol. III, pp.103-107.

Satish K, Gutema Z, Grenier C, Rich PJ, Ejeta G (2012). Molecular tagging and validation of microsatellite markers linked to the low germination stimulant gene (lgs) for Striga resistance in sorghum [*Sorghum bicolor* (L.) Moench]. *Theoretical and Applied Genetics* 124: 989-1003.

Satish K, Srinivas G, Madhusudhana R, Padmaja P, Reddy RN, Mohan SM, Seetharama N (2009). Identification of quantitative trait loci for resistance to shoot fly in sorghum [*Sorghum bicolor* (L.) Moench]. *Theoretical and Applied Genetics* 119: 1425-1439.

Sauvant D, Perez JM and Tran G. 2004. Tables INRA-AFZ de composition et de valeur nutritive des matières premières destinées aux animaux d'élevage: 2ème édition. ISBN 2738011586, 306 p.

Sax K (1923). The association of size differences with seed-coat pattern and pigmentation in *Phaseolus vulgaris*. *Genetics* 8: 552.

Sayed HI and Gadallah AM. 1983. Variation in dry matter and grain filling characteristics in wheat cultivars. *Field Crops Res* 7: 61–71.

Schaffer, J. A. 1980. The effect of planting date and environment on the phenology and modeling of grain sorghum, *Sorghum bicolor* (L.) Moench. Diss. Kansas State University, 1980. Manhattan: Kansas State University.

Schmidt, M. and Bothma, G. 2006. Risk assessment for transgenic sorghum in Africa: Crop-to-crop gene-flow in *Sorghum bicolor* (L.) Moench. *Crop Science* 46: 790-798.

Scifres, C.J. and Bovey, R.W. 1970. Differential resonse of sorghum varieties to picloram. *Agronomy Journal* 62: 775-777.

Seckinger HL and Wolf MJ 1973. Sorghum protein ultrastructure as it relates to composition. *Cereal Chem.* 50: 455-465.

Seetharama, N., Flower, D.J., Jayachandran, R., Krishna, K.R., Peacock, J.M., Singh, S., Soman, P., Usharani, A. and Wani, S.P. 1990. Assessment of genotypic differences in sorghum root characteristics. *Proceedings of International Congress on Plant Physiology*, New Delhi, pp. 215-219.

Seetharama, N., Krishna, K.R., Rego, T.J. and Burford, J. 1988. Prospects for improvement of phosphorus efficiency in sorghum for acid soils. *In: Proceedings of a Workshop on evaluating sorghum for tolerance to Aluminium toxic, tropic soils in Latin America.* Centro International Agricultural Tropicale (CIAT), Cali, Columbia, pp. 229-249.

Seetharama, N., Subba Reddy, B.V., Peacock, J.M., and Bidinger, F.R. 1982. Sorghum improvement for drought resistance. Pages 317-338 In: *Drought resistance in crops, with emphasis on rice.* Los Banos, Philippines: International Rice Research Institute.

Senthil Kumar, S. and Arockiasami, D.I. 1995. VAM fungi in integrated nutrient management. *Indian Journal of Microbiology* 35: 185-188.

Sharda, V.N. and Rattan Singh, 2003. Erosion control measures for improving productivity of farmer's profitability. *Fertilizer News* 48: 71-78.

Sharma, A.K. and Singh, M. 1974. A note on the efficiency of nitrogen fertilizers in relation to time and method of application in hybrid sorghum. *Indian Journal of Agronomy*, 19: 158-160.

Sharma, P.N. and Neto, EBA. (1986). *Agric. Water Management*, 11(2): 169-180.

Sharma, R.P., Dadheech, R.C. and Jat, L.N. 2000. Effect of atrazine and nitrogen on growth and yield of sorghum [(*Sorghum bicolor* (L.) Moench)]. *Indian Journal of Weed Science* 32: 96-97.

Sharma, R.P., Dadheech, R.C. and Vyas, A.K, 2001. Correlation and regression analysis in sorghum and weeds as influenced by weed control and nitrogen levels. *Crop Research* 22: 110-112.

Shelton, D.P., Smith, J.A., Jasa, P.J. and Kanable, R. 1995. Eastimating percent residue covers using calculation method, G 95-1135-A. www.ianr.unl.-edu/pubs/fieldcrops/g135.htm.

Shetty SVR and Rao AN, 1981. Weed management in sorghum/pigeonpea and pearl millet/groundnut intercrop systems-some observations. In: *Proceedings of International Workshop on Intercropping,* 10-13 January, 1979, ICRISAT, Hyderabad, pp. 238-248.

Shetty, S.V.R. and Rao, M.R. 1979. Weed management studies in pigeonpea-based intercropping. In: *Proceedings of VI Asian-Pacific Weed Science Conference*, 11-17 July, 1977. Vol II, pp. 655-672.

Shetty, S.V.R., Sivakumar, M.V.K. and Ram, S.A. 1982. Effect of shading on the growth of some common weeds or the semi-arid tropics. *Agronomy Journal* 74: 1023-1029.

Shinde SH and Umrani NK. 1988. *Indian Journal of Agronomy*, 33: 426-431.

Shinde. S.H. and Umrani, N.K. (1988). *Indian Journal of Agronomy*, 33: 426-431.

Showemimo, F.A., Kimbeng, C.A. and Alabi, S.O. 2002. Genotypic response of sorghum cultivars to nitrogen fertilization in the control of *Striga hermonthica*. *Crop Protection* 21: 867-870.

Shrotriya, G.C. 1998. Balanced fertilization–Indian experience. *Proceedings of Symposium on Plant Nutrition Management for Sustainable Agriculture Growth*. NFDC, Islamabad.

Shull JM, Watterson JJ and Kirleis AW 1992. Purification and immunocytochemical localization of kafirins in *Sorghum bicolor* (L. Moench) endosperm. *Protoplasma* 171: 64-74.

Singh BR and Singh DP. 1995. Agronomic and physiological responses of sorghum, maize and pearl millet to irrigation. *Field Crops Research* 42: 57-67.

Singh M, Chaudhary K, Boora K (2006a). RAPD-based SCAR marker SCA 12 linked to recessive gene conferring resistance to anthracnose in sorghum [*Sorghum bicolor* (L.) Moench]. *Theoretical and Applied Genetics* 114: 187-192.

Singh M, Chaudhary K, Singal H, Magill C, Boora K (2006b). Identification and characterization of RAPD and SCAR markers linked to anthracnose resistance gene in sorghum [*Sorghum bicolor* (L.) Moench]. *Euphytica* 149: 179-187.

Singh MV. 2001.Evaluation of current micronutrient stocks in different agro-ecological zones of India for sustainable crops production. *Fertilizer News* **42**: 25-42.

Singh R and Axtell JD. 1973. High lysine mutant gene (hl) that improves protein quality and biological value of grain sorghum. *Crop Science* 13: 535-539.

Singh R. K. 2007. Indigenous agricultural knowledge in rainfed rice based farming systems for sustainable agriculture: learning from Indian farmers. In: Boon EK, Hens L (eds) Indigenous knowledge systems and sustainable development: relevance for Africa. Kamla Raj Enterprises, New Delhi, pp. 101–110.

Singh, A. and Bains, S.S. 1973. Yield, grain quality and nutrient uptake of CSH 1 and Swarna sorghum at different levels of nitrogen and plant population. *Indian Journal of Agricultural Sciences*, 43: 408-413.

Singh, B.R. and Singh, D.P. 1995. Agronomic and physiological responses of sorghum, maize and pearl millet to irrigation. *Field Crops Research* 42: 57-67.

Singh, H.G. and Sogani, K. 1968. Madras *Agric. Journal.*, 55: 161-167.

Singh, K., Balyan, J.S., 2000. Performance of sorghum-legume intercropping under dierent plant geometries and N levels. *Indian Journal of Agronomy* 45, 64–69.

Singh, M. and Yadav, D.S. 1980. Effect of copper, iron and liming on growth, concentraton and uptake of copper, iron, manganese and zinc in sorghum (*Sorghum bicolor*). *Journal of Indian Society of Soil Science*, 28: 113-118.

Singh, M.V. 2001. Evaluation of current micronutrient stocks in different agro-ecological zones of India for sustainable crops production. *Fertilizer News* **42**: 25-42.

Singh, O.P., Malik, H.P.S. and Ahmad, R.A. 1988. Effect of weed control treatments and nitrogen levels on the growth and yield of forage sorghum. *Indian Journal of Weed Science* 20: 29-34.

Singh, R.M. and Vyas, D.L. 1970. A note on response of grain sorghum to micronutrients. *Indian Journal of Agronomy*, 15: 309-310.

Singh, R.P. and Bajpai, R.P. 1992. Reaction of fodder sorghum varieties to atrazine. *Current Research*, University of Agricultural Sciences Bangalore, India, 21: 44-46.

Singh, R.P. and Singh, O.N. 1999. Integrated weed management in pigeonpea+sorghum intercropping system. In: *Abstracts, 8th Biennial Conference, Indian Society of Weed Science*, Varanasi, February, 5-7, 1999, pp. 103.

Singh, S.P. 1979. Studies on spatial arrangements of sorghum. *In: Proceedings of International Workshop on intercropping*. ICRISAT, Patencheru, A.P. p. 22-24.

Singh, S.P. 1980. Raising jowar in *kharif* and *rabi*. In. *JOWAR*. Indian Council of Agricultural Research, New Delhi, 14-21pp.

Sivakumar, M.V.K. and Virmani, S. M. 1982. The physical environment. *In "Sorghum in the Eightees."* L.R. House, L.K. Mughogo and J.M. Peacock (Eds.). ICRISAT, 83-100 pp.

Smeda, R.J., Corric, R.S. and Rippee, J.H. 2000. Fluazifop-P resistance expressed as a dominant trait in sorghum (*Sorghum bicolor*). *Weed Technology* 14: 397-401.

Smith, B.S., Murry D.S., Green, J.D., Wanyahaya, W.M. and Weeks, D.L. 1990. Interference of three annual grass with grain sorghum (*Sorghum bicolor*). *Weed Technology* 4: 245-249.

Smith, C.W. and Fredricksen, R.A. (Eds.) 2000. *Sorghum: Origin, History, Technology and Production*, New York: John Wiley and Sons.

Sojka, R.E., Karlen, D.L. and Sadler, E.J. 1988. Planting geometries and the efficient use of water and nutrients. In Hargrove WL (ed.) Cropping Strategies for Efficient Use of Water and Nitrogen. ASA Special Publication, Madison, WI, 51: 43-68.

Solaimalai, A. and Muthusankaranarayanan, A. 2000. Effect of sorghum and weed management practices on leguminous intercrops. *Madras Agricultural Journal* 87: 490-491.

Solaimalai, A. and Sivakumar, C. 2002. Evaluation of suitable weed management practices for a sorghum-based intercropping system under irrigated conditions. International *Sorghum and Millets Newsletter* 41: 32-34.

Srinivas G, Satish K, Madhusudhana R, Reddy RN, Mohan SM, Seetharama N (2009). Identification of quantitative trait loci for agronomically important traits and their association with genic-microsatellite markers in sorghum. *Theoretical and Applied Genetics* 118: 1439-1454.

Srinivasarao, Ch., Satyanarayana, T. and Venkateswarlu, B. 2011. Potassium mining in Indian Agriculture: Input and output balance. *Karnataka Journal of Agricultural Sciences*, 24 (1): 20-28.

Srivastava, S. P. and Singh, A. 1969. "Maturity of Hybrid Sorghum as Influenced by Fertilizer Application and Intra-Row Spacings." *Indian Journal of Agricultural Sciences* 40: 1056-060.

Srivastava, S.P. and Singh, Ambika. 1971. Utilization of nitrogen by dwarf sorghum. *Indian Journal of Agricultural Sciences*, 41: 543-546.

Staggenborg, S. A. Vanderlip, R. L. 1996. Sorghum Grain Yield Reductions Caused by Duration and Timing of Freezing Temperatures. *Agronomy Journal* 88: 473-77.

Stahlman, P.W. and Wicks, G.A. 2000. Weeds and their control in sorghum. In: Smith, C.W. and Fredricksen, R.A. (Eds.). *Sorghum: Origin, History, Technology and Production*, New York: John Wiley and Sons, pp. 535-590.

Steiner, J. L. 1986. Dryland grain sorghum water use, light interception, and growth responses to planting geometry. *Agronomy Journal* 78: 720-26.

Stephens, J.C. and Holland, R.F. 1954. Cytoplasmic male-sterility for hybrid sorghum seed production. *Agronomy Journal* 46: 20.

Stephens, J.C.1937. Male sterility in Sorghun: its possible utilization in production of hybrid seed. *Journal of American Society of Agronomy* 29: 690.

Stickler, F. C., and Laude, H. H. 1960. Effect of Row Spacing and Plant Population on Performance of Corn, Grain Sorghum and Forage Sorghum. *Agronomy Journal* 52: 275-77.

Subbarayalu, M. 1982. *Ph.D. Thesis*, Tamil Nadu Agricultural University, Coimbatore.

Subbian, P. and Selvaraju, R. 2000. Effect of row ratio on sorghum (*Sorghum bicolor*) + soybean (*Glycine max*) intercropping system in rainfed Vertisol. *Indian Journal of Agronomy* 45: 526-529.

Subramaniam. V and Jambunathan.R. 1980. Traditional methods of processing sorghum (*Sorghum bicolor*) and Pearl millet (*Pennisetum americanum*) grains in India. Reports of the International Association of Cereal Chemistry (ICC) 10: 115-188.

Subudhi P, Rosenow D, Nguyen H (2000) Quantitative trait loci for the stay green trait in sorghum (*Sorghum bicolor* L. Moench): consistency across genetic backgrounds and environments. *Theoretical and Applied Genetics* 101: 733-741.

Sukumaran S, Xiang W, Bean SR, Pedersen JF, Kresovich S, Tuinstra MR, Tesso TT, Hamblin MT and Yu J. 2012. Association mapping for grain quality in a diverse sorghum collection. *Plant Genome* 5(3): 126-135.

Sundari, A. and Kathiresan, R.M. 2002. Integrated weed management in irrigated sorghum. *Indian Journal of Weed Science* 34: 313-315.

Sundari, A. and Kumar, S.M.S. 2002. Crop-weed competition in sorghum. *Indian Journal of Weed Science* 34: 311-312.

Takeda Y, Hizukuri S, Takeda C and Suzuki A (1987). Structures of branched molecules of amyloses of various origins, and molar fractions of branched and unbranched molecules. *Carbohydrate. Res.* 165: 139-145.

Tamado, T., Ohlander, L. and Milberg, P. 2002. Interference by the weed *Parthenium hysterophorus* L. with grain sorghum: influence of weed density and duration of competition. *International Journal of Pest Management* 48: 183-186.

Tanchev, D. 1989. Study of the doses of simazine herbicide in sorghum growing. *Rasteniev'dni-Nauki* 26: 87-91.

Tandon HLS and Kanwar JS. 1984. *A Review of Fertilizer Use Research on Sorghum in India.* Research Bulletin No. 8. International Crops Research Institute for the Semi-Arid Tropics.

Tandon, H. L. S. and Kanwar, J. S. 1984. *A Review of Fertilizer Use Research on Sorghum in India.* Research Bulletin No. 8. International Crops Research Institute for the Semi-Arid Tropics.

Tao Y, Hardy A, Drenth J, Henzell R, Franzmann B, Jordan D, Butler D, McIntyre C (2003) Identifications of two different mechanisms for sorghum midge resistance through QTL mapping. *Theoretical and Applied Genetics* 107: 116-122.

Tao Y, Henzell R, Jordan D, Butler D, Kelly A, McIntyre C (2000). Identification of genomic regions associated with stay green in sorghum by testing RILs in multiple environments. *Theoretical and Applied Genetics* 100: 1225-1232.

Tao Y, Jordan D, Henzell R, McIntyre C (1998). Identification of genomic regions for rust resistance in sorghum. *Euphytica* 103: 287-292.

Tapia, L.S., Bauman, T.T., Harvey, R.G., Kells, J.J., Kapusta, G., Loux, M.M., Lueschen, W.E., Owen, M.D.K., Hageman, L.H. and Strachan, S.D. 1997. Post-emergence herbicide application timing effects on annual grass control and corn (*Zea mays*) grain yield. *Weed Science* 45: 138-143.

Taylor JRN, Novellie L and Liebenberg NVDW 1984. Sorghum protein body composition and ultrastructure. *Cereal Chem.* 61: 69-73.

Taylor JRN, Schüssler L, Liebenberg NVDW (1985). Protein Body formation in the starchy endosperm of developing *Sorghum bicolor* (L.) Moench seeds. S. Afr. Tydskr. Plantk. 51: 35 - 40.

Tenebe, V.A. and Kamara, H.M. 2002. Effect of *Striga hermonthica* on the growth characteristics of sorghum intercropped with groundnut varieties. *Journal of Agronomy and Crop Science* 188: 376-381.

Tenkouano A, Miller FR, Fredriksen RA, Rosenow DT. 1993. Genetics of non-senescence and charcoal rot resistance in sorghum. *Theor Appl Genet* 85: 644–648.

Thakur, G.S., Dubey, R.K. and Tripathi, A.K. 1990. Screening of herbicides for controlling the weeds in forage sorghum. In: *Abstracts, Biennial Conference, Indian Society of Weed Science*, March 4-5 1990, JNKVV, Jabalpur, India, pp. 54.

Thippeswamy and Alagundagi. S.C. 2001. Effect of intercropping of legumes on forage yield and quality of forage sweet sorghum. *Karnataka Journal of Agricultural Sciences*, 14: 905-909.

Thomas, G.A., French, A.V., Ladewig, J.H. and Lather, C.J. 1980. Row spacing and population density effects on yield of grain sorghum in Central Queensland. *Queensland J. Agric. Anl. Sci.*, 37: 66-67.

Tiryaki, I. and Andrews, D.J., 2001a. Germination and seedling cold tolerance in sorghum: I. Evaluation of rapid screening methods. *Agronomy Journal* 93: 1386-1391.

Tiryaki, I. and Andrews, D.J., 2001b. Germination and seedling cold tolerance in sorghum: II. Parental lines and hybrids. *Agronomy Journal* 93: 1391-1397.

Tiwari, K.N. 2006. Future of Plant Nutrition Research in India. *Indian Journal of Fertilizers* 2: 73-98.

TNAU, 2003. ^{15}N studies: A report. Department of Soil Science and Agricultural Chemistry. Tamil Nadu Agricultural University, Coimbatore. http: // www.tnau.ac.in/scms/ssac/res/sacn151.htm pp. 1-6.

Traore, S., Manson, S.C., Martin, A.R., Mortensen, D.A. and Spotanski, J.J. 2003. Velvetleaf interference effects on yield and growth of grain sorghum. *Agronomy Journal* 5: 1602-1607.

Tuinstra MR, Grote EM, Goldsbrough PB and Ejeta G. 1997. Genetic analysis of post-flowering drought tolerance and components of grain development in *Sorghum bicolor* (L.) Moench. Molecular Breeding 3: 439–448.

Tuinstra, M.R. and Al-Khatib, K. 2007. New herbicide tolerance traits in grain sorghum. In *Proceedings of the 2007 Corn, Sorghum and Soybean Seed Research Conf. and Seed Expo*. Chicago, IL: Am. Seed Trade Assoc.

Tuinstra, M.R., Soumana, S., Al-Khatib, K., Kapran, I., Toure, A., Ast, Av., Bastiaans, L., Ochanda, N.W., Salami, I., Kayentao, M., and Dembele, S. 2009. Efficacy of herbicide seed treatments for controlling *Striga* infestation of sorghum. *Crop Science* 49: 923-929.

Turhollow AF, Webb EG and Downing ME. 2010. Review of Sorghum Production Practices: Applications for Bioenergy, 28.03.11, Available from *http: //info.ornl.gov/ sites/publications/files/Pub22854.pdf*.

Turk, M.A. and Tawah, A.M. 2002. Response of sorghum genotypes to weed management under Mediterranean conditions. *Pakistan Journal of Agronomy* 1: 31-33.

Turkhede, B.B. and Prasad, R. 1978. Effect of rates and timing of nitrogen application on hybrid sorghum. *Indian Journal of Agronomy*, 23: 113-126.

Turner, N.C. 1979. Drought resistance and adaptation to water deficits in crop plants. In. H. Mussell and R.C. Stapler (eds.), *Stress Physiology in Crop Plants*. Wiley, New York, pp. 343-372.

Uleri, A.L. and Ernst, F.F. 1997. Sorghum response to saline industrial cooling water applied at three growth stages. *Agronomy Journal*, 89: 392-396.

Upadhyay, U.C., Lomte, M.H. and Shelke, B.V. 1981. Integrated weed management in sorghum. In: *Proceedings of 8th Asian Pacific Weed Science Society* Conference, Bangalore.

Upadhyaya H, Wang Y, Sharma R, Sharma S (2013a). Identification of genetic markers linked to anthracnose resistance in sorghum using association analysis. *Theoretical and Applied Genetics* Theoretische und angewandte Genetik.

Upadhyaya HD, Wang Y-H, Sharma R, Sharma S (2013b). SNP markers linked to leaf rust and grain mold resistance in sorghum.

Vadez V, Deshpande SP, Kholova J, Hammer GL, Borrell AK, Talwar HS, Hash CT (2011). Stay-green quantitative trait loci's effects on water extraction, transpiration efficiency and seed yield depend on recipient parent background. Functional Plant Biology 38: 553-566.

Vanderlip RL and Reeves HE. 1972. Growth stages of sorghum. *Agronomy Journal* 64: 13-16.

Vanderlip RL. 1993. How a sorghum plant develops. Contribution No. 1203, Agronomy Department, Kansas Agricultural Experiment Station, Manhattan, 66506. (http://www.oznet.ksu.edu).

Vanderlip, R.L. 1972. How a sorghum plant Develops. Cooperative Extension Service, Kansas State University, Manhattan, KS.

Vanderlip, R.L. 1979. How a Sorghum Plant Develops. Circ. S-3. Kansas Cooperative Extension Service, Manhattan, KS.

Vanderlip, R.L. 1993. *How a Sorghum Plant Develops*. Kansas State University. Manhattan, Kansas.

Vanderlip, R.L. and Reeves, H.E. 1972. Growth stages of sorghum. *Agronomy Journal*, 64: 13-16.

Vasimalai, M.P. *et al.* (1981). *Sorghum Newsletter*, 24: 40-41.

Venkatachalam, S., Premanathan, S., Arunachelam G. and Vivekanandan, S. N. 1969. Soil fertility studies in Madras State using radio tracer technique. I. Placement of phosphate to hybrid sorghum. *Madras Agricultural Journal*, 56: 104-109.

Venkateswarlu, K. 1973. Efficiency of nitrogen utilization by hybrid sorghum (CSH 1) and assessment of residual fertility. *Ph.D. Thesis*, G.B. Pant University of Agriculture and Technology, Pantnagar, India.

Venkateswarlu, Sharma, K.C. and Lal, B. 1978. Recovery of fertilizer nitrogen applied to grain sorghum and assessment of residual effect. *Pantnagar Journal of Research* 3: 36-40.

Vessey, J. K. 2003. Plant growth promoting rhizobacteria as biofertilizers. *Plant and Soils* 255: 571-586.

Viets, F.G. 1972. Water deficits and nutrient availability. In T.T. Kozlowski (ed.). *Water deficit and plant growth.* Vol. 3. Plant responses and control of water balance. Academic Press, New York and London.

Vigil, M. F., Henry, W. B., Calderon F. J., Poss, D., Nielsen, D. C., Benjamin, J. G., and Klein, B.2008. A use of skip-row planting as a strategy for drought mitigation in the West Central Great Plains. *Proceedings of the Great Plains Soil Fertility Conference.* Denver, CO. Vol. 12. Pp.101-06.

Vijayalakshmi, K. 1979. Research achievements with special reference to fertilizer use in drylands. *In. Proceedings of the Group discussion on Fertilizer use in Drylands,* Aug. 1979. Fertilizer Association of India, New Delhi. 31-38pp.

Vijayalakshmi, K. 1987. Rain water management in drylands. *In: Technological Advances in Dryland Agriculture,* CRIDA, Hyderabad, pp. 19-45.

Vinall, H. N. and Reed, H. R. 1918. Effect of Temperature and Other Meteorological Factors on the Growth of Sorghums. *Journal of Agricultural Research* 13: 133-47.

Vishnumurthy, T. and Vijayalakshmi, K. 1993. Intercropping sorghum with clusterbean or greengram in Alfisols of Andhra Pradesh. *Indian Journal of Dryland Agriculture Research and Development,* 8: 54-56.

Wade, L. J., and Douglas, A. C. L. 1990. Effect of Plant Density on Grain Yield and Yield Stability of Sorghum Hybrids Differing in Maturity. *Australian Journal of Experimental Agriculture* 30: 257-64.

Watling, J.R. and Press, M.C. 1997. How is the relationship between the C4 cereal *Sorghum bicolor* and the C3 root hemi-parasites *Striga hermonthica* and *Striga asiatica* affected by elevated CO_2? *Plant Cell and Environment* 20: 1292-1300.

Weaver CA, Hamaker BR and Axtell JD (1998). Discovery of grain sorghum germplasm with high uncooked and cooked in vitro protein digestibility. *Cereal Chem.* 75(5): 665-670.

Webb, K.R. and Feez, A.M. 1987. Control of broadleaf weeds with fluroxypyr in sugarcane and grain sorghum in Northern New South Wales and Queensland, Australia. In: *Proceedings, 11th Asian Pacfic Weed Science Society Conference,* 1: 211-217.

Whiteman PC and Wilson GL. 1965. Effects of water stress on the reproductive development of *Sorghum vulgare* Pers. Univ. Queensland Papers, Dept. Botany, 4: 233-239.

Whitney D. 1998. Fertilizer Requirements. *Grain Sorghum Production Handbook.* Manhattan, Kansas: Kansas State University, pp.12-14.

Willey, R.W. 1979. Intercropping-its importance and research needs. Part-1. Competition and yield advantages. *Agronomy Journal* 71: 115-119.

Willey, R.W. 1988. Cropping systems for Dryland. *In. Proceedings of the International Conference on 'Challenges in Dryland Agriculture-a global perspective'.* Amarillo/ Bushland, Texas, USA, 703-709 pp.

Willey, R.W., M. Matarajan, M.S. Reddy, M.R. Rao, P.T.C. Nambiar, J. Kammainan and V.S. Bhatanagar. 1980. Intercropping studies with annual crops. In: *Better Crops for Food*. J.C. Homeless (ed) Ciba Foundation Symp. pp. 83-97.

Willey, R.W., Rao, M.R., Reddy, M.S. and Natarajan, M. 1982. Cropping systems with sorghum. *Sorghum in Eighties, Proceedings of the International Symposium on Sorghum*. November, 2-7, 1981, ICRISAT, Patancheru, A.P., India.

Witt, M. D., Vanderlip, R. L., and Bark, L. D. 1972. Effect of row width and orientation on light intercepted by grain sorghum. *Transactions of the Kansas Academy of Science* 75: 29-40.

Wu Han Wen, Walker, S., Osten, V., Taylor, I. and Sindel, B. 2004. Emergence and persistence of barnyard grass (*Echinichloa colona* (L.) Link) and its management options in sorghum. Weed Management: Balancing people, planet, profit. *In. Proceedings of 14th Australian Weeds Conference*, Wagga, New South wales, Australia, 6-9 September, 2004, pp.538-541.

Wu Y, Huang Y (2008). Molecular mapping of QTLs for resistance to the greenbug *Schizaphis graminum* (Rondani) in *Sorghum bicolor* (Moench). *Theoretical and Applied Genetics* 117: 117-124..

Xu W, Subudhi PK, Crasta OR, Rosenow DT, Mullet JE, Nguyen HT (2000). Molecular mapping of QTLs conferring stay-green in grain sorghum (*Sorghum bicolor* L. Moench). *Genome* 43: 461-469.

Zimdahl, R.L. 1980. *Crop-weed competition: A review*. International Plant Protection Centre, Oregon State University, Corvallis, Oregon 97331, USA.

Ziska, L.H. 2001. Changes in competitive ability between a C_4 and a C_3 weed with elevated carbon dioxide. *Weed Science* 49: 622-627.

Zobel HF (1992). Starch granule structure. Pages 1-36 in: Developments in carbohydrate chemistry. R.J. Alexander and H.F. Zobel, eds. Amer. Assoc. *Cereal Chem.*, St Paul, MN.

Index

www.ingramcontent.com/pod-product-compliance
Lightning Source LLC
Chambersburg PA
CBHW060248230326
41458CB00094B/1541

* 9 7 8 9 3 5 1 3 0 2 9 3 3 *